The Acutely Ill Child
A Ready Reckoner

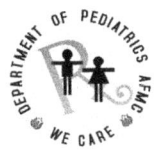

The Acutely Ill Child
A Ready Reckoner

Second Edition

Editors

Biju M John
MD (Pediatrics) Trained in Pediatric Intensive Care
Professor and Head
Department of Pediatrics
Command Hospital (Air Force)
Bengaluru, Karnataka, India

Vishal Sondhi
MD (Pediatrics) DM (Pediatric Neurology)
Professor
Department of Pediatrics
Military Hospital
Srinagar, Jammu and Kashmir, India

Shuvendu Roy
MD (Pediatrics) Trained in Pediatric Neurology
Professor and Head
Department of Pediatrics
Armed Forces Medical College (AFMC)
Pune, Maharashtra, India

G Shridhar
MD (Pediatrics) DM (Neonatology)
Professor
Department of Pediatrics
Armed Forces Medical College (AFMC)
Pune, Maharashtra, India

Foreword
Mukti Sharma

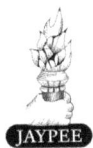

JAYPEE BROTHERS MEDICAL PUBLISHERS
The Health Sciences Publisher
New Delhi | London

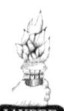 **Jaypee Brothers Medical Publishers (P) Ltd**

Headquarters
Jaypee Brothers Medical Publishers (P) Ltd
EMCA House, 23/23-B
Ansari Road, Daryaganj
New Delhi 110 002, India
Landline: +91-11-23272143, +91-11-23272703
+91-11-23282021, +91-11-23245672
Email: jaypee@jaypeebrothers.com

Corporate Office
Jaypee Brothers Medical Publishers (P) Ltd
4838/24, Ansari Road, Daryaganj
New Delhi 110 002, India
Phone: +91-11-43574357
Fax: +91-11-43574314
Email: jaypee@jaypeebrothers.com

Overseas Office
JP Medical Ltd.
83, Victoria Street, London
SW1H 0HW (UK)
Phone: +44 20 3170 8910
Email: info@jpmedpub.com

EU GPSR Authorised Representative
Logos Europe, 9 rue Nicolas Poussin
17000, La Rochelle, France
Phone: +33 (0) 6 67 93 73 78
E-mail: Contact@logoseurope.eu

Website: www.jaypeebrothers.com
Website: www.jaypeedigital.com

© 2025, Jaypee Brothers Medical Publishers

The views and opinions expressed in this book are solely those of the original contributor(s)/author(s) and do not necessarily represent those of editor(s) or publisher of the book.

All rights reserved. No part of this publication may be reproduced, stored or transmitted in any form or by any means, electronic, mechanical, photocopying, recording or otherwise, without the prior permission in writing of the publishers.

All brand names and product names used in this book are trade names, service marks, trademarks or registered trademarks of their respective owners. The publisher is not associated with any product or vendor mentioned in this book.

Medical knowledge and practice change constantly. This book is designed to provide accurate, authoritative information about the subject matter in question. However, readers are advised to check the most current information available on procedures included and check information from the manufacturer of each product to be administered, to verify the recommended dose, formula, method and duration of administration, adverse effects and contraindications. It is the responsibility of the practitioner to take all appropriate safety precautions. Neither the publisher nor the author(s)/editor(s) assume any liability for any injury and/or damage to persons or property arising from or related to use of material in this book.

This book is sold on the understanding that the publisher is not engaged in providing professional medical services. If such advice or services are required, the services of a competent medical professional should be sought.

Every effort has been made where necessary to contact holders of copyright to obtain permission to reproduce copyright material. If any have been inadvertently overlooked, the publisher will be pleased to make the necessary arrangements at the first opportunity.

Inquiries for bulk sales may be solicited at: jaypee@jaypeebrothers.com

The Acutely Ill Child: A Ready Reckoner

First Edition: 2013

Second Edition: **2025**

ISBN: 978-93-5696-691-8

Dedicated to

All the children, their caregivers, supporting staff, students, nurses, and doctors who passed through the Pediatric Wing of Armed Forces Medical College (AFMC) and Command Hospital Pune, Maharashtra, India

Section Editors

Amit Pathania
MD (Pediatrics) DM (Pediatric Critical Care)
Associate Professor
Department of Pediatrics
Base Hospital
Delhi Cantt, New Delhi, India

Ashwin Arora
MD (Pediatrics) FNB (Pediatric Intensive Care)
Associate Professor
Department of Pediatrics
Military Hospital
Sonitpur, Assam, India

Arvind Kumar
MD (Pediatrics) DM (Pediatric Critical Care)
Associate Professor
Department of Pediatrics
Command Hospital (SC)
Pune, Maharashtra, India

Mithlesh Kumar Tiwari
MD (Pediatrics) DM (Pediatric Critical Care)
Assistant Professor
Department of Pediatrics
Command Hospital (SC)
Pune, Maharashtra, India

Contributors

Abhishek Pandey MD (Pediatrics)
Assistant Professor
Department of Pediatrics
On study leave (PGIMER, Chandigarh, India)

Ajay Beriwal MD (Pediatrics)
Military Hospital
Srinagar, Jammu and Kashmir, India

Amit Devgan MD (Pediatrics)
Professor and Commandant
Department of Pediatrics
Command Hospital
Udhampur, Jammu and Kashmir, India

Amit Pathania
MD (Pediatrics) DM (Pediatric Critical Care)
Associate Professor
Department of Pediatrics
Base Hospital
Delhi Cantt, New Delhi, India

Anjali Gautam MBBS
Resident
Department of Pediatrics
Armed Forces Medical College (AFMC)
Pune, Maharashtra, India

Aradhana Dwivedi
MD (Pediatrics) DM (Medical Genetics)
Associate Professor
Department of Pediatrics
Army Hospital (R&R)
New Delhi, India

Aradhna Aneja
MD (Pediatrics) DM (Pediatric Gastroenterology)
Associate Professor
Department of Pediatrics
Army Hospital (R&R)
New Delhi, India

Arvind Kumar
MD (Pediatrics) DM (Pediatric Critical Care)
Associate Professor
Department of Pediatrics
Command Hospital (SC)
Pune, Maharashtra, India

Arvind Mishra
MD (Pediatrics) FNB (Pediatric Cardiology)
Professor
Department of Pediatrics
Army Institute of Cardio Thoracic Sciences
Pune, Maharashtra, India

Ashwin Arora
MD (Pediatrics) FNB (Pediatric Intensive Care)
Associate Professor
Department of Pediatrics
Military Hospital
Sonitpur, Assam, India

Barnali Mitra MD (Pediatrics)
Associate Professor
Department of Pediatrics
Command Hospital (AF)
Bengaluru, Karnataka, India

Bhaskar Bharadwaj
MD (Pediatrics)
Clinical Tutor
Department of Pediatrics
Armed Forces Medical College (AFMC)
Pune, Maharashtra, India

Biju M John
MD (Pediatrics) Trained in Pediatric Intensive Care
Professor and Head
Department of Pediatrics
Command Hospital (Air Force)
Bengaluru, Karnataka, India

Contributors

Bikash Shreshta
MD (Pediatrics) Fellow Neonatology (NNF)
Associate Professor
Department of Pediatrics
Nepalese Army Institute of Health Sciences
Kathmandu, Nepal

Daljit Singh
MD DNB DM FNNF FIAP
Director General
Armed Forces Medical Services (DGAFMS)
IHQ of Ministry of Defence (Army)
New Delhi, India

G Shridhar
MD (Pediatrics) DM (Neonatology)
Professor
Department of Pediatrics
Armed Forces Medical College (AFMC)
Pune, Maharashtra, India

Gaurav Ray MBBS
Resident
Department of Pediatrics
Armed Forces Medical College (AFMC)
Pune, Maharashtra, India

Giridharan MBBS
Resident
Department of Pediatrics
Armed Forces Medical College (AFMC)
Pune, Maharashtra, India

H Ravi Ramamurthy
MD (Pediatrics) FNB (Pediatric Cardiology)
Professor
Department of Pediatrics
Army Institute of Cardio Thoracic Sciences
Pune, Maharashtra, India

KS Rana
MD (Pediatrics) Fellowship in Pediatric Neurology
Professor
Principal Director (Pediatric Neurology)
Department of Pediatrics
Venkateshwar Super-Specialty Hospital
New Delhi, India

Mithlesh Kumar Tiwari
MD (Pediatrics) DM (Pediatric Critical Care)
Assistant Professor
Department of Pediatrics
Command Hospital (SC)
Pune, Maharashtra, India

Mukti Sharma MD (Pediatrics) DNB FCSI FIAP
Professor and Consultant
Department of Pediatrics
Fortis Medical Centre
Chandigarh, India

Rakesh Gupta MD (Pediatrics) MPhil (HHSM)
Professor and Director
Department of Pediatrics
Government Institute of Medical Sciences
Greater Noida, Uttar Pradesh, India

Ranjit Ghuliani MD (Pediatrics)
Professor
Department of Pediatrics
Additional Medical Superintendent
Sharada University
Greater Noida, Uttar Pradesh, India

Ruchika Jha MD (Pediatrics)
Naval Hospital
Kochi, Kerala, India

Sachendra Badal MD (Pediatrics)
Professor
Department of Pediatrics
Command Hospital (WC)
Panchkula, Haryana, India

Sanjeev Khera
MD (Pediatrics) DM (Pediatric Hematology-Oncology)
Associate Professor
Department of Pediatrics
Army Hospital (R&R)
New Delhi, India

Sarguna K Logen MBBS
Resident
Department of Pediatrics
Armed Forces Medical College (AFMC)
Pune, Maharashtra, India

Sarvesh Kohli
MD (Pediatrics)
Clinical Tutor
Department of Pediatrics
Armed Forces Medical College (AFMC)
Pune, Maharashtra, India

Shuvendu Roy
MD (Pediatrics) Trained in Pediatric Neurology
Professor and Head
Department of Pediatrics
Armed Forces Medical Services
Pune, Maharashtra, India

SK Jatana
MD (Pediatrics)
Professor and Consultant
Pune, Maharashtra, India

Sucheta K Menon MBBS
Resident
Department of Pediatrics
Armed Forces Medical College (AFMC)
Pune, Maharashtra, India

Suprita Kalra
MD (Pediatrics) FNB (Pediatric Nephrology)
Professor
Department of Pediatrics
Command Hospital (SC)
Pune, Maharashtra, India

V Venkateshwar MD (Pediatrics)
Consultant Pediatrician
Department of Pediatrics
NICE Hospital for Women
Newborns, and Children
Hyderabad, Telangana, India

Vinod Dagar MD (Pediatrics)
Associate Professor
Department of Pediatrics
Military Hospital
Pathankot, Punjab, India

Vishal Sondhi
MD (Pediatrics) DM (Pediatric Neurology)
Professor
Department of Pediatrics
Military Hospital
Srinagar, Jammu and Kashmir, India

Foreword

"Medicine is a science of uncertainty and an art of probability."
—William Osler

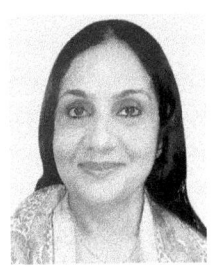

It is not uncommon to find several pediatricians, residents, and nurses surrounding a sick baby in an emergency department or intensive care unit (ICU), attempting to formulate the correct course of management for an acutely ill child. This book is dedicated to such caregivers and anxious parents, who have entrusted their child in our care.

More than a decade has passed since the publication of the first edition and new and improved techniques of monitoring and treatment have since been formulated. Clinical management has become more evidence based, to justify incorporating such modalities. Yet, the scene described above continues to prevail. Hence, this second edition has been prepared to provide comprehensive clinical guidance by incorporating the best evidence in the management of these children and blending such science with the art of experience. Pediatric critical care is a highly dynamic and evolving field and has always been a subject of intense academic and clinical interest. It encompasses a broad range of medical conditions and diseases that affect children, ranging from life-threatening illnesses to traumatic injuries. The field is constantly expanding and adapting as new research and clinical insights emerge. Despite the many challenges and complexities of pediatric critical care, the dedication and expertise of healthcare professionals continue to provide hope and comfort to countless children and their families around the world.

I have had the privilege of contributing to and editing the first edition of *The Acutely Ill Child: A Ready Reckoner* in 2013. The book had been well appreciated by medical students, residents, nurses, and clinicians as a ready reckoner in difficult situations. The second edition of this publication has undergone a significant expansion, with the inclusion of new chapters that cover emerging topics and updating several older ones, to reflect the latest research and clinical protocols. The contributing authors, who are all distinguished clinicians and researchers, have shared their expertise and insights in the care of sick children, which are backed by scientific evidence. Although not exhaustive, this book aims to aid in patient care and serve as a starting point for management, with the possibility of seeking more details elsewhere.

Mukti Sharma
MD (Pediatrics) DNB FCSI FIAP
Professor and Consultant
Department of Pediatrics
Fortis Medical Centre
Chandigarh, India

Preface to the Second Edition

We are extremely pleased to present the second edition of the book, *The Acutely Ill Child: A Ready Reckoner*. The idea of this ready reckoner came about in the year 2010 when we realized its need while handling sick children in an emergency. There was always an immediate requirement for looking at a simplified management approach and verifying the thoughts before putting them into action while handling the emergencies. This was especially required in hospitals and medical colleges where doctors and nurses were being trained in the care of sick children.

Towards this, the Department of Pediatrics at Armed Forces Medical College (AFMC) and Command Hospital, Pune, Maharashtra, India created several protocols for quick and effective handling of emergencies. These protocols then gave way to the concept of this book. It was intended to be a book 'by the residents for the residents' guided by competent faculty. The then residents and faculty of Pune complex contributed immensely to the book content which was published in the year 2013.

The second edition has the updated protocols to bring the management in line with the current standards of evidence-based care and has been vetted by experienced faculty. The chapters in the book cover various common emergencies across different organ systems, each containing a brief and an algorithm to assist with immediate point-of-care management. The last two sections cover common procedures and an array of commonly used charts and scales which we often look for from Internet sources.

This book is dedicated to all those who are involved with taking care of sick children and we hope that their hard work is complimented by the availability of this ready reckoner to be put into use in the initial minutes of a troubled family reporting to the hospital. This book should be of assistance to undergraduates, interns, nurses, residents, and practicing pediatricians who encounter sick children.

We are thankful to all the contributors across the years for sparing their valuable time in creating this simplified algorithmic content.

We are indebted to M/s Jaypee Brothers Medical Publishers (P) Ltd, New Delhi, India.

Finally, as usual, we are forever indebted to our patients and their parents for their belief in us.

Biju M John
Vishal Sondhi
Shuvendu Roy
G Shridhar

Preface to the First Edition

It gives us an immense pleasure to present this comprehensive book on *The Acutely Ill Child: A Ready Reckoner*. The foundation for this book was laid when we felt a need for a handy book for point of care reference in managing children who were having an acute illness but were not critically ill at presentation. We felt that an optimum understanding and interventions carried out by our residents in cases of acute illness would lead to faster recovery and prevent the child from slipping into a critical situation requiring equipment and pediatric intensive care unit (PICU).

In this direction, we produced certain protocols which were easy-to-follow and to implement by the attending physicians. These have provided us our desired results, thereby, encouraging us to write this book. The contributions have been made by experienced faculty in an easy-to-use format, as a ready reckoner for point of care management of acutely ill children. We have tried to cover all the relevant topics including toxicology and inborn errors of metabolism in a short and a comprehensive manner. Moreover, separate sections for the procedures have been included along with a section for charts and scales. All chapters are easy-to-read and assimilate.

This book embodies our hard work in the wards looking after ill children who were our responsibility and aiming to get best results for them and their parents. We feel this book will be very useful for the undergraduates, postgraduates, practising pediatricians and all those doctors who are managing sick children.

We are thankful to all the contributors for sparing their valuable time and stitching together all the management protocols in a lucid algorithmic format for the benefit of the student physicians, teaching physicians and practising physicians.

We are indebted to Shri Jitendar P Vij (Group Chairman), Mr Ankit Vij (Managing Director) and Mr Tarun Duneja (Director-Publishing) of M/s Jaypee Brothers Medical Publishers (P) Ltd, New Delhi, India, for their keen interest in helping us to bring this book to all our readers.

Finally, we are forever indebted to our patients and their families for their belief in us and we dedicate this edition to them.

Mukti Sharma
Biju M John
Vishal Sondhi

Acknowledgments

We wish to extend our sincerest gratitude to Armed Forces Medical College (AFMC), Pune, Maharashtra, India and the office of Director General, Armed Forces Medical Services, New Delhi for allowing us to pursue this project and take it towards publication. We are grateful to the entire fraternity of Residents and Pediatricians in the Armed Forces Medical Services who were responsible for the ideation and culmination of this book across the two editions. We are also indebted to Shri Jitendar P Vij (Group Chairman), Mr Ankit Vij (Managing Director), and Ms Chetna Malhotra (Senior Director—Professional Publishing, Marketing, and Business Development) of M/s Jaypee Brothers Medical Publishers (P) Ltd, New Delhi, India, for accepting our idea and for its successful realization.

Contents

SECTION 1: Supporting a Sick Child

1. **Assessment of a Sick Child** 3
   Daljit Singh, Aradhna Aneja

2. **Hypovolemic Shock** 9
   Aradhna Aneja, Daljit Singh

3. **Cardiogenic Shock** 11
   Aradhna Aneja, SK Jatana, Amit Pathania

4. **Septic Shock** 13
   Aradhna Aneja, Amit Pathania, Biju M John

5. **Anaphylactic Shock** 16
   SK Jatana, Aradhna Aneja, Amit Pathania

6. **Obstructive Shock** 18
   Aradhna Aneja, Daljit Singh

7. **Hyponatremia** 20
   Aradhna Aneja, Biju M John

8. **Hypernatremia** 22
   Aradhna Aneja, Biju M John

9. **Hypokalemia** 24
   Aradhna Aneja, Daljit Singh

10. **Hyperkalemia** 26
    Aradhna Aneja, Daljit Singh

11. **Hypocalcemia** 28
    Aradhna Aneja, Daljit Singh

12. **Approach to Arterial Blood Gas Analysis** 30
    Amit Pathania, Biju M John

13. **Sedation and Analgesia in Children** 36
    Aradhna Aneja, Biju M John

14. **Nutrition in a Critically Ill Child** 39
    Aradhna Aneja, Biju M John, Amit Pathania

SECTION 2: Respiratory Disorders

15. **Approach to a Child with Respiratory Distress**... 47
    Amit Pathania, Rakesh Gupta

16. **Acute Respiratory Failure** 49
    Amit Pathania, Rakesh Gupta

17. **Pediatric Acute Respiratory Distress Syndrome** 52
    Amit Pathania, Rakesh Gupta, Biju M John

18. **Croup**.. 56
    Rakesh Gupta, Amit Pathania

19. **Foreign Body Aspiration**.. 58
    Amit Pathania, Rakesh Gupta

20. **Acute Bronchiolitis**... 60
    Amit Pathania, Rakesh Gupta

21. **Acute Severe Asthma**... 62
    Rakesh Gupta, Amit Pathania

22. **Mechanical Ventilation** 65
    Amit Pathania, Biju M John

SECTION 3: Cardiovascular Disorders

23. **Approach to Cyanotic Infant** 73
    Arvind Mishra, Aradhana Dwivedi, Mukti Sharma

24. **Cyanotic Spells or "Tet Spells"**... 77
    Aradhana Dwivedi, Mukti Sharma, Arvind Mishra

25. **Congestive Cardiac Failure** 79
    Mukti Sharma, Aradhana Dwivedi, Arvind Mishra

26. **Hypertensive Emergencies in Children** 84
    Aradhana Dwivedi, Mukti Sharma, Arvind Mishra

SECTION 4: Hematological and Oncological Disorders

27. **Disseminated Intravascular Coagulation**.. 91
    Amit Devgan, Barnali Mitra

28. **Febrile Neutropenia**... 93
    Vishal Sondhi, Barnali Mitra

29. **Tumor Lysis Syndrome**... 95
    Barnali Mitra, Vishal Sondhi

30. **Hemophilia Emergencies** 99
    Barnali Mitra, Amit Devgan

31. **Acute Transfusion Reactions** 101
    Barnali Mitra, Vishal Sondhi

32. **Acute Illness in a Child with Sickle Cell Disease** 104
    Barnali Mitra, Vishal Sondhi

33. **Bleeding Disorders** 107
    Vishal Sondhi

SECTION 5: Endocrine Disorders

34. **Diabetic Ketoacidosis** 111
    Bikash Shreshta, V Venkateshwar, Biju M John

35. **Hypoglycemia** 114
    Bikash Shreshta, V Venkateshwar

36. **Syndrome of Inappropriate Antidiuretic Hormone Secretion** 116
    V Venkateshwar, Bikash Shreshta

37. **Adrenal Crisis** 118
    Bikash Shreshta, V Venkateshwar

38. **Diabetes Insipidus** 120
    Bikash Shreshta, V Venkateshwar

SECTION 6: Renal Disorders

39. **Acute Kidney Injury** 125
    V Venkateshwar, Bikash Shreshta, Suprita Kalra

40. **Hemolytic Uremic Syndrome** 130
    Bikash Shreshta, V Venkateshwar, Suprita Kalra

41. **Renal Replacement Therapy** 133
    Bikash Shreshta, V Venkateshwar, Suprita Kalra

SECTION 7: Gastrointestinal Tract and Liver Disorders

42. **Acute Abdomen** 139
    Vinod Dagar, Amit Devgan

43. **Gastrointestinal Bleed** 143
    Vinod Dagar, Amit Devgan

44. Intestinal Obstruction 148
    Vinod Dagar, Amit Devgan

45. Button Battery Ingestion.. 151
    Sarvesh Kohli

46. Approach to Acute Liver Failure 153
    Vinod Dagar, Amit Devgan

SECTION 8: Neurological Disorders

47. Approach to Coma 161
    Arvind Mishra, KS Rana

48. Status Epilepticus.. 164
    Vishal Sondhi

49. Increased Intracranial Pressure 169
    Arvind Mishra, KS Rana

50. Head Injury in Children 172
    Arvind Mishra, KS Rana

51. Acute Flaccid Paralysis.. 175
    H Ravi Ramamurthy, KS Rana

52. Febrile Encephalopathy... 180
    Vishal Sondhi

53. Autoimmune and Demyelinating Disorders... 183
    Ruchika Jha, Vishal Sondhi

SECTION 9: Neonatal Disorders

54. Respiratory Distress in Neonates.. 189
    G Shridhar

55. Neonatal Sepsis... 192
    G Shridhar

56. Neonatal Seizures 196
    G Shridhar

57. Inborn Errors of Metabolism 199
    Suprita Kalra

58. Approach to a Child with Ambiguous Genitalia 202
    Sarguna K Logen

SECTION 10: Infections

59. Severe Dengue 209
    Anjali Gautam
60. Complicated Malaria 211
    Sucheta K Menon
61. Rickettsial Disease 213
    Giridharan

SECTION 11: Toxicology and Environmental Hazards

62. Clinical Approach to a Suspected Case of Poisoning 217
    Sachendra Badal, Shuvendu Roy
63. Hydrocarbon Poisoning 222
    Sachendra Badal, Shuvendu Roy
64. Acetaminophen Toxicity 224
    Sachendra Badal, Shuvendu Roy
65. Organophosphorus Poisoning 227
    Sachendra Badal, Shuvendu Roy
66. Iron Poisoning 230
    Sachendra Badal, Shuvendu Roy
67. Snake Bite Treatment Protocol 233
    Sachendra Badal, Shuvendu Roy
68. Approach to Scorpion Bite 237
    Sachendra Badal, Shuvendu Roy
69. Drowning 240
    Suprita Kalra, Ranjit Ghuliani
70. Burns 242
    Ranjit Ghuliani, Suprita Kalra
71. Electrical Injuries 245
    Sarvesh Kohli

SECTION 12: Procedures

72. Use of Bedside Ultrasonography in PICU 251
    Arvind Kumar
73. Endotracheal Intubation 254
    Sanjeev Khera

74. Rapid-sequence Intubation 257
    Sanjeev Khera

75. Central Venous Line (Femoral Vein) 259
    Sanjeev Khera

76. Intraosseous Cannulation 262
    Sanjeev Khera

77. Peripherally Inserted Central Catheter Insertion 265
    Sanjeev Khera, Gaurav Ray

78. Radial Artery Cannulation 268
    Sanjeev Khera

79. Umbilical Vein Catheterization 271
    Sanjeev Khera, Gaurav Ray

80. Intercostal Drainage Tube Insertion 274
    Mithlesh Kumar Tiwari

81. Thoracocentesis: Needle Aspiration of Pneumothorax 276
    Sanjeev Khera

82. Abdominal Paracentesis 278
    Sanjeev Khera

SECTION 13: Charts and Scales

Section Editors: *Vinod Dagar, Abhishek Pandey, Sarvesh Kohli, Ajay Beriwal, Bhaskar Bharadwaj*

83. Pediatric Advanced Life Support Algorithms 283
84. Pediatric Early Warning Score 291
85. Triage 292
86. Ventilator Illustration 294
87. Noninvasive Ventilation Illustration 295
88. Sedation Withdrawal 296
89. Rapid-sequence Intubation 298
90. Maintenance Intravenous Fluids in Children 300
91. Total Parenteral Nutrition and Enteral Nutrition 301
92. Edema in Nephrotic Syndrome 305
93. Coma and Pain Scales 307

94.	Catheter and Tube Sizes	309
95.	Blood Component Replacement	313
96.	Abnormal Sodium	315
97.	Transudate versus Exudate	316
98.	Steroids and Efficacy	317
99.	Emergency Drug Preparation	318
100.	Important Formulae	319
101.	Glucose-6-phosphate Dehydrogenase and Drugs	321
102.	Drug Levels	322
103.	Electrocardiogram Values	326
104.	Intravenous Compatibility Charts	328
105.	Sample Collection	336
106.	Laboratory Values	337
107.	Computed Tomography Scan and Lesions	344
108.	Common Pediatric Applications	346
109.	Pediatric Neuroimaging Primer	347
110.	Pediatric Neurology Charts	352

Suggested Reading *357*
Index *361*

Introduction

The response of healthcare providers in the initial and immediate few minutes of a sick child reporting to the medical facility has extremely important connotation towards a successful outcome in the management of sick children. The process of learning the art and science of pediatric acute care is tedious and requires years of dedication and hard work. The senior clinicians can often guide this process. However, they are not always available as the first point of contact. Hence, the individuals in the chain of care are likely to be benefited with quick references on management of sick children. It is with this background, that this book, *The Acutely Ill Child: A Ready Reckoner* was created. The residents and faculty from the Department of Pediatrics, Armed Forces Medical College (AFMC), Pune, Maharashtra, India complex including its affiliated hospitals have contributed immensely towards both the editions of this book over more than a decade.

The book retains the extremely popular format from the first edition with all the necessary updates. The first section deals with supporting a sick child across several physiological derangements. Sections 2 to 8 deal with common emergencies covering different systems. Sections 9 to 11 cover neonatology, infections, toxicology and environmental hazards. Section 12 deals with procedures and Section 13 deals with a compendium of useful information, charts, and scales. Each of the emergencies described carries a brief text on the topic with a simple and algorithmic management approach placed next to it.

Everyone involved in the management of sick children irrespective of their position in the chain of care is likely to find this ready reckoner a very useful addition to their toolkit for a quick and effective emergency medical response.

Daljit Singh
MD DNB DM FNNF FIAP
Director General
Armed Forces Medical Services (DGAFMS)
IHQ of Ministry of Defence (Army)
New Delhi, India

SECTION 1

Supporting a Sick Child

- **Assessment of a Sick Child**
  Daljit Singh, Aradhna Aneja
- **Hypovolemic Shock**
  Aradhna Aneja, Daljit Singh
- **Cardiogenic Shock**
  Aradhna Aneja, SK Jatana, Amit Pathania
- **Septic Shock**
  Aradhna Aneja, Amit Pathania, Biju M John
- **Anaphylactic Shock**
  SK Jatana, Aradhna Aneja, Amit Pathania
- **Obstructive Shock**
  Aradhna Aneja, Daljit Singh
- **Hyponatremia**
  Aradhna Aneja, Biju M John
- **Hypernatremia**
  Aradhna Aneja, Biju M John
- **Hypokalemia**
  Aradhna Aneja, Daljit Singh
- **Hyperkalemia**
  Aradhna Aneja, Daljit Singh
- **Hypocalcemia**
  Aradhna Aneja, Daljit Singh
- **Approach to Arterial Blood Gas Analysis**
  Amit Pathania, Biju M John
- **Sedation and Analgesia in Children**
  Aradhna Aneja, Biju M John
- **Nutrition in a Critically Ill Child**
  Aradhna Aneja, Biju M John, Amit Pathania

CHAPTER 1

Assessment of a Sick Child

Daljit Singh, Aradhna Aneja

The assessment follows a rapid systematic approach for management of a seriously ill/injured child. This is described in following steps:
- *Initial impression:* It is the first, quick visual and auditory observation of the child's consciousness, breathing, and color (CBC).
  - *Consciousness:* Level of consciousness may be characterized as unresponsive, irritable, or alert.
  - *Breathing:* Check for increased work of breathing, use of accessory muscles, absent/decreased respiratory effort, abnormal breath sounds, or abnormal breathing pattern.
  - *Color:* Look for abnormal skin color—pallor, cyanosis, and mottling, suggesting poor perfusion, poor oxygenation, or both.
- *Based on the initial assessment, determine if the child's problem is life-threatening or not.*
  - If it is a life-threatening problem, immediately begin appropriate interventions.
  - If it is not a life-threatening, continue with the systematic approach.
  - If the child is unresponsive and not breathing/only gasping, shout for help/activate emergency response. Check to see if there is a pulse.
    - *If no pulse:* Start cardiopulmonary resuscitation (CPR), follow pediatric cardiac arrest algorithm.
    - If pulse present, provide rescue breathing.
    - If, despite adequate oxygenation and ventilation, the heart rate <60 beats/min with signs of poor perfusion, provide chest compressions and ventilations. Proceed according to pediatric cardiac arrest algorithm.
    - If heart rate >60 beats/min, begin the evaluate–identify–intervene sequence.
  - If child is breathing adequately, proceed with the evaluate–identify–intervene sequence.
- *Evaluate-identify-intervene sequence:* Evaluate the child by primary assessment, secondary assessment, and diagnostic tools. After evaluation, identify the problem by type and severity and then, intervene with appropriate actions.

Evaluation: It includes primary assessment, secondary assessment, and diagnostic tools. These are as described below:
- *Primary assessment:* Follow ABCDE approach described as follows:

  A: Airway—Check for airway patency, which is done by:
  - Look for movement of chest or abdomen.

- Listen for breath sounds.
- Feel the movement of air at the nose/mouth.

Based on above evaluation, classify airway as:
- *Clear:* Airway is open and unobstructed.
- *Maintainable:* Airway can be maintained by simple measures (e.g., head tilt–chin lift)
- *Not maintainable:* Airway cannot be maintained without advanced interventions (e.g., intubation)

Simple measures:
- Comfortable positioning
- Use head tilt–chin lift to open airway (in case of cervical spine injury, open the airway using a jaw thrust without neck extension)
- Suction the nose/oropharynx
- Foreign body airway obstruction relief measures:
  - *<1 year:* Back slaps and chest thrusts
  - *>1 year:* Abdominal thrusts

Advanced measures:
- Endotracheal intubation
- Foreign body removal with laryngoscopy
- Continuous positive airway pressure (CPAP)
- Cricothyrotomy

B: Breathing—Assessment of breathing includes evaluation of:
- *Respiratory rate:* Count the number of times chest rises in 30 seconds and multiply it by 2 to determine the respiratory rate and assess as tachypnea/bradypnea/apnea
- *Respiratory effort:* Signs of increased respiratory effort include nasal flaring/retractions/open-mouth breathing, and head bobbing/see-saw respiration.
- *Tidal volume:* Check for:
  - Magnitude of chest wall excursion
  - Auscultate for distal air movement
- *Airway and lung sounds:* Stridor/grunting/wheezing/gurgling/crackles
- *Pulse oximetry:* Oxygen saturation >94% indicates adequate oxygenation.

C: Circulation—Assessment of circulation includes evaluation of:
- *Cardiovascular functions:*
  - Skin color
  - Heart rate
  - Heart rhythm
  - Blood pressure
  - Pulses (central and peripheral)
  - Capillary refill time
- *End-organ functions:*
  - Brain perfusion (mental status)
  - Skin perfusion
  - Renal perfusion (urine output)

D: Disability—Disability assessment includes quick evaluation of cerebral cortex and brain stem evaluation, which includes:
- *AVPU pediatric response scale:* System for rating child's level of consciousness and response to stimuli
  - *A:* Alert
  - *V:* Voice
  - *P:* Painful
  - *U:* Unresponsive
- Glasgow Coma Scale
- Pupillary response to light

The causes of decreased level of consciousness in children include:
- Poor cerebral perfusion
- Meningitis, encephalitis
- Hypoglycemia
- Hypoxemia, hypercarbia
- Traumatic brain injury
- Drugs

E: Exposure—Undress the child to facilitate a focused physical examination. Check for hypothermia, bleeding, petechiae/purpura, and abdominal distension.
- *Secondary assessment:* It is done after the primary assessment and stabilization of the child. It includes focused history and detailed physical examination.
  - *Focused history:* Use the SAMPLE pneumonic to identify important aspects of child's history and presenting complaints.
    - *S:* Signs and symptoms
    - *A:* Allergies
    - *M:* Medications
    - *P:* Past medical history
    - *L:* Last meal
    - *E:* Events
  - *Detailed physical examination:* Perform a thorough head-to-toe physical examination.
- *Diagnostic tests:* These consist of ancillary studies to detect and identify the presence and severity of respiratory and circulatory abnormalities.
  - Assessment of respiratory abnormalities:
    - Arterial blood gas
    - Venous blood gas
    - Hemoglobin concentration
    - Pulse oximetry
    - Chest X-ray
    - Exhaled CO_2 monitoring
    - Capnography
    - Peak expiratory flow rate

- Assessment of circulatory abnormalities:
    - Arterial blood gas
    - Venous blood gas
    - Central venous oxygen saturation
    - Total serum CO_2
    - Arterial lactate
    - Hemoglobin concentration
    - Invasive arterial pressure monitoring
    - Chest X-ray
    - Central venous pressure monitoring
    - Echocardiography
- Identify the type and severity of child's problem as follows:

Respiratory:

Type	Severity
Upper airway obstruction	Respiratory distress
Lower airway obstruction	Respiratory failure
Lung tissue disease	
Disordered control of breathing	

Circulatory:

Type	Severity
Hypovolemic shock	Compensated shock
Distributive shock	Hypotensive shock
Cardiogenic shock	
Obstructive shock	

- Cardiopulmonary failure
- Cardiac arrest
- *Intervene:* On the basis of identification of child's problem, intervention steps include:
    - Positioning the child to maintain patent airway
    - Activate emergency response
    - Start CPR
    - Place the child on monitors (cardiac, pulse oximeter)
    - Oxygen and ventilation
    - Medications and fluids
- The sequence of *evaluate-identify-intervene* continues until the child is stable.

The pediatric advanced life support (PALS) systematic approach algorithm is given in **Flowchart 1**.

CHAPTER 1: Assessment of a Sick Child

Flowchart 1: Pediatric advanced life support (PALS) systematic approach algorithm.

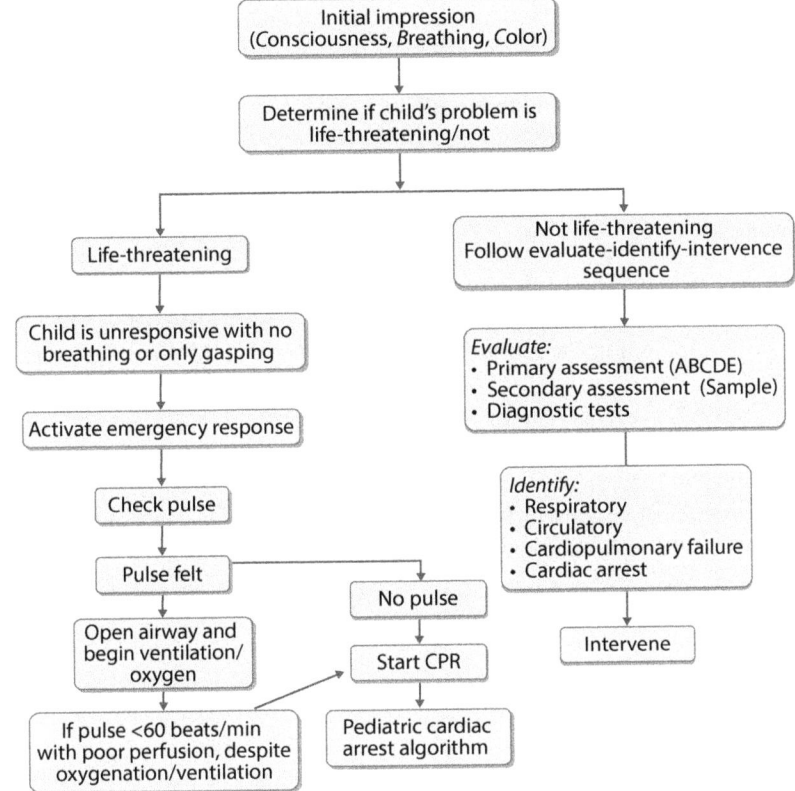

The PALS—Evaluate, Identify, and Intervene cycle is shown in **Table 1**.

TABLE 1: Pediatric advanced life support (PALS)—evaluate, identify, and intervene cycle.			
Evaluate	*Identify*		*Intervene*
Airway: • Open • Maintainable • Not maintainable	• Maintainable with simple maneuvers • Not maintainable		• Positioning and suction • Head tilt, chin lift, and jaw thrust • Oropharyngeal airway • LMA • Intubate
Breathing: • Respiratory rate and pattern • Respiratory effort • Chest expansion • Lung sound • SpO$_2$	Severity: • Respiratory distress • Respiratory failure	Type: • Upper airway • Lower airway • Parenchymal disease • Disordered control breathing	Oxygen: • If stridor, adrenaline nebulization + Inj Dexamethasone if indicated • Nebulization with salbutamol if wheeze • Antibiotics if fever • If grunt, ventilation with PEEP

Contd...

Contd...

Evaluate	Identify		Intervene
Circulation: • HR and rhythm • Pulses (central and peripheral) • CRT • Skin color and temperature • BP	*Severity:* • Shock • Compensated • Hypotensive	*Type:* • Hypovolemic • Obstructive • Distributive • Cardiogenic	• IV cannula • IV fluids • Blood products • Inotropes • Remove obstruction if obstructive
Disability: • AVPU • Pupils • Blood glucose	• Decreased consciousness • Hypoglycemia • Pupillary abnormality/raised ICP		• IV glucose • Ventilation • ICP lowering measures
Exposure: • Temperature and skin (rash, bleeding, trauma)	• Temperature • Skin injury/rash/bleed		• Antipyretics • Hemostasis

(AVPU: alert, voice, painful, unresponsive; BP: blood pressure; CRT: capillary refill time; HR: heart rate; ICP: intracranial pressure; IV: intravenous; LMA: laryngeal mask airways; PEEP: positive end-expiratory pressure; SpO_2: peripheral oxygen saturation)

CHAPTER 2

Hypovolemic Shock

Aradhna Aneja, Daljit Singh

- Hypovolemic shock is the most common cause of shock in infants and children.
- It is defined as a decrease in the intravascular blood volume to an extent that effective tissue perfusion cannot be maintained.
- It is characterized by decreased preload leading to reduced stroke volume and low cardiac output.
- *Etiology:*
  - *Whole blood loss:*
    - Hemorrhage (external and internal)
  - *Fluid and electrolyte loss:*
    - Vomiting and diarrhea
    - Excessive diuretic use
    - *Endocrine:* Diabetic ketoacidosis (DKA), diabetes insipidus
  - *Plasma loss:*
    - Burns
    - *Capillary leak syndromes:* Sepsis, anaphylaxis
    - *Protein-losing syndromes:* Nephritic syndrome, intestinal obstruction
- *Clinical features*:
  - Tachycardia
  - Tachypnea
  - Normal blood pressure or hypotension with a narrow pulse pressure
  - Prolonged capillary refill
  - Cool extremities
  - Weak or absent peripheral pulses, weak central pulses
  - Oliguria
  - Changes in mental state
  - The dehydration can be classified as mild (3%—30 mL/kg), moderate (6%—60 mL/kg), and severe (9%—90 mL/kg) for older children and similarly for an infant, mild (5%), moderate (10%), and severe (15%).
  - *Management* of hypotensive shock is given in **Flowchart 1**.

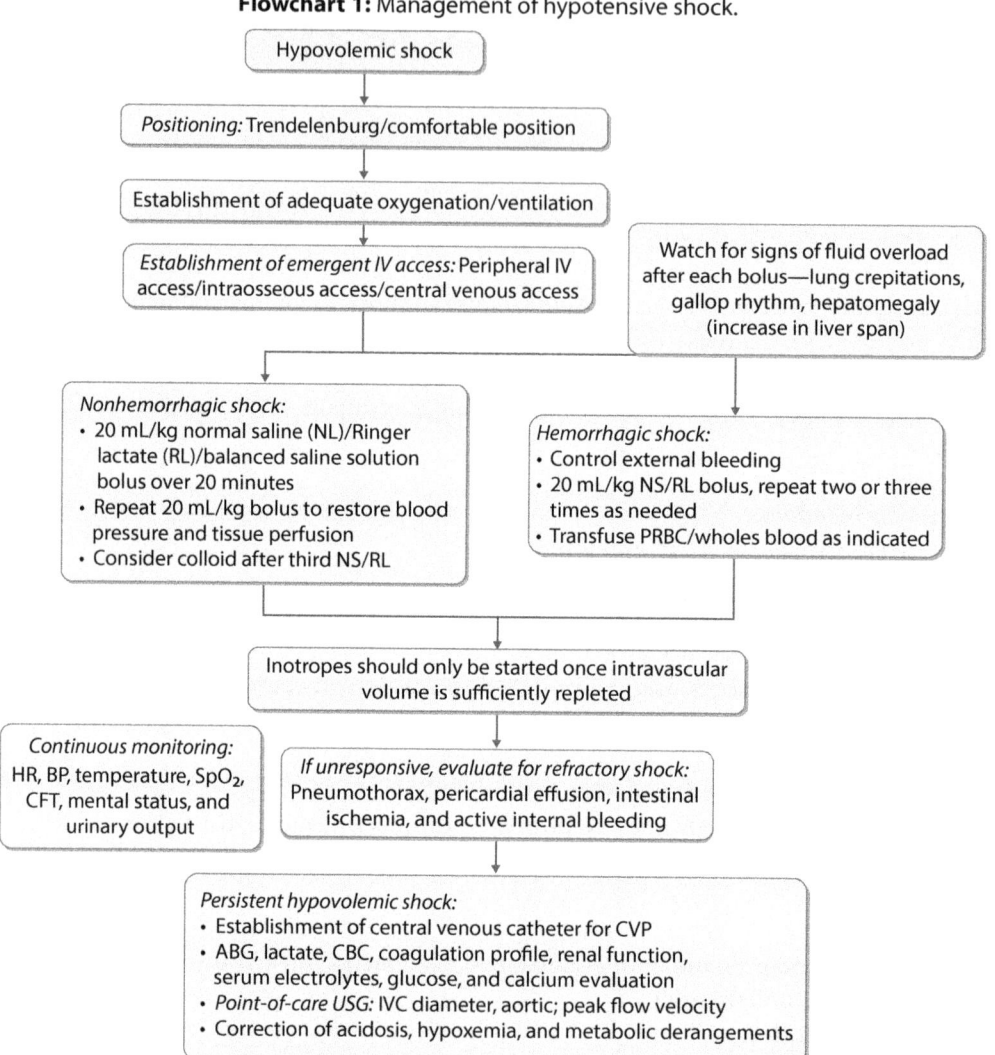

Flowchart 1: Management of hypotensive shock.

(ABG: arterial blood gas; BP: blood pressure; CBC: complete blood count; CFT: capillary filling time; CVP: central venous pressure; HR: heart rate; IV: intravenous; IVC: inferior vena cava; PRBC: packed red blood cell; SpO$_2$: peripheral oxygen saturation; USG: ultrasonography)

CHAPTER 3

Cardiogenic Shock

Aradhna Aneja, SK Jatana, Amit Pathania

- Cardiogenic shock is a condition of inadequate tissue perfusion resulting from myocardial dysfunction.
- Myocardial dysfunction can be caused by pump failure (poor contractility), congenital heart disease, or rhythm abnormalities.
- *Etiology of cardiogenic shock:*
  - *Heart rate abnormalities:*
    - Supraventricular tachycardia
    - Bradycardia
    - Ventricular dysrhythmias
  - *Cardiomyopathy/carditis:*
    - *Infectious:* Viral, bacterial, fungal, rickettsial, sepsis
    - *Metabolic:* Hypoglycemia, glycogen storage disorder, carnitine deficiency, mucopolysaccharidoses
    - *Connective tissue disorders:* Systemic lupus erythematosus (SLE), juvenile rheumatoid arthritis (JRA), Kawasaki disease, polyarteritis nodosa
    - *Neuromuscular disorders:* Duchenne muscular dystrophy, spinal muscular atrophy
    - Hypoxic/ischemic events
    - Poisoning/drug toxicity
  - Congenital heart disease
  - Trauma
- Cardiogenic shock is characterized by decreased cardiac output, marked tachycardia, and high systemic vascular resistance.
- *Clinical features:*
  - Features of congestive heart failure (pulmonary edema, hepatomegaly, jugular venous distension)
  - Cyanosis with cyanotic congenital heart disease (CCHD)
  - *Features of shock:* Tachycardia, tachypnea, normal or low blood pressure with a narrow pulse pressure, weak peripheral/central pulses, delayed capillary refill time, cool extremities, diaphoresis, oliguria, changes in mental status
- *Management includes:*
  - Cautious fluid administration and monitoring
  - Laboratory and nonlaboratory studies
  - Pharmacologic support

Management of cardiogenic shock is shown in **Flowchart 1**.

SECTION 1: Supporting a Sick Child

Flowchart 1: Management of cardiogenic shock.

```
                        ┌─────────────────────┐
                        │  Cardiogenic shock  │
                        └──────────┬──────────┘
                                   ▼
        ┌──────────────────────────────────────────────────┐
        │ Minimize myocardial oxygen demands:              │
        │  • Supplemental oxygen/mechanical ventilation    │
        │  • Maintain normal core temperature              │
        │  • Provide sedation                              │
        │  • Correct anemia                                │
        └──────────────────────┬───────────────────────────┘
                               ▼
┌────────────────────────────────────────────────────────────────┐
│ Administer fluid resuscitation cautiously:                     │
│  • 5–10 mL/kg isotonic crystalloid infusion                    │
│  • Deliver slowly, over 30–60 minutes and reassess for         │
│    response after each bolus                                   │
└──────────────────────┬─────────────────────────────────────────┘
                       ▼
┌──────────────────────────────────────────────────────────┐
│ Order laboratory and nonlaboratory studies to determine  │
│ cause:                                                   │
│  • ABG, hemoglobin, lactate, cardiac enzymes             │
│  • Chest X-ray, ECG, echocardiogram                      │
└──────────────────────────────────────────────────────────┘
```

- **CHD/myocarditis/cardiomyopathy/poisoning**
  - *Optimize preload:* Diuretics
  - *Increase contractility:*
    - IV dobutamine (@2–20 µg/kg/min), only if BP is normal for the age
    - Epinephrine (0.05–3.0 µg/kg/min)
  - *Decrease afterload:*
    - Nitroprusside (3–4 µg/kg/min), ACE inhibitors (enalapril @ 0.01 mg/kg/dose 8 hourly)
    - Milrinone (0.5–0.75 µg/kg/min)

- **Bradyarrhythmias/tachyarrhythmias**
  - Management algorithms:
    - Bradycardia
    - Tachycardia with poor perfusion (refer to arrhythmia algorithm)

Deteriorating cardiogenic shock
- Left ventricular assist devices; biventricular assist devices/ECMO
- Cardiac transplantation

(ABG: arterial blood gas; ACE: angiotensin-converting enzyme; BP: blood pressure; CHD: congenital heart disease; ECG: electrocardiogram; ECMO: extracorporeal membrane oxygenation; IV: intravenous)

CHAPTER 4: Septic Shock

Aradhna Aneja, Amit Pathania, Biju M John

- Septic shock is defined as sepsis and cardiovascular dysfunction despite administration of isotonic intravenous fluid boluses >40 mL/kg in 1 hour.
- *Phoenix Sepsis criteria* **(Table 1):**

TABLE 1: The Phoenix Sepsis Score

	0 Point	1 Point	2 Points	3 Points
Respiratory (0–3 points)	PaO$_2$:FiO$_2$ ≥400 Or SpO$_2$:FiO$_2$ ≥292	PaO$_2$:FiO$_2$ < 400 on any respiratory support Or PaO$_2$:FiO$_2$ <292 on any respiratory support	PaO$_2$:FiO$_2$ 100–200 with invasive mechanical ventilation Or PaO$_2$:FiO$_2$ 148–220 with invasive mechanical ventilation	PaO$_2$:FiO$_2$ <100 with invasive mechanical ventilation Or PaO$_2$:FiO$_2$ <148 with invasive mechanical ventilation
Cardiovascular (0–6 points)		1 point each (up to 3 points):	2 points each (up to 6 points):	
	No vasoactve medications	1 vasoactive medication	≥2 vasoactive we medications	
	Lactate <5 mmol/L	Lactate 5–10.9 mmol/L	Lactate ≥11 mmol/L	
Age-based mean arterial pressure mm Hg (0–2 points)				
<1 month	>30	17–30	<17	
1–11 months	>38	25–38	<25	
1–<2 years	>43	31–43	<31	
2–<5 years	>44	32–44	<32	
5–<12 years	>48	36–48	<36	
12–17 years	>51	38–51	<38	
Coagulation (0–2 points)		1 point each (up to 2 points)		
	Platelets ≥100 × 10^3/µL INR ≤1.3 D-dimer ≤2 mg/L FEU Fibrinogen ≥100 mg/dL	Platelets <100 × 10^3/µL INR >1.3 D-dimer >2 mg/L FEU Fibrinogen <100 mg/dL		
Neurological (0–2 points)	Glasgow Coma Scale >10; pupils reactive	Glasgow Coma Scale score ≤10	Fixed pupils bilaterally	

(FEU: fibrinogen equivalent unit; FiO$_2$: fraction of inspired oxygen; INR: international normalized ratio; PaO$_2$: partial pressure of arterial oxygen; SpO$_2$: peripheral oxygen saturation)

- *Sepsis:* Suspected infection and Phoenix Sepsis Score ≥2 points
- *Septic shock:* Sepsis with ≥1 cardiovascular point
■ *Septic shock is a combination of three classic types of shock:* Hypovolemic, cardiogenic, and distributive.
■ Clinical manifestation could be either warm shock (increased cardiac output and decreased systemic vascular resistance) or cold shock (decreased cardiac output and increased systemic vascular resistance).
■ *Early recognition of septic shock in children:* A crucial step: Early recognition is crucial for successful treatment and improved outcomes. Unlike adults, children may not exhibit the classic signs of shock, making early detection more challenging. Here are some of the key signs to watch for:
  - *Altered mental status:* Confusion, drowsiness, or unusual behavior
  - *Abnormal vital signs:* Rapid breathing (tachypnea), rapid heart rate (tachycardia), and abnormal temperature (hypothermia or hyperthermia)
  - *Decreased urine output:* Reduced urination frequency or wet diapers
  - *Changes in skin perfusion:* Cold, clammy, or pale skin
  - *Metabolic abnormalities:* Increased blood lactate levels indicating potential organ dysfunction
■ *Investigations*: Hematologic abnormalities, positive sepsis screen, raised lactate, hypoalbuminemia with electrolyte disturbance, prolonged PT/PTTK (prothrombin time/partial thromboplastin time with kaolin), elevated fibrin split products, chest X-ray, culture of body fluids [blood, urine, cerebrospinal fluid (CSF), peritoneal fluid etc.].
■ *Management:* The principles of management of septic shock may be broadly classified as:
  - Goal-directed therapy
  - Antimicrobial therapy and source removal
  - Interventions to enhance host responses
  - Management of organ dysfunction
■ *Therapeutic endpoints* of resuscitation of septic shock (as shown in **Flowchart 1**)

Flowchart 1: Management of septic shock.

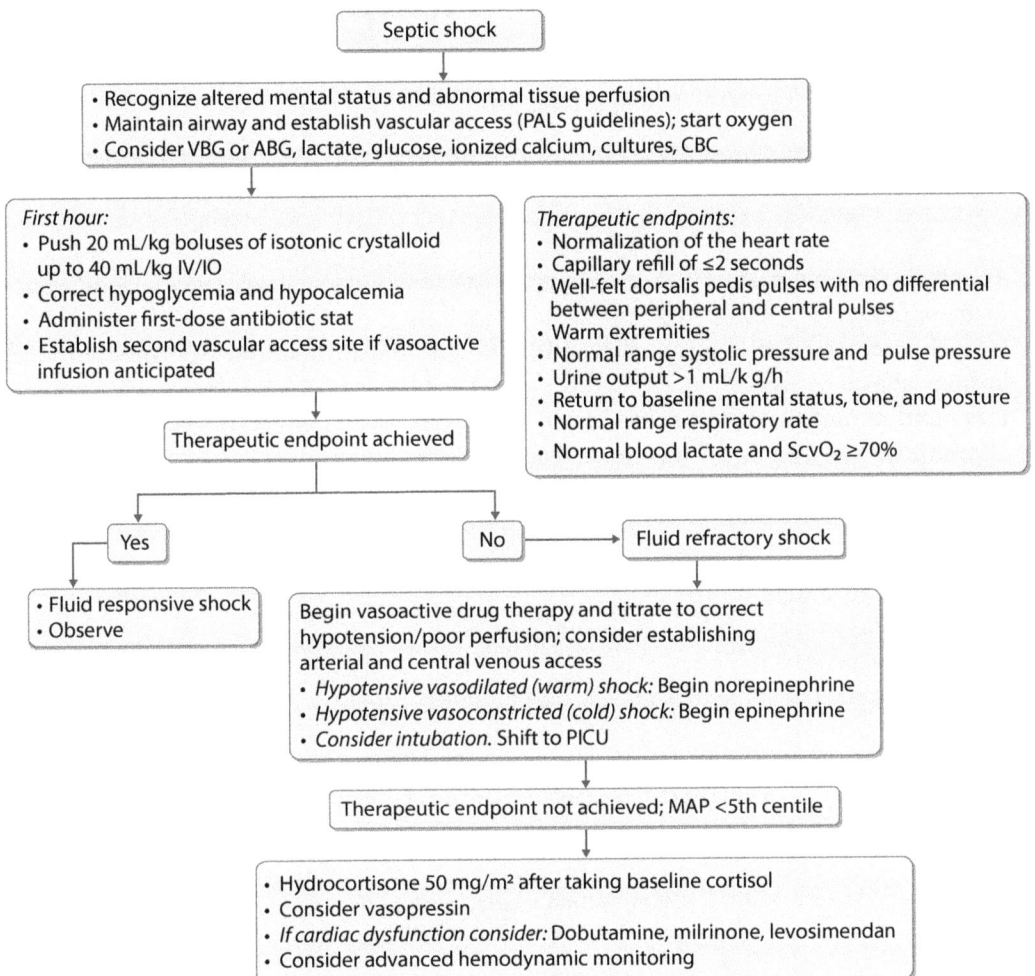

(ABG: arterial blood gas; CBC: complete blood count; IO: intraosseous; IV: intravenous; MAP: mean arterial pressure; PALS: pediatric advanced life support; PICU: pediatric intensive care unit; ScvO$_2$: central venous oxygen saturation; VBG: venous blood gas)

CHAPTER 5: Anaphylactic Shock

SK Jatana, Aradhna Aneja, Amit Pathania

- Anaphylactic shock results from a serious allergic reaction to a drug, vaccine, food, venom, toxin, or plant.
- It is characterized by systemic vasodilation, increased capillary permeability, and bronchospasm.
- It is rapid in onset, causing acute-phase symptoms, which typically begin 5-10 minutes after exposure, sometimes, may cause death.
- It occurs due to sudden release of potent biologically active mediators from mast cells and basophils.
- *Clinical features:*
  - Pruritus around mouth/face
  - Anxiety/agitation
  - Flushing, urticaria
  - Angioedema (swelling of face, lips, and tongue)

Flowchart 1: Management of anaphylactic shock.

```
Anaphylactic shock
        ↓
Ensure ABC resuscitation, euglycemia
Do not allow to sit or walk
        ↓
Inj epinephrine in dose of 0.01 mg/kg IM (maximum 0.5 mg)—can
be repeated in 5–15 minutes; switch to IV infusion if >3 doses required
        ↓
• Fluid bolus of 20 mL/kg of isotonic crystalloid over 20 minutes
• Nebulize with beta-2 agonist (salbutamol @ 0.15 mg/kg in 3 mL NS)
• Nebulization with adrenaline for airway edema
• Corticosteroids: IV methylprednisolone 1–2 mg/kg (maximum 125 mg)
  or IV hydrocortisone @ 5 mg/kg/dose
• Antihistamines: H₁ blockade, diphenhydramine (1.25 mg/kg PO) or
  cetirizine (0.25 mg/kg PO) + H₂ blockade IV ranitidine 1–2 mg/kg up to 50 mg
        ↓  ← No response
• Epinephrine infusion (IV infusion @ 0.1 µg/kg/min)
• Vasopressors (IV vasopressin @ 1 mU/kg/min)
```

(ABC: airway, breathing, circulation; IV: intravenous; NS: normal saline)

- Tightness in throat, dry staccato cough
- Respiratory distress with stridor/wheezing
- Nausea, vomiting, abdominal cramps
- Tachycardia
- Hypotension
- Altered sensorium/loss of consciousness
■ *Diagnosis*: This is based on clinical features developing in seconds to minutes after exposure.
■ Management involves **(Flowchart 1)**:
  - Treatment of life-threatening cardiorespiratory problems
  - Blockade of allergic mediators

CHAPTER 6

Obstructive Shock

Aradhna Aneja, Daljit Singh

- Obstructive shock is a condition of impaired cardiac output caused by physical obstruction to the blood flow.
- *Etiology:*
  - Cardiac tamponade
  - Tension pneumothorax
  - Pulmonary/systemic hypertension
  - Massive pulmonary embolism
  - Duct-dependent congenital heart lesions
- *Clinical features:* These depend on the cause of obstructive shock given as follows—
  - *Cardiac tamponade:* It is caused by accumulation of fluid, blood, or air in the pericardial space. As cardiac output becomes restricted, a child may have features of congestive cardiac failure (CCF), but lungs are usually clear. Specific physical signs include:
    - Pulsus paradoxus
    - Narrowed pulse pressure
    - Distended neck veins
    - Muffled heart sounds/pericardial rub
  - *Tension pneumothorax:* This is caused by entry of air into the pleural space. It is to be suspected in the victim of chest trauma or in an intubated child, who suddenly deteriorates during positive pressure ventilation (including bag and mask ventilation). Specific signs are:
    - Rapid deterioration in perfusion
    - Tracheal deviation to opposite side
    - Distended neck veins
    - Diminished breath sounds on affected side
    - Hyperresonance on affected side
  - *Duct-dependent cardiac lesions:* It is of two types—
    1. Duct dependent for pulmonary blood flow (cyanotic congenital heart disease):
       - Present with cyanosis
    2. Duct dependent for systemic blood flow/left ventricular outflow tract obstruction
       - For example coarctation of aorta, interrupted aortic arch, critical aortic stenosis, hypoplastic left heart syndrome; these present as:
       - Rapidly progressive deterioration in systemic perfusion
       - Congestive heart failure
       - Differential cyanosis
       - Differential blood pressure

- Absence of femoral pulses
- Rapid deterioration in mental status
- Respiratory failure with signs of pulmonary edema
- *Pulmonary embolism:* This is caused by total/partial obstruction of pulmonary artery. It is to be suspected in presence of underlying predisposing conditions such as central venous catheters, sickle cell disease, disorders of coagulation, and malignancy. Clinical features include:
  - Tachycardia
  - Hypotension
  - Cyanosis
  - Features of right heart failure
- *Investigations and management*: These depend on the specific cause, on the basis of clinical suspicion **(Flowchart 1)**.

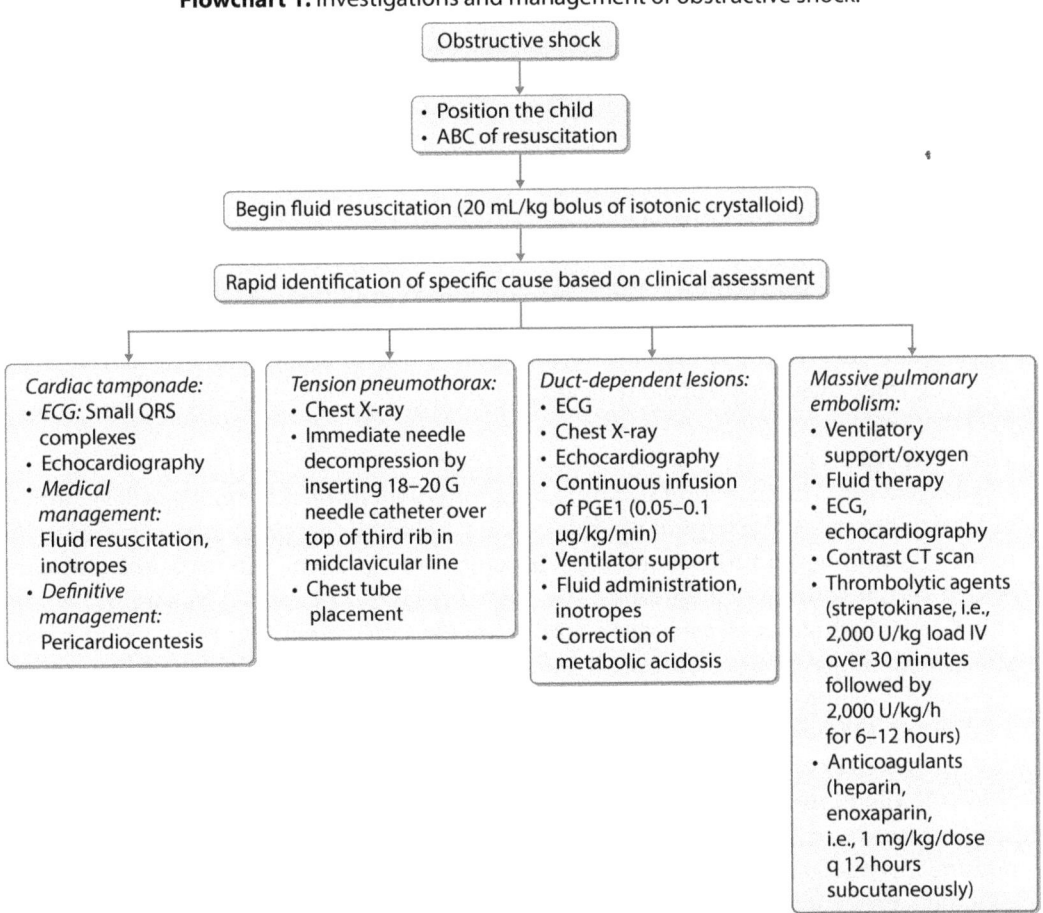

Flowchart 1: Investigations and management of obstructive shock.

(ABC: airway, breathing, circulation; CT: computed tomography; ECG: electrocardiogram; IV: intravenous; PGE1: prostaglandin E1)

CHAPTER 7

Hyponatremia

Aradhna Aneja, Biju M John

- Hyponatremia is defined as serum sodium of <135 mEq/L.
- *Causes of hyponatremia* are as follows:
  - *Decreased total body sodium:*
    - *Renal causes:*
      - *Diuretics:* Thiazides, mannitol, loop diuretics
      - Tubulointerstitial diseases
      - Obstructive uropathy
      - Renal tubular acidosis, chronic pyelonephritis
      - Cerebral salt wasting
    - *Extrarenal causes:*
      - Vomiting/diarrhea
      - Septicemia, peritonitis, burns
      - Ventriculostomy drainage
  - *Increased total body sodium:*
    - Congestive heart failure, cirrhosis, nephritic syndrome, renal failure
  - *Normal total body sodium:*
    - Syndrome of inappropriate antidiuretic hormone secretion (SIADH), hypothyroidism, glucocorticoid deficiency
  - *Pseudohyponatremia:*
    - Hyperglycemia, hyperlipidemia
- *Clinical features:* The severity of signs and symptoms depend on the rapidity of development of hyponatremia. Acute hyponatremia features include lethargy, apathy, disorientation, nausea, vomiting, and muscle cramps. Most patients present with seizures and coma have a serum sodium <120 mEq/L. The signs are generally related to cerebral edema. Other signs include decreased deep tendon reflexes, pseudobulbar palsy, and Cheyne-Stokes respiratory pattern. Chronic hyponatremia may be asymptomatic or present with nonspecific symptoms of nausea, vomiting, and lethargy.
- *Treatment* **(Flowchart 1)***:* The management of hyponatremia is based on the pathophysiology of the specific etiology (hypovolemic, euvolemic, or hypervolemic) as shown in the **Flowchart 1**. It requires a slow correction with judicious monitoring. It is important to avoid "overtly rapid" correction of hyponatremia, because it may cause central pontine myelinolysis (CPM). The calculation of fluid correction for 24 hours is as follows:
  - Calculate sodium requirement, i.e., sodium deficit + sodium maintenance:
    - *Sodium deficit:* (135 − measured sodium) × weight × 0.6
    - *Sodium maintenance:* 2–4 mEq × weight (per 24 hours)

CHAPTER 7: Hyponatremia

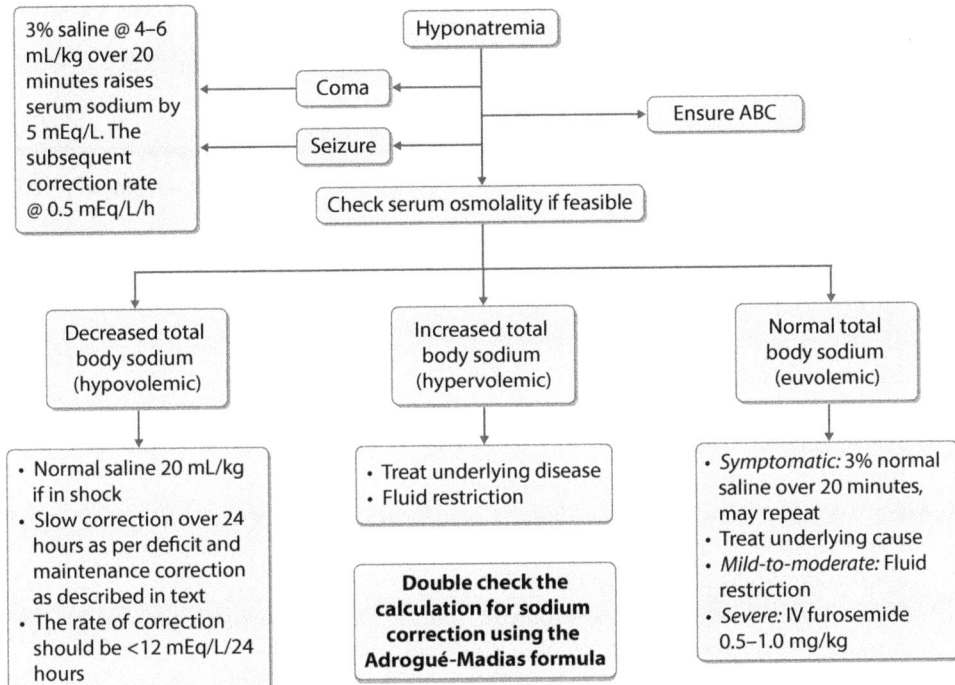

Flowchart 1: Treatment of hyponatremia.

(ABC: airway, breathing, circulation; IV: intravenous)

- Determine the fluid requirement for 24 hours, i.e., fluid deficit + fluid maintenance:
  - Fluid deficit: 10 mL/kg/% dehydration
- Based on above calculations, calculate the sodium concentration of the replacement fluid (i.e., by dividing sodium requirement by fluid requirement).

CHAPTER 8

Hypernatremia

Aradhna Aneja, Biju M John

- Hypernatremia is defined as sodium concentration >145 mEq/L.
- *Causes of hypernatremia*:
  - *Excessive sodium:*
    - Improperly mixed formula
    - Intravenous hypertonic saline/excess sodium bicarbonate
    - Hyperaldosteronism
    - Ingestion of seawater/sodium chloride
  - *Water deficit:*
    - Central diabetes insipidus
    - Nephrogenic diabetes insipidus
    - *Increased insensible losses:* Premature infants, radiant warmers, phototherapy
    - *Inadequate intake:* Ineffective breastfeeding, adipsia
  - *Water and sodium deficits:*
    - *Gastrointestinal losses:* Diarrhea, emesis, nasogastric suction
    - *Cutaneous losses:* Burns, excessive sweating
    - *Renal losses:* Diabetes mellitus, chronic kidney disease (dysplasia and obstructive uropathy), polyuric phase of acute tubular necrosis
- *Clinical features:* Features of hypernatremic dehydration are given as follows—
  - Doughy feel of skin irritability
  - Lethargy
  - Restlessness
  - High-pitched cry
  - Fever
  - Hyperglycemia, hypocalcemia
- *Complications:* These include brain hemorrhage (seizure and coma), central pontine myelinolysis, and thrombotic complications.
- *Diagnosis:* This involves history, clinical examination, serum sodium levels, with combined sodium and water deficits; urine analysis differentiates between renal and nonrenal etiologies.
- *Management* **(Flowchart 1):** Hypernatremia should not be corrected rapidly. The goal is to decrease serum sodium by 12 mEq/L every 24 hours @ 0.5 mEq/h. Frequent monitoring of serum sodium is required.

The calculation of free water deficit is by following formula:

Water deficit: Body weight × 0.6(1 − 145/current sodium) which is equivalent to 3–4 mL of water/kg for each 1 mEq of sodium above 145 mEq.

CHAPTER 8: Hypernatremia

Flowchart 1: Management of hypernatremia.

```
                        Hypernatremia
                              │
    ┌─────────────────────────┼─────────────────────┐
    │                         │                     │
 Seizures                    ...              Ensure ABC
    │                         │
Refer to management         Shock
of seizure on page            │
                       Protocol for shock
                          management
                              │
                       Assess hydration
                              │
            ┌─────────────────┴─────────────────┐
   Hypovolemic/euvolemic                   Hypervolemic
```

Hypovolemic/euvolemic:
- *Low total body sodium:*
  - *Renal:* Osmotic diuresis, obstructive uropathy
  - *Extrarenal:* Diarrhea, burns
- *Normal total body sodium (free water loss):*
  - *Renal:* DI
  - *Extrarenal:* Central DI, sweating

- Restore intravascular volume, i.e., NS @ 20 mL/kg over 20 minutes
- Determine time for correction on basis of initial sodium concentration:
  - *145–157 mEq/L:* 24 hours
  - *158–170 mEq/L:* 48 hours
  - *171–183 mEq/L:* 72 hours
  - *184–196 mEq/L:* 84 hours
- Administer fluid, i.e., 0.5 NS with 5% dextrose @ 1.25–1.5 times maintenance over time as above

Double check the calculation for sodium correction using the Adrogué-Madias formula

Hypervolemic:
- *High total body sodium:*
  - Salt poisoning
  - Improper feeding
  - Hypertonic solutions

- Consider loop diuretics
- Peritoneal dialysis if poor renal function or CHF

Complications:
- *Seizures, cerebral edema:* Treat with hypertonic (3%) saline infusion @ 4–6 mL/kg
- *Hypocalcemia:* Refer to Chapter on same
- *CHF, pulmonary edema:* Oxygen + diuretics

(ABC: airway, breathing, circulation; CHF: congestive heart failure; DI: diabetes insipidus; NS: normal saline)

CHAPTER 9

Hypokalemia

Aradhna Aneja, Daljit Singh

- Hypokalemia is defined as serum potassium <3.5 mEq/L.
- *Causes of hypokalemia* are as follows:
    - *Spurious:*
        - High white blood cell count
    - *Transcellular shifts:*
        - Alkalosis
        - Insulin
        - Hypokalemic periodic paralysis, thyrotoxic periodic paralysis
        - *Drugs:* Beta-adrenergic agonists, theophylline
    - *Decreased intake:*
        - Malnutrition, anorexia nervosa
    - *Extrarenal losses:*
        - Diarrhea
        - Laxative abuse
        - Sweating
        - Vomiting/nasogastric suction
    - *Renal losses:*
        - Renal tubular losses (proximal/distal)
        - Ureterosigmoidostomy
        - Diabetic ketoacidosis
        - Interstitial nephritis—postobstructive diuresis
        - Diuretic phase of acute tubular necrosis
        - *Tubular toxins:* Amphotericin, aminoglycosides
        - Bartter syndrome, Gitelman syndrome
    - *Endocrinal:*
        - Cushing syndrome, hyperaldosteronism
- *Clinical features:* These are mentioned as follows—
    - Muscle weakness, hypotonia, paralysis, respiratory paralysis
    - *Cardiac:* Arrhythmias (supraventricular tachycardia, ventricular tachycardia, heart block)
    - Constipation, urinary retention
    - In patients with liver disease, it exacerbates encephalopathy
- *Diagnosis:*
    - History and clinical features
    - Serum and urinary potassium assay

- *Electrocardiogram (ECG) changes:* Flattened T wave, depressed ST-segment, prominence of U wave, arrhythmias
- *Management (Flowchart 1):* Factors affecting treatment include potassium level, clinical symptoms, renal function, and ongoing losses.

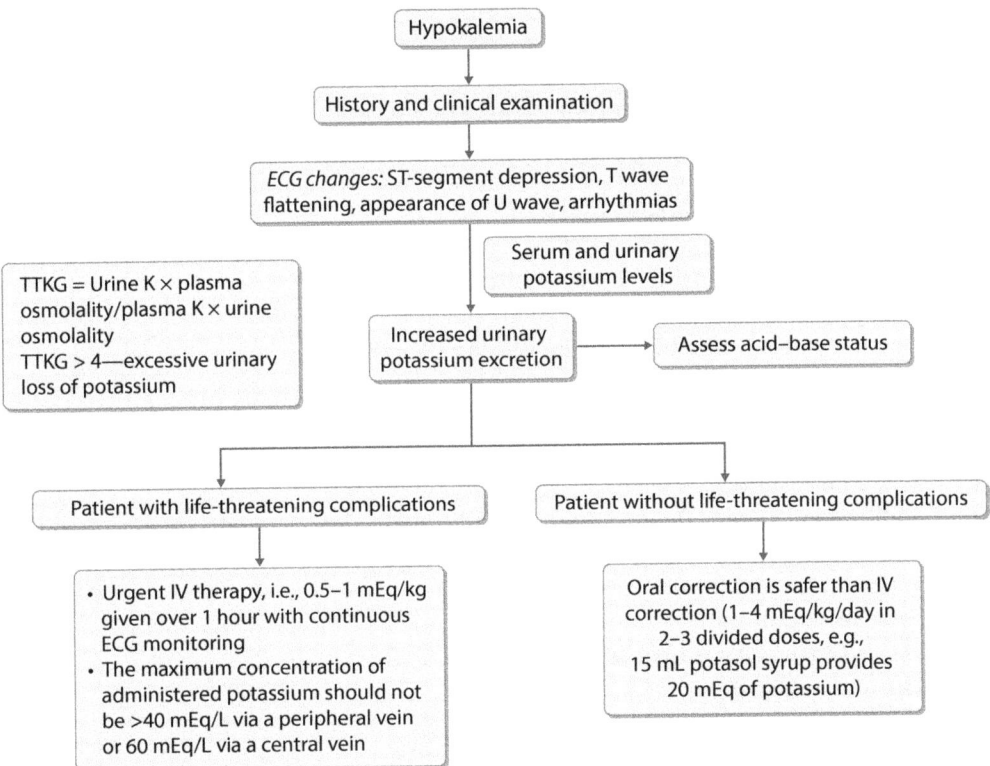

Flowchart 1: Management of hypokalemia.

(ECG: electrocardiogram; IV: intravenous; TTKG: transtubular potassium concentration gradient)

CHAPTER 10

Hyperkalemia

Aradhna Aneja, Daljit Singh

- Hyperkalemia is defined as a serum potassium level of >5.5 mEq/L in a nonhemolyzed sample.
- Causes of hyperkalemia:
  - *Spurious laboratory value:*
    - Hemolysis
    - Tissue ischemia during blood withdrawing
    - Thrombocytosis (platelets >100,000/mm^3)
    - Leukocytosis [white blood cells (WBC) >100,000/mm^3]
  - *Increased intake:*
    - Intravenous or oral
    - Blood transfusions
  - *Transcellular shifts:*
    - Acidosis
    - Rhabdomyolysis
    - Tumor lysis syndrome
    - Tissue hemolysis
    - *Digitalis*/fluoride intoxication
    - Insulin deficiency
    - Malignant hyperthermia
    - Exercise
  - *Decreased excretion:*
    - *Renal failure:* Dehydration/shock
    - Primary adrenal disease
    - Hypoaldosteronism
    - Renal tubular disease
  - *Drugs:*
    - Angiotensin-converting enzyme inhibitors/angiotensin 2 blockers
    - Beta blockers
    - Potassium-sparing diuretics
    - NSAIDs (nonsteroidal anti-inflammatory drugs)
- *Clinical features (Table 1):* These are due to the role of potassium in membrane stabilization.
- *Management (Flowchart 1):* The treatment has two basic goals, i.e., to stabilize the heart to prevent life-threatening arrhythmias and to remove potassium from the body.
  - The first step is to stop all sources of additional potassium [oral or intravenous (IV)]
  - Treatment depends on the level of plasma potassium.

CHAPTER 10: Hyperkalemia

TABLE 1: Potassium levels and changes.

Serum potassium (mEq/L)	ECG changes	Symptoms
2.5	Prominent U waves, AV conduction defects, ventricular arrhythmias, ST-segment depression	Apathy, weakness, paresthesia
7.5	Peaked T waves	Weakness, paresthesia
8.0	Loss of P wave, widening of QRS complex	–
9.0	ST-segment depression, further widening of QRS complex	Tetany
10.0	Bradycardia, sine wave QRS-T, first degree AV block, ventricular arrhythmias, cardiac arrest	–

(AV: atrioventricular; ECG: electrocardiogram)

Flowchart 1: Management of hyperkalemia.

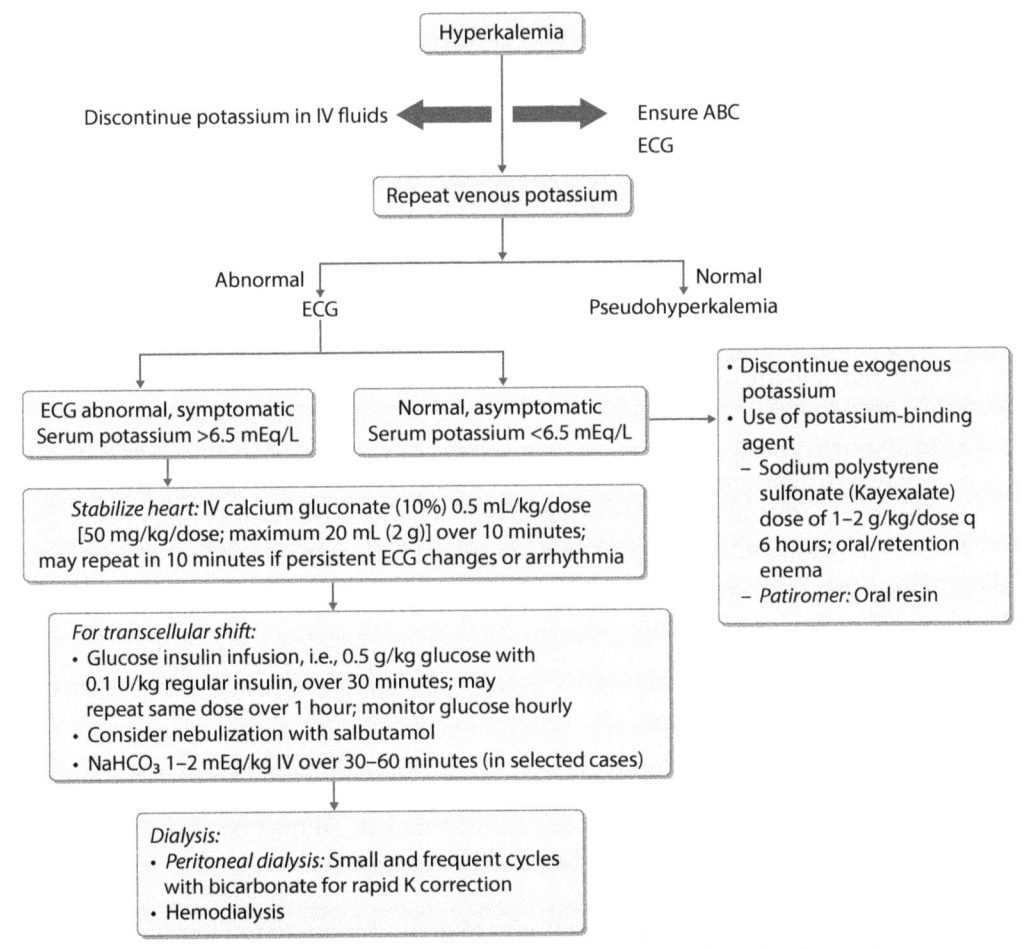

(ECG: electrocardiogram; IV: intravenous; NaHCO$_3$: sodium bicarbonate)

CHAPTER 11

Hypocalcemia

Aradhna Aneja, Daljit Singh

- Hypocalcemia is defined as serum ionized calcium <4 mg/dL or total serum calcium <8 mg/dL
- *Forms of calcium in the body:* Approximately 40% of calcium is bound to proteins (albumin), 10% is complexed with anions, and remaining 50% exists in ionized form.
- *Etiology:*
  - Inadequate intake/malabsorption
  - *Parathyroid hormone (PTH)-related:*
    - Congenital agenesis/dysgenesis of parathyroid gland
    - Trauma
    - Radiation
    - *Parathyroid gland destruction:* Wilson disease, thalassemia, hemochromatosis
  - Insensitivity to PTH
  - DiGeorge syndrome
  - *Suppression of PTH release:*
    - Hypomagnesemia
    - Maternal hypermagnesemia
    - Sepsis
    - Calcium-sensing receptor mutation
  - *Vitamin D-related:*
    - Inadequate intake
    - Decreased absorption
    - *Impaired activation:* Renal disease, liver failure, hyperphosphatemia
  - *Drugs:* Phenytoin, phenobarbital, carbamazepine, rifampicin, calcitonin
- *Clinical features:*
  - *Overt features:*
    - *Nervous system:* Tetany, convulsions, carpopedal spasm, muscle cramps and twitching, paraesthesia of perioral region, finger and toes, myoclonic jerks, laryngeal stridor, apnea in newborn
    - *Cardiovascular system:* Hypotension, congestive cardiac failure, arrythmia, myocardial depression
    - *Other changes:* Dry coarse skin, eczema, brittle hair with alopecia, brittle nails with smooth transverse grooves, dental enamel hypoplasia
  - Signs of latent hypocalcemia:
    - *Chvostek sign:* Provoked facial muscle twitching (percussion of nerve anterior to external auditory meatus)

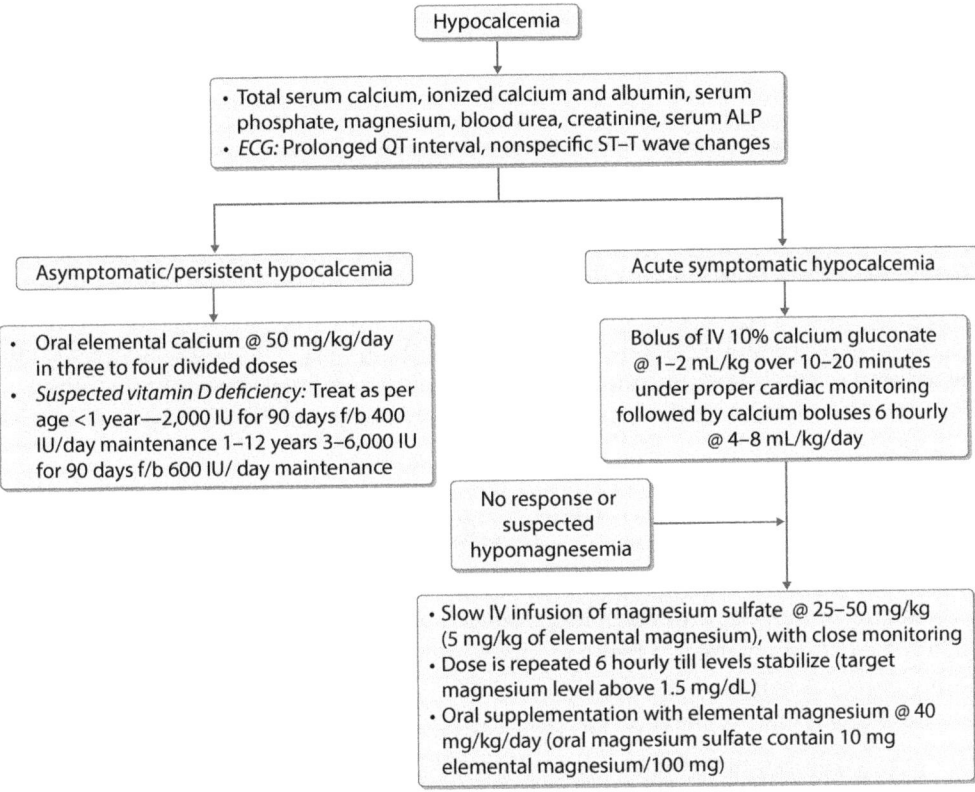

Flowchart 1: Management of hypocalcemia.

(ALP: alkaline phosphatase; ECG: electrocardiogram; f/b: followed by; IV: intravenous)

- *Trousseau sign:* Provoked carpopedal spasm with ischemia (compression of arm/leg with blood pressure cuff to a pressure above systolic pressure for 3 minutes)
- Diagnosis:
  - Determination of free ionized calcium
  - Check serum proteins as reduction of serum albumin by 1 g/dL produces fall of protein-bound calcium fraction of 0.8 mg/dL
  - *Electrocardiogram (ECG) changes:* Prolonged QT interval, nonspecific ST–T wave changes.

CHAPTER 12: Approach to Arterial Blood Gas Analysis

Amit Pathania, Biju M John

- *Ensure correctness of sampling and correctness of report:* Look at the clinical profile and amount of oxygen being delivered [fraction of inspired oxygen (FiO$_2$)]. Send blood gases and electrolytes (with bicarbonate if available) at same time. This will help in ascertaining the validity of the blood gas report (blood gas machine measures only the blood gases and pH). The serum bicarbonate and blood gas bicarbonate should be matching. Also remember:

$$(H^+) = \frac{24 \times pCO_2}{(HCO_3^-)}$$

(H) = 80 − XY (pH is 7 × XY when pH is in range of 7.20–7.50)

The sample must be processed immediately, preferably within 20 minutes and must be sent on ice pack as blood is a living medium and cells consume O$_2$ and CO$_2$ is produced. Homogenize the sample before processing.

The changes of arterial blood gas (ABG) every 10 minutes in vitro are given in **Table 1**.

TABLE 1: Changes of arterial blood gas (ABG) every 10 minutes in vitro.

	37°C	4°C
pH	0.01	0.001
pO$_2$ (mm Hg)	0.1	0.01
pCO$_2$ (mm Hg)	1	0.1

(pCO$_2$: partial pressure of carbon dioxide; pO$_2$: partial pressure of oxygen)

- *Identify the dominant disorder:* Normal range pH 7.35–7.45, partial pressure of carbon dioxide (pCO$_2$) 35–45 mm Hg, HCO$_3^-$ 22–26 mEq/L; for calculations take pH 7.4, pCO$_2$ 40, and HCO$_3^-$ 24 as normal.

Primary disorder and direction of changes are given in **Table 2**.

TABLE 2: Primary disorder and direction of changes.

Primary disorder	Initial change	Compensatory change
Metabolic acidosis	↓ HCO$_3^-$	↓ PaCO$_2$
Metabolic alkalosis	↑ HCO$_3^-$	↑ PaCO$_2$
Respiratory acidosis	↑ PaCO$_2$	↑ HCO$_3$
Respiratory alkalosis	↓ PaCO$_2$	↓ HCO$_3$

(PaCO$_2$: partial pressure of arterial carbon dioxide)

- Calculate compensation and its appropriateness **(Table 3)**.

TABLE 3: Primary disorder and compensation.

Disorder	pH	Primary change	Compensatory response	Equation for compensatory response
Metabolic acidosis	↓	↓ HCO_3^-	↓ pCO_2	$\Delta pCO_2 = 1.2 \times \Delta HCO_3^-$
Metabolic alkalosis	↑	↑ HCO_3^-	↑ pCO_2	$\Delta pCO_2 = 0.7 \times \Delta HCO_3^-$
Respiratory acidosis	↓	↑ pCO_2 (partial pressure of carbon dioxide)	↑ HCO_3^-	• Acute: $\Delta HCO_3^- = 0.1 \times \Delta pCO_2$ • Chronic: $\Delta HCO_3^- = 0.3 \times \Delta pCO_2$
Respiratory alkalosis	↑	↓ pCO_2	↓ HCO_3^-	• Acute: $\Delta HCO_3^- = 0.2 \times \Delta pCO_2$ • Chronic: $\Delta HCO_3^- = 0.5 \times \Delta pCO_2$

- *For metabolic acidosis*: Calculate anion gap (AG), corrected AG, delta AG, and bicarbonate gap.
  - AG = $Na^+ - (Cl^- + HCO_3^-)$; normal ~12 mmol/L
  - Corrected AG: Correct for albumin—for every 1 g/dL below 4.0 g/dL, AG increases by 2.5.
  - AG adjusted = AG + 0.25 (normal albumin − observed albumin) (normal albumin = 4 g/dL)
  - Δ AG = AG − 12
  - $\Delta HCO_3^- = 24 - HCO_3^-$
    - $\Delta AG = \Delta HCO_3^-$: Pure high AG metabolic acidosis
    - $\Delta AG > \Delta HCO_3^-$: High AG metabolic acidosis + Metabolic alkalosis
    - $\Delta AG < \Delta HCO_3^-$: High AG metabolic acidosis + Non-AG acidosis (hyperchloremic metabolic acidosis)

"USEDCARP versus MUDPILES" for causes of metabolic acidosis are given in **Table 4**.

TABLE 4: "USEDCARP versus MUDPILES" for causes of metabolic acidosis.

Normal AG metabolic acidosis	Increased AG metabolic acidosis
Ureteroenterostomy	Methanol
Small-bowel fistula	Uremia
Extra chloride	DKA
Diarrhea	Paraldehyde
Carbonic anhydrase inhibitor use	Iron/INH/inhalants (CO, CN)
Adrenal insufficiency	Lactic acidosis
Renal tubular acidosis	Ethanol/ethylene glycol
Pancreatic fistula	Salicylate/starvation/solvents

(AG: anion gap; DKA: diabetic ketoacidosis; INH: isoniazid)

Normal AG acidosis (hyperchloremic metabolic acidosis) is given in **Table 5**.

TABLE 5: Normal anion gap acidosis (hyperchloremic metabolic acidosis).

• Urine Cl⁻ >Urine Na⁺ + K⁺ • Urine pH <5.5 • *GI:* Losses—diarrhea, small bowel/pancreatic drainage • *Renal losses:* Proximal RTA • Miscellaneous—adrenal insufficiency, carbonic anhydrase	• Urine Cl⁻ <Urine Na⁺ + K⁺ • Urine pH >5.5 Distal RTA

(GI: gastrointestinal; RTA: renal tubular acidosis)

Treatment of metabolic acidosis is essentially treatment of cause and maintenance of perfusion and oxygenation. 1 mEq/kg sodium bicarbonate over 30-60 minutes in an emergency is prescribed. The deficit (usually corrected when bicarbonate <10 mEq/L) is 0.6 × body weight × (desired bicarbonate − actual bicarbonate). Other available drugs are THAM and Carbicarb.

- For metabolic alkalosis:
  - *Compensation:* Hypoventilation and elevation of partial pressure of arterial carbon dioxide ($PaCO_2$) (maximal $PaCO_2$ rarely exceeds 55 mm Hg)
  - Need to do urinary electrolytes to decide on response to fluids **(Table 6)**.

TABLE 6: Urinary electrolytes and response to fluids.

Urine electrolyte	Saline sensitivity	Saline resistant
Cl	<10 mEq/L (unless on diuretics)	>20 mEq/L
Na	<20 mEq/L (unless recent vomiting)	>20 mEq/L
K	May be high if high distal Na (diuretics or recent vomiting)	Usually high as aldosterone is acting

- *Knowing about other values on your ABG:*
  - *Total CO_2 (TCO_2):* "Total CO_2" is a value often reported on blood gas slips. TCO_2 is defined as the sum of the carbonic acid and the bicarbonate.

$$TCO_2 = (H_2CO_3) + (HCO_3^-)$$

  As the normal ratio of bicarbonate to carbonic acid at physiologic pH is around 20:1, TCO_2 will therefore be about 5% higher than serum bicarbonate. When you observe a difference between TCO_2 and bicarbonate that is larger than 5%, the patient will be acidotic. The TCO_2 is not particularly informative by itself. However, it will be abnormal in cases of chronic (compensated) acid–base disorders, such as when chronically elevated carbon dioxide levels cause bicarbonate retention.
  - *Base excess:* The "buffer base" is the total of all the anionic buffer components in the blood such as bicarbonate, sulfates, and phosphates. The base excess is the amount of deviation of the patient's buffer base from normal, in other words, how much extra basic (anionic) chemicals the patient has in his blood, expressed in milliequivalents per liter. The base excess is also defined as the amount of acid (in mEq/L) that would have to be added to the patient's blood to bring it to normal pH of 7.4. Base excess

can be a negative value. Although many physicians use the difference between the patient's bicarbonate and an average bicarbonate of 24 as an indication of the patient's need for bicarbonate replacement, the base excess is a more accurate measure, because it also takes into account other buffers such as phosphate and hemoglobin. It remains accurate in cases where the buffering capacity of hemoglobin is decreased due to anemia.
- *Base excess of extracellular fluid (ECF):* The base excess of blood does not truly indicate the base excess of the total ECF. Because of different protein contents and the absence of hemoglobin, ECF has a different buffering capacity. In addition, each ECF (e.g., CSF vs. interstitial fluid) has a different buffer status. Clinical determination of the amount of bicarbonate required for treatment of severe acidosis is usually based on the base excess of the blood. There is an unavoidable inaccuracy, however, due to several factors as follows:
  - The time course of the acidosis makes the blood acid poorly reflect the total body acid burden in many cases.
  - Depending on the state of hydration, body fluid distribution varies.
  - ECF as a percent of body weight varies with age and fat content (and thus the correction formula for bicarbonate often uses $0.1 - 0.3 \times$ body weight (desired bicarbonate − actual bicarbonate).
- *Standard and actual bicarbonate:* Standard bicarbonate indicates the status of bicarbonate, which would be there if CO_2 compensation did not happen.
  - The standard bicarbonate indicates a metabolic acidosis or alkalosis:
    - When the standard bicarbonate is low, this is a sign of metabolic acidosis.
    - When the standard bicarbonate is high, this is a sign of metabolic alkalosis.
  - The difference between the actual bicarbonate and the standard bicarbonate indicates a respiratory acidosis or alkalosis.
    - When the actual bicarbonate is higher than the standard bicarbonate, this is a sign of respiratory acidosis.
    - When the actual bicarbonate is lower than the standard bicarbonate, this is a sign of respiratory alkalosis.
  - When the actual bicarbonate and the standard bicarbonate are equal, this indicates respiratory balance.
    - When both are low and equal, it indicates uncompensated metabolic acidosis.
    - When both are high and equal, it indicates uncompensated metabolic alkalosis.
- What do you do with partial pressure of arterial oxygen (PaO_2)?
Tells us about oxygenation:
  - Calculate the alveolar-arterial oxygen gradient. Some machines will give you the gradient if you feed the FiO_2 correctly.

  $$PaO_2 = FiO_2 (Patm - pH_2O) - PaCO_2/R$$

  where Patm is atmospheric pressure, pH_2O is partial pressure of water, and R is respiratory quotient
  - Look at the PaO_2/FiO_2 ratios

- If child is on ventilator, calculate oxygenation index (OI) (MAP × FiO_2/PaO_2) where MAP is mean airway pressure

  Normal A-a gradient:
  - A-a = Age in years/4 +4
  - *Young person at sea level*: A-a increases 5–7 mm Hg for every 10% increase in FiO_2 (room air: 10–20 mm Hg, 100% O_2: 60–70 mm Hg)
  - A-a gradient changes with age (20 years: 4–17 mm Hg, 40 years: 10–24 mm Hg, 60 years: 17–31 mm Hg)

Oxyhemoglobin relation is given in **Table 7**.

TABLE 7: Oxyhemoglobin relation.

PaO_2 mm Hg	SpO_2%
60	90
40	75
26	50

(PaO_2: partial pressure of arterial oxygen; SpO_2: peripheral oxygen saturation)

- *Remember*:
  - Anaerobic collection
  - Avoid excess heparin
    - May in itself reduce pH; 0.05 mL of heparin per 1 mL of blood (<1:20)
  - No delay in processing (or cool to 4°C)
    - Can be refrigerated for a maximum of 2 hours

The difference between arterial blood gas and venous blood gas is given in **Table 8**.

TABLE 8: Difference between arterial blood gas (ABG) and venous blood gas (VBG).

	Arterial	Venous
pH	7.35–7.45	0.04 units less
PaO_2	95 mm Hg	40 mm Hg
$PaCO_2$	35–45 mm Hg	5–7 mm Hg more
SaO_2	97%	75%

($PaCO_2$: partial pressure of arterial carbon dioxide; PaO_2: partial pressure of arterial oxygen; SaO_2: arterial oxygen saturation)

Management of arterial blood gas is given in **Flowchart 1**.

CHAPTER 12: Approach to Arterial Blood Gas Analysis

Flowchart 1: Management of arterial blood gas.

```
                              Arterial blood gas
                                     │
                                 Check pH
                        ┌────────────┴────────────┐
                   pH <7.35                    pH >7.45
                   Acidosis                    Alkalosis
                       │                            │
          Check partial pressure of        Check pCO₂ and HCO₃
          carbon dioxide pCO₂ and HCO₃      ┌─────────┴─────────┐
           ┌─────────┴─────────┐       Increased HCO₃      Decreased pCO₂
      Decreased HCO₃    Increased pCO₂        │
      Metabolic acidosis                Metabolic alkalosis
             │                                 │
    Check expected compensation     Check expected compensation
    Compared with expected pCO₂     Compared with expected pCO₂
      ┌──────┼──────┐                  ┌──────┼──────┐
    Lower  Normal  Higher            Lower  Normal  Higher
    pCO₂   pCO₂    pCO₂              pCO₂   pCO₂    pCO₂
```

Under acidosis branch (metabolic acidosis compensation):
- Lower pCO₂ → Mixed metabolic acidosis and respiratory alkalosis
- Normal pCO₂ → Simple metabolic acidosis
- Higher pCO₂ → Mixed metabolic acidosis and respiratory acidosis

Under acidosis branch (Increased pCO₂):
- Respiratory acidosis
- Check expected compensation, Compared with expected HCO₃
  - Lower HCO₃ → Mixed respiratory acidosis and metabolic acidosis
  - Normal HCO₃ → Simple respiratory acidosis
  - Higher HCO₃ → Mixed respiratory acidosis and metabolic alkalosis

Under alkalosis branch (metabolic alkalosis compensation):
- Lower pCO₂ → Mixed metabolic alkalosis and respiratory alkalosis
- Normal pCO₂ → Simple metabolic alkalosis
- Higher pCO₂ → Mixed metabolic alkalosis and respiratory acidosis

Under alkalosis branch (Decreased pCO₂):
- Respiratory alkalosis
- Check expected compensation, Compared with expected HCO₃
  - Lower HCO₃ → Mixed respiratory alkalosis and metabolic acidosis
  - Normal HCO₃ → Simple respiratory alkalosis
  - Higher HCO₃ → Mixed respiratory alkalosis and metabolic alkalosis

CHAPTER 13

Sedation and Analgesia in Children

Aradhna Aneja, Biju M John

- The ability to provide safe and effective sedation and analgesia is an important skill for pediatric emergency care.
- Procedural sedation is the delivery of sedating agent to produce a state of depressed consciousness.
- Analgesia is loss of sensation to painful stimuli, without affecting the sensorium.
- Common indications of procedural sedation and analgesia (PSA) are given as follows:
  - Wound dressing changes
  - Burn care
  - Orthopedic manipulation
  - Lumbar puncture
  - Chest tube insertion
  - Eye injuries
  - Central line placement
  - Abscess incision and drainage
  - Bone marrow aspiration and biopsy
  - Computed tomography (CT) scan and magnetic resonance imaging (MRI)
  - Ultrasound
  - Echocardiography
  - Electroencephalogram (EEG)
- *Levels of sedation*:
  - *Minimum sedation:* Patient responds to verbal commands, with no effect on cognitive function, respiratory, and cardiovascular function.
  - *Moderate sedation and analgesia:* Patient responds to verbal commands, impairment of cognitive function, with no effect on respiratory/cardiovascular function.
  - *Deep sedation and analgesia:* Patient cannot be easily aroused, spontaneous ventilation may be inadequate, with no effect on cardiovascular system.
  - *General anesthesia:* Loss of consciousness, adequate airway cannot be maintained, and cardiovascular system may be impaired.
- *Preparation before PSA*:
  - Appropriate patient selection is vital as severe systemic diseases/life-threatening conditions are contraindications to PSA.
  - A thorough history and clinical examination is crucial before sedation. Important aspects of history include past medical history, chronic illnesses, allergies, current medications, and last oral intake.
  - Detailed explanation regarding procedure and sedation including risks, benefits, and potential side effects.

- Informed consent by legally responsible person
- Following equipment to be kept ready before sedation and analgesia:
  - High-flow oxygen source
  - Suction apparatus
  - Vascular access
  - *Airway management supplies:* Bag and mask, endotracheal tubes, laryngoscopes
  - Pulse oximetry, blood pressure device, electrocardiogram (ECG)
  - Resuscitation drugs [intravenous (IV) fluids], reversal drugs like naloxone and flumazenil

- *Commonly used drugs for sedation and analgesia:* These are mentioned in **Table 1**.

TABLE 1: Commonly used drugs for sedation and analgesia.

Analgesics class	Analgesics name	Dose/route	Peak	Duration
Opiates	Morphine	0.1–0.2 mg/kg IV	15 minutes	2–4 hours
	Fentanyl	1–2 µg/kg IV	10 minutes	30–60 minutes
Sedatives:				
Benzodiazepines	Midazolam	0.02–0.1 mg/kg IV	5 minutes	1–2 hours
		0.2–0.5 mg/kg IN	20–30 minutes	60–90 minutes
		0.5–0.75 mg/kg PO	20–30 minutes	60–90 minutes
Barbiturates	Pentobarbital	2–5 mg/kg PR (maximum 150 mg)	15–60 minutes	1–3 hours
		1–3 mg/kg IV (maximum 150 mg)	1 minute	15 minutes
Hypnotics	Propofol	1 mg/kg IV, then 0.5 mg/kg IV over 30–60 minutes	6–7 minutes	5–10 minutes
	Etomidate	0.1–0.2 mg/kg IV	30 seconds	5–10 minutes
Dissociative:				
	Ketamine	1–2 mg/kg IV	5 minutes	30–60 minutes
		3–5 mg/kg IM	10 minutes	1–2 hours
Adjuvants for ketamine	Atropine	1 mg/kg IM/IV, minutes 0.1 mg (maximum 0.5 mg)	–	–
	Midazolam	0.05 mg/kg IV	–	–
Inhaled	Nitrous oxide	30–50% N_2O, mixed with O_2	3–5 minutes	5–10 minutes
Reversal agents:				
Opioid reversal	Naloxone	<5 years or <20 kg: 0.1 mg/kg IV/IO/IM/SC	1–2 hours	–
		>5 years or >20 kg: 2 mg IV/IO/IM/SC	1–2 hours	–
Benzodiazepine reversal	Flumazenil	0.02 mg/kg IV q 1 minute (maximum 1 mg)	–	–

(IM: intramuscular; IO: intraosseous; IN: intranasal; IV: intravenous; SC: subcutaneous)

The sedation protocol is given in **Flowchart 1**.

Flowchart 1: Sedation protocol.

Informed consent before sedation
↓

Nil per orally as:

Ingested material	Minimum fasting period
• Light meals	• 6 hours
• Formula feeds	• 6 hours
• Breast milk	• 4 hours
• Clear fluids	• 2 hours

↓

Reevaluation should be done just prior to sedation in terms of informed consent, NPO status, URI/fever, medication status

↓

Preparation for a sedation procedure, follow the acronym SOAPME:
- S: Suction apparatus and suction catheters
- O: Oxygen and flowmeters
- A: Airway—bag and mask, ET tubes, laryngoscopes
- P: Pharmacy, i.e., drugs
- M: Monitors
- E: Equipment for anesthesia, resuscitation, good lighting

↓

Painless procedures:
- Chloral hydrate @ 50–100 mg/kg PO
- Diazepam @ 0.25–0.3 mg/kg PO
- Diphenhydramine @ 5 mg/kg/day q 6 hours PO
- Midazolam @ 0.5–0.75 mg/kg PO

Sedation and analgesia for painful procedures of short duration:
- EMLA (eutectic mixture of local anesthetics): Lidocaine 2.5%, prilocaine 2.5% topically
- EMLA + Midazolam @ 0.1 mg/kg IV
- LET (Lidocaine 4% + Epinephrine 0.1% + Tetracaine 0.5%) topically
- TAC (Tetracaine 0.25–0.5% + Adrenaline 0.025–0.05% + Cocaine 4–11.8%) topically
- Lidocaine 2% topically and injectable (0.5–2%) locally with maximum dose 5 mg/kg
- Midazolam @ 0.1 mg/kg IV + IV ketamine @ 0.25 mg/kg
- Midazolam @ 0.1 mg/kg IV × 3 doses + Fentanyl 1µg/kg IV × 3 doses

Deep sedation and analgesia:
- Midazolam @ 0.1 mg/kg IV + IV ketamine @ 0.25 mg/kg
- Midazolam @ 0.1 mg/kg IV × 3 doses + Fentanyl 1µg/kg IV × 3 doses
- Midazolam @ 0.1 mg/kg × 3 doses + Ketamine @ 0.25 mg/kg × 1 dose + atropine 0.02 mg/kg × 1 dose
- Propofol @ 1 mg/kg followed by 0.5 mg/kg IV (only for use by expert airway managers)
- Midazolam @ 0.1 mg/kg IV + Morphine @ 0.1 mg/kg/dose IV

(ET: endotracheal; IV: intravenous; NPO: nothing by mouth; URI: upper respiratory infections)

CHAPTER 14

Nutrition in a Critically Ill Child

Aradhna Aneja, Biju M John, Amit Pathania

- Critically illness is a catabolic phase with increased caloric needs, urinary nitrogen loss, inadequate intake, loss of protein stores, and gluconeogenesis. There is increased energy expenditure due to fever, pain, increased work of breathing, anxiety, infection, and starvation, which leads to negative nitrogen balance, morphological changes in gut, enzymatic changes, decreased cellular, and humoral immunity.
- It is important to provide appropriate nutritional support to a critically ill child to prevent/treat macro/micronutrient deficiency and prevent complications.
- There are *two modes of nutrition*:
  1. Enteral
  2. Parental
- *Enteral nutrition is superior* to parenteral nutrition as:
  - Trophic effects on intestinal villus
  - Reduces bacterial translocation
  - Supports gut-associated lymphoid tissue
  - Promotes secretory immunoglobulin A (IgA) secretion and function
  - Less risk of infection
  - Lower cost
- Initiation of enteral nutrition should begin as early as possible, usually within 24 hours in severe trauma, burns, and catabolic states.
- *Contraindications to enteral nutrition*:
  - Nonfunctional gut, anatomic disruption, gut ischemia
  - Severe peritonitis
  - Severe shock states
- Routes of enteral feeding are nasogastric, transpyloric, percutaneous/surgical placement [percutaneous endoscopic gastrostomy (PEG), jejunostomy].
- *Fluid requirements*: Maintenance requirement + Deficit correction + Replacement of ongoing losses; maintenance fluid requirement is as per Holliday–Segar formula.
- *Nutrition requirement* is calculated on basis of total energy requirements.
  - Total daily energy requirement (kcal/day) = Resting energy expenditure (REE) + REE × Total factors
  - *REE*: World Health Organization (WHO) equation (kcal/day)

0–3 years	3–10 years	10–18 years
Male: 60.9 × weight − 54	*Male:* 22.7 × weight + 495	*Male:* 12.2 × weight + 746
Female: 61 × weight − 51	*Female:* 22.4 × weight + 499	*Female:* 17.5 × weight + 651

- Factors adding to REE are:

Factor	Multiplication factor
Maintenance	0.2
Activity	0.1–0.25
Fever	0.13 per degree >38°C
Simple trauma	0.2
Multiple injuries	0.4
Burns	0.5–1
Sepsis	0.4
Growth	0.5

Aim: Attain 65–70% of caloric goal (WHO REE for age) within first week. The caloric goal cannot be met on day 1. Both carbohydrates and lipids should be gradually increased as tolerated till caloric goal is reached.

- *Caloric intake*: The desired goal for nonprotein caloric intake for normal children is given as follows:

Age	Energy requirement (kcal/kg/day)
Premature infants	70–90
Full term to 1 year	80–95
2–9 years	60–70
10–13 years	50–60
Adolescents	40

- *Carbohydrates*: It constitutes 60–70% of nonprotein calories It may be given in form of polysaccharides/disaccharides/monosaccharides. 1 g of dextrose gives 3.4 kcal of energy. The daily intake calculations as shown follows:

Age	First day	Subsequent day
Neonates	5 g/kg/day	2 g/kg/day
Infants >1 month of age	10 g/kg/day	5 g/kg/day
Older children/adolescents	10% dextrose	Increased by 2.5–5% daily

- *Lipids*: These constitute 30–40% of nonprotein calories. 1 g of lipids provide 9 kcal, 20% (2 g/mL) lipid solution in glycerol provides 2 kcal/mL. The lipid intake calculations are shown below:

Age	First day	Subsequent days
Premature/low-birth-weight (LBW) infants	0.5 g/kg/day	Increase by 0.5 g/kg/day to maximum of 3 g/kg/day
Infants, children, adolescent	1 g/kg/day	Increase by 0.5–1 g/kg/day to maximum of 3 g/kg/day

- *Protein intake*: Begin at 1-1.5 g/kg/day, gradually advance to calculated dose given as follows:

Age	Protein requirement (g/kg/day)
Premature infants	2.0–3.5
Birth to 1 year	2.0–2.5
2–9 years	1.5–2.0
10–13 years	1.5–2.0
Adolescents	1.0–1.5

Nonprotein calorie to nitrogen ratio: The calories and proteins must be provided in proportion to maintain ratio of 150-250:1 to enhance use of proteins for anabolism. Patients on restricted protein intake should be provided with ratio of 300-350:1.

Ratio = Nonprotein calories/gram of nitrogen (6.25 g of protein = 1 g of nitrogen)

- *The guidelines for initiation and maintenance of parenteral nutrition* is shown in **Table 1**.

TABLE 1: Guidelines for initiation and maintenance of parenteral nutrition.

Substrate	Initiation	Advancement	Goals	Comments
Dextrose	10%	2–5%/day	25%	Increase as tolerated, consider insulin if hyperglycemic
Amino acid	1 g/kg/day	0.5–1 g/kg/day	2–3 g/kg/day	Maintain calorie–nitrogen ratio at 200:1
20% lipids	1 g/kg/day	0.5–1 g/kg/day	2–3 g/kg/day	Only use 20%

- Calculations
  Dextrose:
  - - g/100 mL dextrose × - mL/day = - g/day
  - - g/day divided by (weight × 1.44) = - mg/kg/day
  - - g/kg/day × 3.4 kcal/g = - kcal/kg/day

  Fat: 20 g/100 mL fat × - mL/day = - g/day
  - - g/kg/day × 9 kcal/g = - kcal/kg/day

  Proteins:
  - Grams of proteins divided by 6.25 = - nitrogen
  - Nonprotein calorie/nitrogen = Calorie:Nitrogen ratio

- Electrolytes

Sodium	2–4 mEq/kg/day
Potassium	2–3 mEq/kg/day
Magnesium	0.25–0.5 mEq/kg/day
Calcium	• *Neonate*: 50–100 mg/kg • *Infant*: 100–200 mg/kg • *Adolescent*: 50–100 mg/kg
Phosphate	30–70 mg/kg/day

Other trace elements and multivitamin supplements are added depending on clinical condition.

- Monitoring of patients on total parenteral nutrition (TPN)

Monitoring parameter	Frequency
Weight, intake/output	Daily
Blood glucose	Twice daily initially, then once daily
Hemogram	Once weekly
Urine glucose	Once daily
Electrolytes (sodium, potassium, chloride)	Every 24–48 hourly initially, once weekly later
Serum calcium, magnesium, phosphorus	Every 24–48 hourly initially, once weekly later
Triglycerides	Daily initially, then once weekly
Albumin, liver function test (LFT)	Weekly
Length, head circumference	Weekly
Blood urea, serum creatinine	Every 48–72 hourly, once weekly later

Algorithm for enteral nutrition is given in **Flowchart 1**.

CHAPTER 14: Nutrition in a Critically Ill Child

Flowchart 1: Algorithm for enteral nutrition.

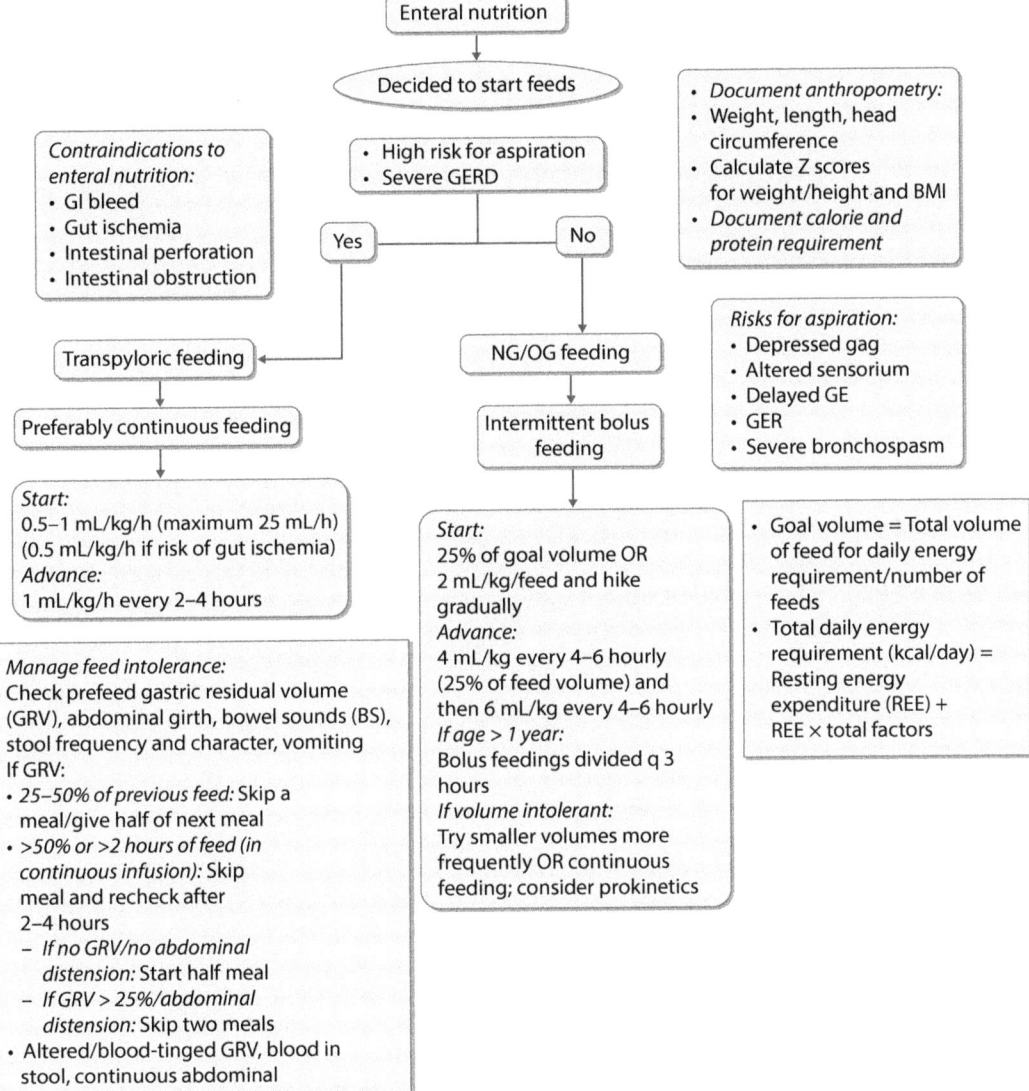

(BMI: body mass index; GE: gastric emptying; GER: gastroesophageal reflux; GERD: gastroesophageal reflux disease; GI: gastrointestinal; NG: nasogastric; OG: orogastric)

SECTION 2

Respiratory Disorders

- **Approach to a Child with Respiratory Distress**
  Amit Pathania, Rakesh Gupta
- **Acute Respiratory Failure**
  Amit Pathania, Rakesh Gupta
- **Pediatric Acute Respiratory Distress Syndrome**
  Amit Pathania, Rakesh Gupta, Biju M John
- **Croup**
  Rakesh Gupta, Amit Pathania
- **Foreign Body Aspiration**
  Amit Pathania, Rakesh Gupta
- **Acute Bronchiolitis**
  Amit Pathania, Rakesh Gupta
- **Acute Severe Asthma**
  Rakesh Gupta, Amit Pathania
- **Mechanical Ventilation**
  Amit Pathania, Biju M John

CHAPTER 15
Approach to a Child with Respiratory Distress

Amit Pathania, Rakesh Gupta

- *Respiratory distress* is a clinical state characterized by tachypnea and increased respiratory effort (resulting in nasal flaring, retractions, and use of accessory muscles).
- Respiratory distress can be classified depending on the site of involvement into upper airway obstruction, lower airway obstruction, lung parenchymal disease, pleural disease, disordered control of breathing, and nonpulmonary causes.
- Physical examination targets toward localizing the site of distress and includes assessment of respiratory rate, retractions, work of breathing, chest wall excursion, pattern of breathing, SpO_2 and abnormal sounds (grunting, stridor, and wheeze).
- *Common causes of respiratory distress are:*
  - *Upper airway respiratory obstruction (outside the thorax):* Foreign body, swelling of tissue linings of upper airway, falling back of tongue, thick secretions, and mass lesion pharyngeal/peritonsillar abscess.
  - *Lower airway respiratory obstruction* (lower trachea, bronchi, and bronchioles): Bronchial asthma and bronchiolitis
  - *Parenchymal (lung tissue/alveolar capillary unit):* Pneumonias, pulmonary edema, acute respiratory distress syndrome (ARDS), pulmonary contusion, and other lung tissue disease such as allergic reaction, toxins, vasculitis, and infiltrative disease.
  - *Pleural:* Pneumothorax, pleural effusion, empyema, and hemothorax
  - *Disordered control of breathing:* Neurological disorders [e.g., seizures, central nervous system (CNS) infection, head injury, brain tumor, hydrocephalus, and neuromuscular disease]
  - *Nonpulmonary causes:* Congestive cardiac failure, acidosis, anemia, inborn error of metabolism, and functional causes such as hyperventilation
- *Clinical findings:*
  - *Upper airway respiratory obstruction:* Typical signs observed predominantly during inspiration and includes tachypnoea, inspiratory retractions, hoarseness, seal-like cough, stridor, poor chest rise, and poor air entry.
  - *Lower airway respiratory obstruction:* Typical signs occur during expiration and include tachypnea, wheezing, and increased expiratory effort (i.e., expiration is active rather than a passive process).
  - *Parenchymal:* Marked tachypnea, tachycardia, grunting, hypoxemia, crepitations, and increased respiratory effort
  - *Pleural:* On involved side—hemithorax movement reduced, decreased breath sound, dull percussion in effusion, hyper-resonant in pneumothorax, mediastinal shift to other side if massive.
  - *Disordered control of breathing:* Irregular respiration, tachypnoea alternating with bradypnea, variable respiratory effort, shallow breathing, and central apnea.

SECTION 2: Respiratory Disorders

- *Nonpulmonary causes:* Tachypnea is usually silent (i.e., tachypnoea with no/minimal retractions).
- Investigations are done to localize the pathology and assess the severity of distress. Common test includes imaging studies, sepsis screen, and arterial blood gas (ABG).

Approach to a child with respiratory distress is given in **Flowchart 1**.

Flowchart 1: Approach to a child with respiratory distress.

Signs	Upper respiratory tract	Lower respiratory tract	Parenchymal	Pleural	Central	Non-respiratory
Tachypnea	+	++	+++++	++	Funny respiration bradypnea/apnea	Silent tachypnea
Retractions	++++ Inspiration effortful	++ Expiration prolonged	++	+	No retractions Shallow breathing	No retractions
Stridor	+++++	-	-	-	-	-
Hoarseness/snoring	+	-	-	-	-	-
Grunting	+/-	+	++++	-	-	-
Wheezing	+/-	++++	+/-	-	-	-
Crepitations	-	-	+++	-	-	-
Air entry	-	-	-	Decreased	-	-

Upper airway obstruction:
- Cool mist
- Epinephrine nebulization (0.5 mL/kg of 1:1000. Maximum: 5 mL)
- Injection Dexa (0.6 mg/kg IM)

If excessive secretions consider:
- Ipratropium nebulization
- Glycopyrrolate

No improvement, consider:
- ET intubation/tracheostomy
- Identify possible cause
  - Foreign body
  - Croup
  - Anaphylaxis*

Lower airway obstruction
- Nebulization with Salbutamol (0.15 mg/kg/dose)
- Bronchiolitis*
- Bronchial asthma*

Start oxygen
Head box/prongs/mask/HFNC

Management: Ensure ABC airway:
- Allow child to assume position of comfort
- Make airway patent by—head tilt, chin lift, jaw thrust, and head extension
- If cervical spine injury—only jaw thrust and no head extension
- Clear the airway—remove foreign body/suction
- Use airway adjunct—oropharyngeal/nasopharyngeal airway as indicated

Consider: | Not maintainable
- Application of CPAP
- Endotracheal tube insertion
- Cricothyrotomy/tracheostomy

*Nonpulmonary:**
- "Silent tachypnea"
- Metabolic cause
- Anemia
- Congestive cardiac failure

} Treat the cause

*See respective chapters

Lung parenchymal disease (alveolar capillary unit damage)
- Start appropriate antibiotics—hypoxemia refractory to O_2
- Consider: CPAP/BiPAP
- Mechanical ventilation with PEEP
- Identify possible cause: Pneumonia—infection/chemical/aspiration
- Pulmonary edema-Fluid overload/CCF*/sepsis/ARDS*

Pleural causes:
- Needle thoracostomy (in emergency for pneumothorax)
- Chest tube drainage—for pneumothorax, hemothorax, empyema, massive effusions

Disordered breathing:
- Treatment options: BiPAP (if respiratory trigger +)
- Mechanical ventilation
- Identify possible cause
- Raised ICP
- Altered consciousness
- Poisoning
- Neuromuscular disease
- Mechanical ventilation

(ABC: airway, breathing, and circulation; BiPAP: biphasic positive airway pressure; CPAP: continuous positive airway pressure; HFNC: high-flow nasal cannula; IM: intramuscular; PEEP: positive end-expiratory pressure)

CHAPTER 16
Acute Respiratory Failure

Amit Pathania, Rakesh Gupta

- *Respiratory failure* is defined as inability of the respiratory system to fulfil the gas exchange needs of the patient, i.e., oxygenation and ventilation are insufficient to meet the metabolic demands of the body.
  In absence of intra-cardiac shunt: PaO_2 <60 mm Hg; $PaCO_2$ >50 mm Hg
  Patient's general state, respiratory efforts, and potential for impending exhaustion is more important indicator than blood gases.
- *Pathophysiology:* Respiratory failure can be due to failure of ventilation, impaired pulmonary perfusion, ventilation-perfusion mismatch, impaired gas transfer across the capillary membrane, and uptake by the tissues. Classified into two types: Type I (non-ventilatory/normocapnic respiratory failure—low PaO_2, normal/low $PaCO_2$) Type II (ventilatory/hypercapnic respiratory failure—high $PaCO_2$ with variable hypoxemia).
- *Causes:*

Type I (mismatch of alveolar ventilation relative to perfusion)	Type II (respiratory pump failure)
• Pneumonias • Pulmonary edema • Bronchiolitis • Acute respiratory distress syndrome (ARDS) • Aspiration • Radiation • Interstitial lung disease (ILD) • Sepsis	• *Airway obstruction:* Croup, asthma, foreign body (FB) • *Chest wall restriction:* Kyphoscoliosis, diaphragmatic hernia, massive effusion • *Respiratory muscle weakness:* Guillain–Barré (GB) syndrome, Duchenne muscular dystrophy (DMD), spinal muscular atrophy (SMA), fatigue of muscles • *Central control abnormality:* Infections, drugs, toxins, stroke, sleep apnea

- *Clinical evaluation:* Respiratory failure should be anticipated rather than recognized. Evaluation should always start with a rapid assessment of the adequacy of ventilation, including the presence and vigor of respiratory movements, breathing rate, presence of cyanosis, SpO_2, state of consciousness, and the presence of probable site of airway obstruction.
- *Investigation:* After initial stabilization. Directed to find the cause
  ABG–look for hypoxemia, hypercarbia, acidosis
  - *(A-a) DO_2:* Alveolar- arterial oxygen difference
    Index of the efficiency of gas exchange by lung. Normal 5–10 mm Hg at room air. It increases as the FiO_2 increases and about 200 at FiO_2 1 in normal individuals. (A-a) DO_2 increases in presence of V/Q mismatch, right to left shunt, and diffusion defect
    $PaO_2 = P_iO_2 - (P_aCO_2/R)$
    P_iO_2 – calculated by $F_iO_2 \times$ (atmospheric pressure – water vapor pressure)
    $R = 0.8$ = flow of CO_2 molecule/flow of O_2 across alveolar membrane/min

- *a/A ratio—arterial to alveolar pO_2 ratio:* It does not change with varying FiO_2 healthy infant – 0.8; RDS – 0.1–0.2; value <0.22 in neonate is indication for surfactant.
- P_aO_2/FiO_2 *ratio:* Indicator of impairment of oxygenation
  200–300 = Acute lung injury
  <200 = ARDS
- *Oxygenation index:* Indicator of oxygenation in mechanically ventilated patients
  OI = Mean airway pressure MAP × FiO_2 × $100/P_aO_2$
- *Principles of treatment:* Early support of respiratory function when respiratory failure is imminent or already established and treat the underlying etiology.
- FiO_2 *delivered by various devices:*

	FiO_2 delivered	Flow required
Nasal cannula	24–50%	2–4 L/min
Face mask	40%	4–5 L/min
Venturi mask	40–60%	4–5 L/min
Nonrebreathing mask	80%	6–8 L/min
Under hood	95%	10 L/min
Heated humidified high flow nasal canula (HHHFNC)	21–100%	2–60 L/min

- *Rapid sequence intubation:* Preoxygenate with 100% oxygen. Give atropine 0.02 mg/kg (minimum 0.1 mg). Administer sedation and muscle relaxant. Put endotracheal tube after visualizing the glottis (perform Sellick's maneuver to prevent aspiration). Confirm the tube in place and secure with tape.
- *Choice of sedative-options:*

Unspecified	Normotensive	Thiopentone 4–7 mg/kg
Head injury	Hypotensive	• Lignocaine 1–2 mg/kg • Fentanyl 2–5 µg/kg
	Normotensive	• Lignocaine 1–2 mg/kg • Thiopentone 4–7 mg/kg
Shock	Mild	• Midazolam 0.1 mg/kg, • Ketamine 1 mg/kg, • Thiopentone 1–2 mg/kg
	Severe	None/Fentanyl 1 µg/kg
Acute asthma		Ketamine 2–4 mg/kg

Choice of muscle relaxant—vecuronium 0.1–0.2 mg/kg; succinylcholine 1–2 mg/kg
- *Indications of mechanical ventilation*—mainly clinical (blood gas though important but not absolutely necessary; PaO_2 <60 mm Hg; $PaCO_2$ >50 mm Hg despite FiO_2 = 1)
  - When hypoxemia or significant hypoventilation persist despite noninvasive support.
  - Maintaining airway patency who have the potential for airway compromise, e.g., neurological deterioration.
  - Severe shock
  Acute respiratory failure is shown in **Flowchart 1**.

Flowchart 1: Acute respiratory failure.

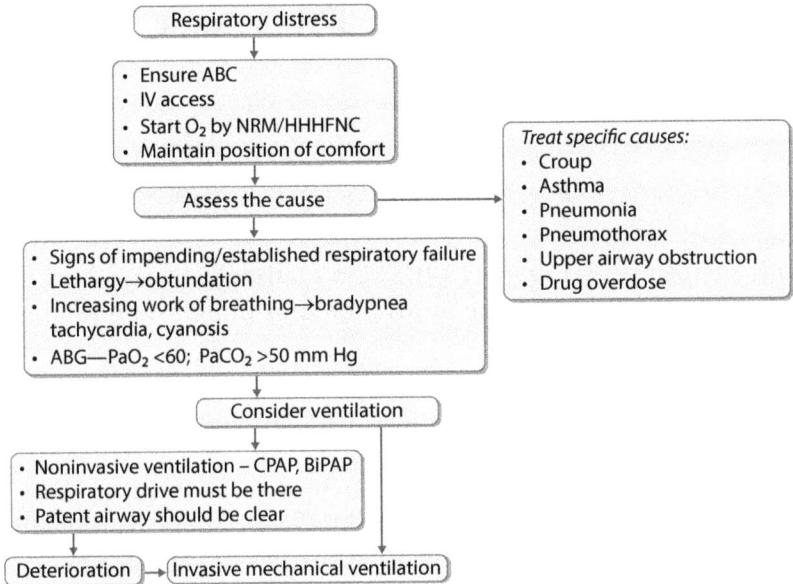

(ABC: airway, breathing, and circulation; BiPAP: biphasic positive airway pressure; CPAP: continuous positive airway pressure; HHHFNC: heated humidified high flow nasal cannula; IV: intravenous; NRM: non-rebreather mask)

CHAPTER 17: Pediatric Acute Respiratory Distress Syndrome

Amit Pathania, Rakesh Gupta, Biju M John

- Acute respiratory distress syndrome (ARDS) is a syndrome of acute lung inflammation characterized by alveolar leukocyte infiltration and protein-rich pulmonary edema resulting in acute respiratory failure.
- *Diagnostic criteria include:*
  - *Pediatric:* 29 days–18 years of life (excluding perinatal lung condition)
  - *Acute:* Within 7 days of known clinical insult
  - *Respiratory:* Diffuse pulmonary inflammation (bilateral infiltrates on chest radiograph). Pulmonary edema (not fully explained by cardiac failure or fluid overload)
  - *Distress:* Severe arterial hypoxemia resistant to oxygen therapy alone

Age	Exclude patients with perinatal-related lung disease			
Timing	Within 7 days of known clinical insult			
Origin of edema	Respiratory failure not fully explained by cardiac failure or fluid overload			
Chest imaging	Chest imaging findings of new infiltrate(s) consistent with acute pulmonary parenchymal disease			
Oxygenation	**Noninvasive mechanical ventilation**	**Invasive mechanical ventilation**		
	PARDS (No severity stratification)	**Mild**	**Moderate**	**Severe**
	Full face-mask bilevel ventilation or CPAP ≥5 cmH$_2$O • PF ratio ≤300 • SF ratio ≤264	• 4 ≤ OI <8 • 5 ≤ OSI <7.5	• 8 ≤ OI <16 • 7.5 ≤ OSI <12.3	• OI ≥16 • OSI ≥12.3
	Special populations			
Cyanotic heart disease	Standard criteria above for age, timing, origin of edema and chest imaging with an acute deterioration in oxygenation not explained by underlying cardiac disease			
Chronic lung disease	Standard criteria above for age, timing, and origin of edema with chest imaging consistent with new infiltrate and acute deterioration in oxygenation from baseline which meet oxygenation criteria above[3]			
Left ventricular dysfunction	Standard criteria for age, timing and origin of edema with chest imaging changes consistent with new infiltrate and acute deterioration in oxygenation which meet criteria above not explained by left ventricular dysfunction			

- *Pathophysiology* involves increased permeability/edema of alveoli, thrombotic obstruction of pulmonary microvasculature followed by interstitial fibrosis. The host inflammatory response is a key feature in the pathogenesis of this disease.

- *Etiology:* Pneumonia, sepsis, aspiration, severe trauma, massive transfusion, burns, near drowning, drug overdose, and re-perfusion injuries.

Acute respiratory distress syndrome commonly progresses through three stages:
- *Exudative phase:* Acute development of decreased pulmonary compliance and arterial hypoxemia leading to tachypnea, dyspnea, agitation. ABG-hypoxemia. CXR-diffuse alveolar infiltrates.
- *Fibroproliferative stage:* Chronic inflammation and scarring of the alveolar-capillary unit leads to increased alveolar dead space and refractory pulmonary hypertension.
- *Recovery phase*: Restoration of the alveolar epithelial barrier, gradual improvement in pulmonary compliance and resolution of arterial hypoxemia. Eventual return to premorbid pulmonary function.
- *Treatment modalities*
  - Control of causative factors (sepsis, shock, etc.)
  - Respiratory management
    - Noninvasive ventilation—CPAP/BiPAP/HFNC—initial trial. Observe for worsening and consider early invasive ventilation within 0-6 hours.
    - Invasive mechanical ventilation
      - Controlled oxygen exposure (FiO_2)
      - Avoidance of volutrauma (low tidal volume) and atelectrauma (appropriate PEEP)
      - Mechanical ventilation settings strategies:
        - *Tidal volume:* 4-6 mL/kg (Baby Lung Concept); never above 8 mL/kg
        - *Peak inspiratory pressure (PIP)/plateau pressure (Pplat):* Pplat <28 cmH_2O. Driving pressure up to 15. Pplat never above 32 cmH_2O
        - *Positive end-expiratory pressure (PEEP):* High PEEP requirement up to 10 cmH_2O. May go up to 15 cmH_2O before considering high-frequency oscillation (HFO). Monitor cardiopulmonary interactions.
        - *Target SpO_2:* Permissive hypoxemia—mild/moderate—92-97%, severe 88-92%
        - Permissive hypercapnia—pCO_2 up to 55 and pH ≥7.2
    - Nonconventional ventilation
      - *High frequency oscillatory ventilation (HFOV):* Consider if OI >16 and not maintaining on high settings of conventional ventilation.
      - *Extra corporeal membrane oxygenation (ECMO):* VV ECMO if OI >40 and good cardiac function.
    - Ancillary pulmonary-specific treatments
      - *Prone ventilation:* Recommended for pediatric acute respiratory distress syndrome (PARDS) with hypoxemia not responding to other ventilatory intervention. Consider with invasive and HFO both.
      - *Inhaled Nitric oxide:* It is a pulmonary vasodilator and used if document RV dysfunction (POCUS—interventricular septum ballooning to left, severe TR jet) and resistant hypoxemia to high settings.
      - *Lung recruitment maneuver*—not recommended
      - *Surfactant:* Against routine use

- Corticosteroids and other anti-inflammatory agents—methylprednisolone—use only in established ARDS in selected population only. Improves oxygenation, compliance and shortens duration of vasoactive infusions. No increase in infectious complications. No change in mortality. Some benefit were shown in COVID patients.

Flowchart 1: Acute respiratory distress syndrome (ARDS) management.

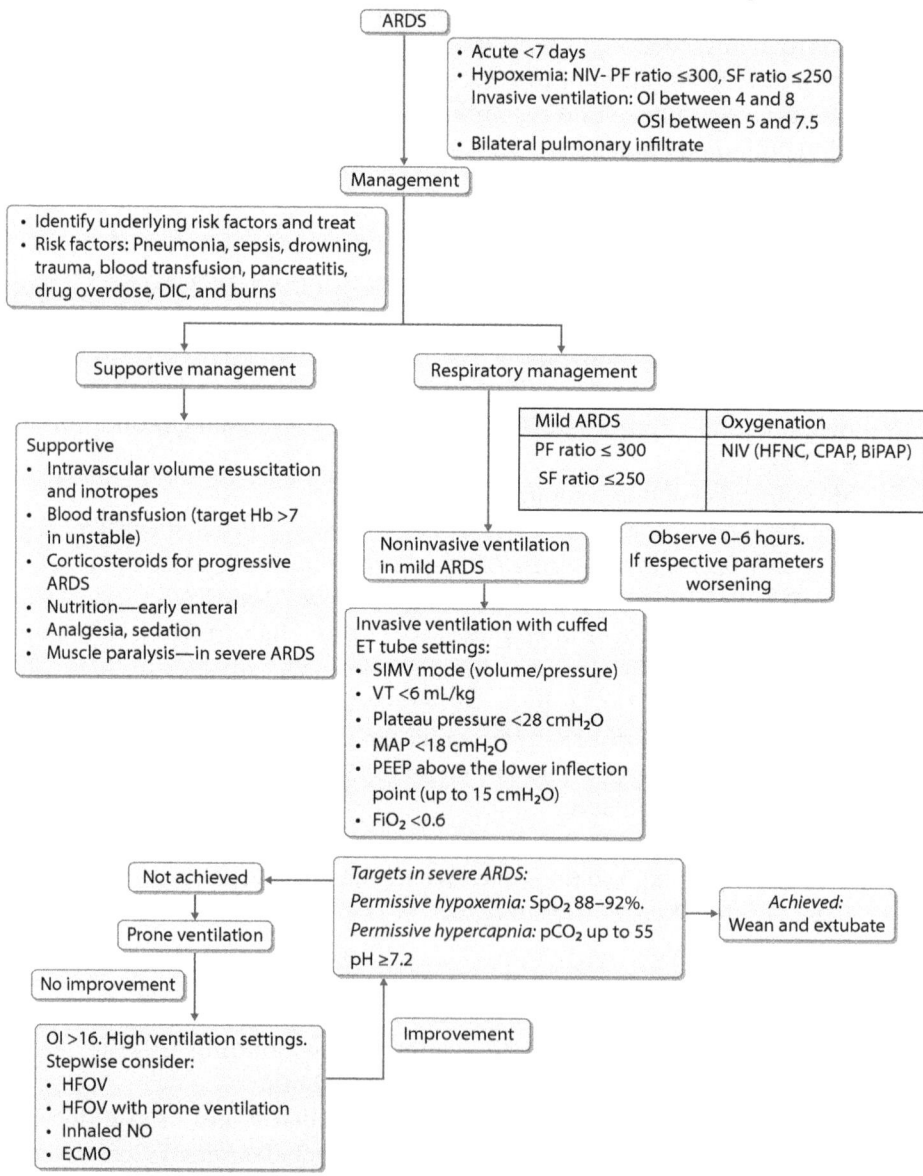

(ARDS: acute respiratory distress syndrome; BiPAP: bilevel positive airway pressure; CPAP: continuous positive airway pressure; ECMO: extracorporeal membrane oxygenation; HFNC: high flow nasal cannula; HFOV: high frequency oscillatory ventilation)

- Supportive therapies
  - *Careful fluid administration:* Two-thirds to three-fourths of maintenance. Titration with perfusion and urine output. Overzealous fluid therapy must not be given as it adds to pulmonary edema, may consider vasoactive drugs early.
  - *Nutrition:* Early enteral nutrition (must start within 72 hours if no contraindication). Protein @ 1.5 g/kg/day
  - *Sedation/analgesia:* Titrate to minimum and effective dose. Drug break of 2 hours daily.
  - *Muscle paralysis:* In severe ARDS consider muscle paralysis to prevent self-inflicted lung injury (SILI) and if protective ventilation not achieved by sedation alone.
  - *Transfusion:* Consider packed red blood cell (PRBC) transfusion when Hb <7 g/dL
  - *Airway clearance therapy and mucolytics:* Not routinely recommended. Frequent suctioning with N-acetyl cysteine (NAC), mucolytics, saline not advised as PEEP get lost. To be done on SOS basis.

Acute respiratory distress syndrome (ARDS) management is shown in **Flowchart 1**.

CHAPTER 18

Croup

Rakesh Gupta, Amit Pathania

- Croup or laryngotracheobronchitis (LTB) is a clinical syndrome characterized by:
  - Barking or brassy cough
  - Hoarse voice
  - Inspiratory stridor and suprasternal retraction
  - Respiratory distress
    - Common cause of upper airway obstruction
    - Usually, mild and self-limiting, mainly a viral infection, BUT is also the commonest cause of potentially life-threatening airway obstruction in childhood.
- *Typical presentation*—preceded by low-grade fever and coryza. As the illness progresses, hoarseness, and characteristic "croupy" or barking cough will develop. Other symptoms include dyspnea, stridor, and wheezing. Symptoms are worse at night, peak between 24 and 48 hours and generally resolve within 1 week.
- *Examination:* Throat examination should be gentle and if epiglottitis is suspected examination should be attempted where emergency tracheostomy can be done.
- *Differential diagnosis*—spasmodic laryngitis, acute epiglottitis, retropharyngeal abscess, bacterial tracheitis, diphtheritic croup, and foreign body.
- Investigations (blood test, radiograph neck) cause anxiety leading to further distress and obstruction. If done reveals tapering of subglottic trachea (steeple sign).
- Treatment modalities
  - Oxygen therapy—to maintain SpO_2 >92%
  - Mist therapy
  - *Epinephrine:* Dose 0.5 mL/kg of 1:1,000 dilution (maximum: 2.5 mL up to 4 years; 5 mL >4 years)
  - Repeat 30 minutes → 2–4 hours interval till stridor subsides
  - Steroids—oral or intramuscular—dexamethasone 0.6 mg/kg IM stat or nebulization—budesonide 2 mg BD
  - Symptomatic
  - Fever control
  - Coryza—if bothersome, antihistaminic
  - Nasal blockade—normal saline nasal drops
  - Sedatives—should not be administered.

The details of croup is given in **Flowchart 1**.

Flowchart 1: Croup.

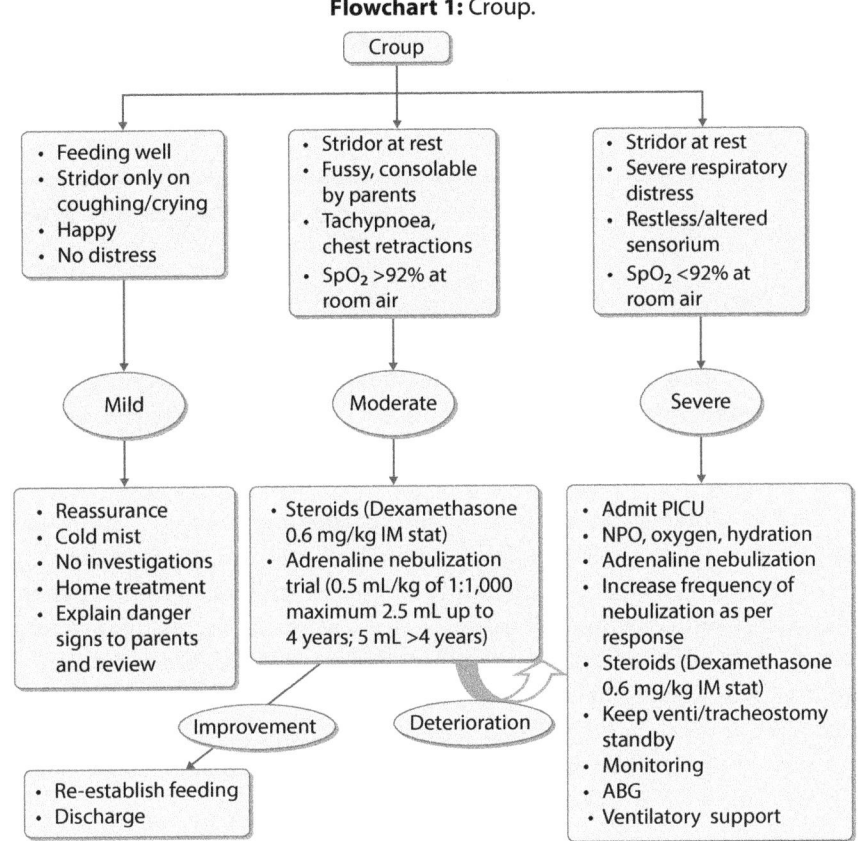

CHAPTER 19

Foreign Body Aspiration

Amit Pathania, Rakesh Gupta

- Foreign body (FB) aspirations are a common pediatric accident.
- A total of 90% of foreign bodies are seen <3 years of age as infants and toddlers use their mouths to explore their surroundings. Foods (mainly nuts) and toys account for 90% of FB.
- Manifestations depend on size, composition, location of FB, degree, and duration of obstruction. Three stages of symptoms may result from aspiration of an object into the airway:
  - *Initial event:* Violent paroxysms of coughing, choking, gagging, stridor, and possibly airway obstruction occur immediately when the foreign body is aspirated.
  - *Asymptomatic interval:* Foreign body becomes lodged, fatigue sets in, and the immediate irritating symptoms subside. This stage is most treacherous and accounts for a large percentage of delayed diagnoses and overlooked foreign bodies.
  - *Complications*—include fever, cough, hemoptysis, pneumonia, and atelectasis due to obstruction, erosion, or infection caused by underlying FB.
- *Examination*—clinical triad of wheezing, coughing, and diminished breath sounds in 40%; although 75% may have one of these abovementioned findings.
- *Investigations:*
  - *X-ray*—posterior anterior/lateral (PA/Lat) view neck and chest only 10% FB are radio opaque.
    - Changes are seen secondary to obstruction of airway.
    - May reveal unilateral hyperlucency, resorption atelectasis, compensatory emphysema of contralateral lung, pneumonia, pneumothorax, and shift of mediastinum.
  - *Fluoroscopy*: Difference in inspiration and expiration inflation of lung.
  - *CT scan*—more informative
  - *Virtual bronchoscopy*—three dimensional (3D) computed tomographic (CT) pulmonary images. Diagnostic but not therapeutic.
  - *Bronchoscopy*—diagnostic and therapeutic.
- *Emergency management:* Basic life support (BLS) with search for foreign body. Suspect, if respiratory distress has had a sudden onset or if the chest does not rise when ventilation is first attempted in an unconscious, apneic infant.
  - *Treatment:* Open airway by head-tilt/chin-lift maneuver, and ventilation is attempted. Attempts to remove a foreign body are indicated. Age <1 year combination of five back blows and five chest thrusts are administered. The foreign body is removed if it is seen. If no foreign body is visualized, repeat the above steps. Age >1 year—administered a

series of five abdominal thrusts (the *Heimlich maneuver*) with the child standing or siting. If unconscious, then in lying position. After the abdominal thrusts, examine airway for a foreign body and remove if visualized. If no foreign body is seen, repeat the above steps after repositioning the head.
- *Definitive treatment:* Bronchoscopic removal of FB or surgical removal if bronchoscopy fails.

Foreign body aspiration is given in **Flowchart 1**.

Flowchart 1: Foreign body aspiration.

```
                        Foreign body aspiration
                                 |
           ┌─────────────────────┴─────────────────────┐
      Acute choking                        Gagging episode followed by bout of cough
                                                  Witnessed/unwitnessed
```

- Excessive irritability→ collapse
- Signs of imminent respiratory failure
- Universal choking sign

Symptomatic (67%)

Asymptomatic (33%) Present after lag period

- Heimlich maneuver or
- Chest thrust and back blows with head down position
- Look for FB. Try removal if visible; no blind sweep

Symptoms:
- Local irritation—cough, hoarseness, shortness of breath
- Airway obstruction—stridor, unilateral wheeze, decreased breath sounds

Chest X-ray:
- Only 10% FB radiopaque
- 50–75%—partially obliterated air column
- CT scan—more sensitive
- Virtual bronchoscopy—diagnostic

- Complications
- Pneumonitis
- Bronchiectasis

FB in main bronchus—rigid bronchoscopy/ETT with flexible bronchoscopy and removal by dormia basket removal

Bronchoscopic removal

FB in peripheral segments/ failure of bronchoscopic removal PED SURG for bronchotomy and removal of FB

(ETT: endotracheal tube; FB: foreign body; PED SURG: pediatric surgery)

CHAPTER 20: Acute Bronchiolitis

Amit Pathania, Rakesh Gupta

- Bronchiolitis is an acute inflammation of the lower respiratory tract involving smallest bronchioles, usually due to a viral infection [commonest—respiratory syncytial virus (RSV)/Adeno/influenza] seen in children of 6 months–2 years.
- *Pathophysiology:* Bronchiolar narrowing due to edema, mucus, and cellular debris leading to air trapping, overinflation or atelectasis and consequent V/Q mismatch resulting into hypoxemia, hypercapnia, and acidosis.
- *Typical presentation:* Usually begins as a prodrome with mild coryza, running nose, and cough over a period of 2–3 days, followed by increasing respiratory distress with a "tight" wheezy cough.
- Symptoms are out of proportion of signs.
- Diagnosis is clinical. Investigation is usually not required. X-ray chest may show hyperinflation.
- *Differential diagnosis:*
  - Bronchopneumonia
  - Bronchial asthma
- Treatment—self-limiting disease
  - Oxygen—warmed and humidified. Target SpO_2 >92%. High-flow nasal cannula (HFNC), continuous positive airway pressure (CPAP), Vent as per indication. CPAP most effective but HFNC tolerated best.
  - Ensure hydration—IV fluids as per RDA
  - Nebulization (trial→continue if improvement)
    - Saline nebulization: 3 mL, 2–4 hourly (3% hypertonic saline preferred)
    - *Bronchodilators*
      - *Nebulized adrenaline*
        Dose: 0.5 mL/kg of 1:1,000 (maximum 2.5 mL up to 4 years; 5 mL >4 years)
      - *Salbutamol*
        >6 months of age, family history of asthma and atopy
        Dose: 0.15 mg/kg/dose, continue only if objective improvement
  - Feeds—oral feeds—(if RR <60, SpO_2 >92%), IV fluids—if RR >80/min
  - Steroids—NO role
  - Antibiotics—NO role
  - Sedation—NO. Attempt to calm the child by nasal clearing, fever control, and position of maximum comfort.

- *Not recommended:*
  - Cool mist
  - Chest physiotherapy
- *Ribavirin:* Expensive and teratogenic for healthcare professionals no clear benefit, may be tried in immunocompromised and high-risk situation.
- *Monoclonal antibodies:* Palivizumab is given 15 mg/kg monthly during RSV season for maximum 5 doses for prophylaxis in special situations. Newer m Ab- second generation motavizumab, third generation Numax-YTE.
  - Preterm infants with chronic lung disease
  - Acyanotic congenital heart disease on decongestive therapy and moderate-to-severe pulmonary hypertension
  - Infants with neuromuscular disease with impaired cough.

Acute bronchiolitis is given in **Flowchart 1**.

Flowchart 1: Acute bronchiolitis.

```
                    Acute bronchiolitis
        ┌──────────────────┼──────────────────┐
        ▼                  ▼                  ▼
• Feeds normally    • Shortness of breath    • Unable to feed
• No respiratory      during feeds           • Severe respiratory
  distress          • Moderate respiratory     distress with marked
• SpO₂ >92%           distress—some chest      retractions nasal
                      wall retraction and      flaring grunting/apnea
                      nasal flaring          • SpO₂ <92%
                    • SpO₂ <92%                (Not correctable
                      (Correctable with O₂)    with O₂)
        ▼                  ▼                  ▼
      Mild              Moderate             Severe
        ▼                  ▼                  ▼
• Reassurance       • Admit                • Admit PICU
• No investigations • Oxygen               • Oxygen (keep SpO₂ 92%)
• Home treatment    • Hydration (IV fluids) • Nasal Prong/Mask
• Nose clearing     • Hypertonic saline          ▼
• Explain danger      nebulization         • Heated high flow (HFNC)
  signs to parents  • Adrenaline nebulization    ▼
  and review          trial 0.5 mL/kg of    • Continuous PAP (CPAP)
                      1:1,000 (maximum 2.5       ▼
                      mL up to 4 years;    • Ventilatory support
                      5 mL >4 years)       • Hydration (IV fluids)
                                           • Hypertonic saline
          Improvement ◄── ──► Deterioration  nebulization
                ▼                          • Adrenaline nebulization
• Re-establish feeding
• Stop O₂
• Discharge
```

CHAPTER 21

Acute Severe Asthma

Rakesh Gupta, Amit Pathania

- *Acute severe asthma* is defined as severe asthma that fails to respond to inhaled β_2-agonists, oral or IV steroids and oxygen.
- *Pathophysiology:* Bronchial hyperreactivity causes airway obstruction, hyperinflation, and air trapping thus leading to ventilation/perfusion mismatch and hypoxemia.
- *Triggers:* Air pollutants, weather condition, viral infections (RSV or rhino virus) or allergen exposure and exercise.
- *"Red Flag" or dangerous signs in a case of severe asthma*
  - Increased respiratory effort
  - Agitation or dyspnea followed by altered level of consciousness
  - Inability to lie down or inability to speak
  - Distant or absent breath sounds ("silent chest")
  - Cyanosis
  - Pulsus paradoxus
  - PEFR <30% of predicted
  - Oxygen saturation <90%
- *Assessment of severity:* The severity of exacerbation is assessed by evaluating history, vital parameters, use of accessory muscles, and ability to complete sentence and SpO_2. MPIS helps in categorizing the patient and monitoring after therapy starts.

Modified Pulmonary Index Score for asthma

MPIS groups	0	1	2	3
SpO_2%	>95	93–95	90–92	<90
Accessory muscle use	None	Mild	Moderate	Severe
Inspiratory/expiratory ratio	2:1	1:1	1:2	1:3
Wheezing	None	End expiratory	Inspiratory/expiratory wheezing, good aeration	Inspiratory/expiratory wheezing, decreased aeration
Heart rate:				
• <3 years old	<120	120–140	141–160	>160
• >3 years old	<100	100–120	121–140	>140
Breathing frequency (breaths/minute):				
• <6 years old	<30	31–45	46–60	>60
• >6 years old	<20	21–35	36–50	>50

- *Investigations:*
  - *X-ray chest:* Limited role but may be indicated when there is suspected air leak, pneumonia, first time wheezer or the underlying cause of wheezing is in doubt.
  - *Arterial blood gas*—at base line and subsequently as indicated. PaO_2 <60 mm Hg, or $PaCO_2$ ≥50 mm Hg—indicates respiratory failure and plan mechanical ventilation.
  - *Other investigations*—blood count, electrolytes, as indicated.
- *Treatment:* Primary goals of asthma management include correction of hypoxemia, rapid improvement of airflow obstruction, and prevention of progression or recurrence of symptoms.
  - *General treatment:* Hospitalization in pediatric intensive care unit (PICU), IV access, continuous pulse oximetry, and cardiorespiratory monitoring. Avoid sedation.
  - *Oxygen:* Humidified oxygen (maintain SpO_2 >95%)
  - *IV fluid:* Poor intake, vomiting, and increased loss of insensible fluids may cause dehydration. Fluid replacement should be aimed toward euvolemia. Isotonic fluid is used to correct dehydration. Be cautious of hypokalemia due to use of β_2-agonists.
    - *Bronchodilators:*
      - β_2-*agonists* remain the mainstay of therapy and first-line treatment for acute asthma. They are administered via inhaled, intravenous, subcutaneous, or oral routes. Salbutamol or terbutaline are preferred due to relative β_2-selectivity. Treatment with β_2-agonist causes generalized pulmonary vasodilation even in those segments of lung which are atelectatic thus exacerbating V/Q mismatch and worsening hypoxemia. Therefore, O_2 should always be given along with β_2-agonist.
        - *Inhaled short acting β_2-agonists*—(salbutamol) continuous or intermittent nebulization in doses of 0.15 mg/kg/dose (0.5–1 mg/kg/h).
        - *Intravenous β_2-agonists* (e.g., terbutaline) are considered in patients unresponsive to standard treatment as well as those in whom nebulization is not feasible (intubated patients, patients with poor air entry). Terbutaline 10 µg/kg IV loading dose followed by continuous infusion of 0.1–10 µg/kg/min.
        - *Anticholinergic agents:* Ipratropium bromide inhalation. 125–500 µg. (4–8 puff every 20 minutes × 3 times)
    - *Steroids:* Short-course systemic corticosteroid therapy is recommended for use in severe asthma exacerbations to hasten recovery and prevent recurrence of symptoms. Oral prednisolone or IV hydrocortisone or methylprednisolone is equally effective in acute management of status asthmaticus.
    - *Magnesium sulphate*—leads to smooth-muscle relaxation secondary to inhibition of calcium uptake. Dose 25–50 mg/kg in 30 minutes every 6–8 hours. Watch for hypotension, muscle weakness, arrhythmia, and CNS and respiratory depression.
    - *Theophylline*—role in the treatment of children with severe, life-threatening asthma exacerbations. *Dose:* Loading 5–7 mg/kg over 20 minutes followed by maintenance 0.5–0.9 mg/kg /h.
    - *Mechanical ventilation*
      - *Rapid sequence intubation*—histamine releasing agents (morphine, atracurium) to be avoided. Ketamine has additional advantage of bronchodilation.
      - *Goals of ventilation* to maintain adequate oxygenation, allow permissive hypercarbia as long as pH >7.2. Preferred ventilator settings—low RR, short

inspiratory time, minimum positive end-expiratory pressure (PEEP) and prolonged I:E ratio.
- *Sedation*—ketamine preferred in asthma patients on mechanical ventilation, due to its muscle relaxation property. *Dose:* 1 mg/kg/hour infusion.
- *Leukotriene inhibitor*—no role.
- *Antibiotics*—no role in acute asthma unless secondary infection.

The details of acute severe asthma are given in **Flowchart 1.**

Flowchart 1: Acute severe asthma.

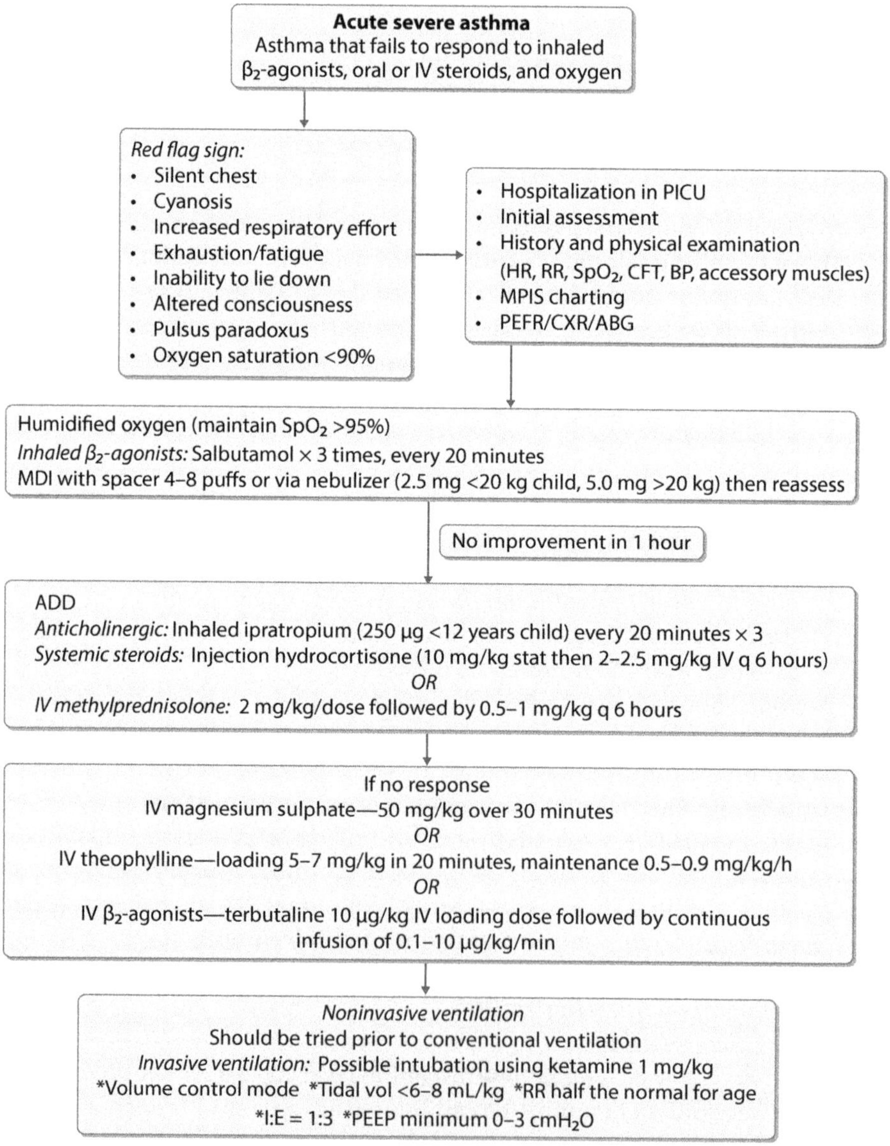

Acute severe asthma
Asthma that fails to respond to inhaled β_2-agonists, oral or IV steroids, and oxygen

Red flag sign:
- Silent chest
- Cyanosis
- Increased respiratory effort
- Exhaustion/fatigue
- Inability to lie down
- Altered consciousness
- Pulsus paradoxus
- Oxygen saturation <90%

- Hospitalization in PICU
- Initial assessment
- History and physical examination (HR, RR, SpO_2, CFT, BP, accessory muscles)
- MPIS charting
- PEFR/CXR/ABG

Humidified oxygen (maintain SpO_2 >95%)
Inhaled β_2-agonists: Salbutamol × 3 times, every 20 minutes
MDI with spacer 4–8 puffs or via nebulizer (2.5 mg <20 kg child, 5.0 mg >20 kg) then reassess

No improvement in 1 hour

ADD
Anticholinergic: Inhaled ipratropium (250 μg <12 years child) every 20 minutes × 3
Systemic steroids: Injection hydrocortisone (10 mg/kg stat then 2–2.5 mg/kg IV q 6 hours)
OR
IV methylprednisolone: 2 mg/kg/dose followed by 0.5–1 mg/kg q 6 hours

If no response
IV magnesium sulphate—50 mg/kg over 30 minutes
OR
IV theophylline—loading 5–7 mg/kg in 20 minutes, maintenance 0.5–0.9 mg/kg/h
OR
IV β_2-agonists—terbutaline 10 μg/kg IV loading dose followed by continuous infusion of 0.1–10 μg/kg/min

Noninvasive ventilation
Should be tried prior to conventional ventilation
Invasive ventilation: Possible intubation using ketamine 1 mg/kg
*Volume control mode *Tidal vol <6–8 mL/kg *RR half the normal for age
*I:E = 1:3 *PEEP minimum 0–3 cmH_2O

(ABG: arterial blood gas; CXR: chest X-ray; PEFR: peak expiratory flow rate; PICU: pediatric intensive care unit)

CHAPTER 22

Mechanical Ventilation

Amit Pathania, Biju M John

- A ventilator is a device which gives positive support to the breath and thus is indicated in the pathologies where ventilation is impaired, control of breathing is decreased, or work of breathing required to be reduced.
- *Basic concepts and important terminologies*
  - *Equation of motion*
    - Pressure gradient is required to move air from one point to another.
    - *Movement of air is opposed by:* Flow resistance of airways
      - Elastic property of alveoli and lung

    Compliance (C_L) = Δ Volume/Δ Pressure (distensibility)
    Elastance = $\Delta P/\Delta V$ (property of a substance to oppose deformation)
    Resistance = $\Delta P/\Delta$ flow (opposition to generation of flow)
    Airway pressure (Paw) = P elastic + P resistive + P inert (negligible thus ignored)
    = Elastance × volume + flow × resistance
    = Volume/compliance + flow × resistance
  - *Time constant (K_T)*—is the time taken for the transthoracic pressure change to be transmitted as volume change in the lungs. 3 K_T is required for 95% and 5 K_T for 99% inflation or deflation of lung.

  At the beginning of breath atmospheric/ventilatory pressure is higher than alveolar pressure resulting in movement of air in alveoli and during expiration alveolar pressure is higher, so exhalation takes place. Time constant is time for equilibrium of pressure between atmosphere and alveoli.

  K_T depends on compliance and resistance. $K_T \propto C_L \times R$
  - *Implications:*
    - Disease with decreased compliance (stiff lung) = reduced K_T
      Both K_T (inspiratory) and K_T (expiratory) reduced because stiffer alveoli recoil with greater force. Therefore, small V_T (tidal volume) to be given to prevent ventilator-induced lung injury (VILI).
    - Disease with increased resistance = increased K_T.
      In intrathoracic airway obstruction—airway narrowing is much more pronounced during expiration. K_T (expiratory) prolonged.
      Therefore, ventilator setting should be—low rates V_T and long expiratory time.

- *Basic ventilation variables:*

Phase variable	Terminology	Options
Starting the ventilation	Trigger	Time, flow, pressure
Sustaining the ventilation	Limit	Volume, pressure, time, flow
Stopping the ventilation	Cycle	Flow, time, volume

- *Modes of ventilators:* There are four basic breath types:

Breath type	Phase variables		
	Trigger	Limit	Cycle
Mandatory	Machine (M)	M	M
Assisted	Patient (P)	M	M
Supported	P	M	P
Spontaneous	P	P	P

- *Ventilator parameters:*

Abbreviation	Term	Definition
PIP	Peak inspiratory pressure	Point of maximum airway pressure
PEEP	Peak end expiratory pressure	Pressure maintained in airways at the end of exhalation
V_T	Tidal volume	Volume of gas entering patient lung during inspiration (6–8 mL/kg)
Ti	Inspiratory time	Duration of time in inspiration
T_E	Expiratory time	Duration of time in expiration
MAP	Mean airway pressure	Average of the pressure in the airway throughout the respiratory cycle

(MAP: mean airway pressure; PEEP: positive end expiratory pressure; PIP: peak inspiratory pressure)

- *Two primary methods for positive pressure ventilation:*

	Pressure ventilation	Volume ventilation
Parameter set by operator	• PIP, PEEP, Ti, RR, FiO_2 • MAP—can be controlled	• V_T, RR, PEEP, Ti, FiO_2 • MV—can be controlled
Advantage	• Lower PIP for same V_T because of decelerating flow pattern • Being protective for noncompliant lung	MV guarantee
Disadvantage	• V_T can change as patient compliance changes • If endotracheal tube obstruction—delivers less V_T • Minute ventilation not guaranteed	• No limit on PIP • Square wave result in higher PIP for same V_T
Our choice	• *Children <10 kg:* As small tidal volumes difficult to regulate • Stiff lung	Good starting point for most ventilation especially normal lungs

(MAP: mean airway pressure; MV: minute volume; PEEP: positive end expiratory pressure; PIP: peak inspiratory pressure; RR: respiratory rate)

- *Goals of assisted ventilation:* Oxygenation and CO_2 elimination.
  Oxygenation—depend on FiO_2 and mean airway pressure (MAP). MAP automatically calculated by ventilator and various steps to increase MAP are shown in diagram here.

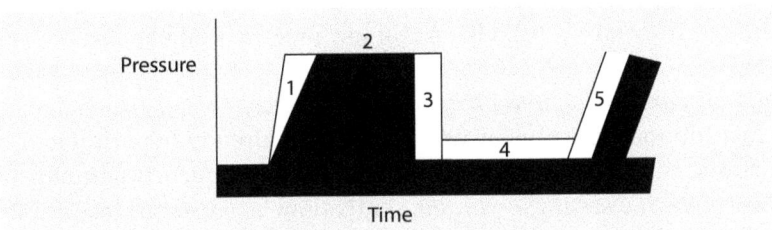

(1) Increased inspiratory flow rate, (2) Increased preset pressure limit, (3) Increased inspiratory time, (4) Increased PEEP, and (5) Increased ventilator rate. Note that with each maneuver, the area under the curve increases. Area under the curve represents mean airway pressure.

Carbon dioxide elimination: CO_2 diffuses easily across alveolar membrane, so its elimination depends on total volume of gas coming in contact with alveoli (alveolar ventilation). Minute volume (MV) = RR × (V_T – dead space)

- *Initial settings in neonatology:*

Disease	PIP	PEEP	Ti	I:E ratio	RR	FiO_2
Moderate RDS	18–20	4–5	0.4	1:2	40–50	0.5
Severe RDS	23–25	5	0.4	1:2	40–50	0.9–1.0
Apnea of prematurity	12–14	3–4	0.4–0.5	1:2	30–40	0.21–0.3
MAS	16–20	2–3	0.4–0.5	1:3-4	30	0.9–1.0

(MAS: meconium aspiration syndrome; PEEP: positive end expiratory pressure; PIP: peak inspiratory pressure; RDS: respiratory distress syndrome; RR: respiratory rate)

- *Blood gas and ventilator changes:*

PaO_2	pCO_2	Diagnosis	Action
N	↑	Low MV, nMAP	↑RR
N	↓	High MV, nMAP	↓RR
↓	↑	Low MV, low MAP	↑PIP
↑	↓	High MV, high MAP	↓PIP
↓	↓	High MV, low MAP	↑PEEP
↑	↑	Low MV, high MAP	↓PEEP
↓	N	↓ PaO_2, nMAP, nMV ↓ MAP, nMV, nPAO_2	↑FiO_2 ↑PIP and PEEP
↑	N	↑ PaO_2, nMAP, nMV ↑ MAP, nMV, nPAO_2	↓FiO_2 ↓PIP and PEEP

(MAP: mean airway pressure; MV: minute volume; PEEP: positive end expiratory pressure; PIP: peak inspiratory pressure : RR: respiratory rate)

- *Disease-specific ventilation in pediatrics:* The pressure gradient that inflates the lung must overcome the pulmonary mechanics of the patient respiratory system.

- *Primary respiratory muscle failure (respiratory pump failure)*—spontaneous breath is encouraged to reduce chances of disuse atrophy.

  Assisted ventilation is a useful mode because trigger sensitivity can be increased to exercise the respiratory muscle.

  Ideal settings: Normal V_T, RR, $FiO_2 = 0.3$, low positive end expiratory pressure (PEEP) 3–5 cmH_2O

- *Disorder with airway obstruction:* Bronchiolitis, asthma

  Problems: Institution of positive airway pressure to already hyperinflated lung leads to decreased cardiac output, hypotension, impaired venous return, pulmonary hypertension.

  Therefore, preferred settings—volume ventilation: $V_T = 6-8$ mL/kg, I:E 1:2–4, so that no air trapping (to prevent pneumothorax, barotrauma)

  If expiratory time is less—small volume of air keeps on accumulating resulting in inadvertent PEEP. Thus, PEEP also has to be lower. Time constants (expiratory) should be kept high. Rates should be low.

- *Parenchymal lung disease:* Pneumonia, acute respiratory distress syndrome (ARDS)

  Problems: Reduction in functional residual capacity (FRC) and diffuse subsegmental atelectasis leading to V/Q mismatch and intrapulmonary shunting.

  Aim is to maintain lung volumes above closing volume throughout the respiratory cycle. *Options:* SIMV (Volume/Pressure) mode. $V_T < 6$ mL/kg, plateau pressure <30 cmH_2O, MAP <18 cmH_2O, PEEP above lower inflection point, $FiO_2 < 0.6$.

- *Weaning:* Timing depends on primary pathology and goals achieved.
  - Prerequisites:
    - Hemodynamic stability
    - Off sedation
    - *Neurological control:* Gag present
    - Ventilator settings to be near physiological and improvement in primary pathology

Thereafter three ways—put on spontaneous mode and gradually decrease $P_{support}$ and PEEP/ put on T piece/reduce ventilatory rate and also reduce $P_{support}$ appropriately.

Acceptable $P_{support}$ for extubation:

Endotracheal tube size	3–3.5	4–4.5	>5
$P_{support}$	10	8	6

Mechanical ventilation is given in **Flowchart 1**.

CHAPTER 22: Mechanical Ventilation

Flowchart 1: Mechanical ventilation.

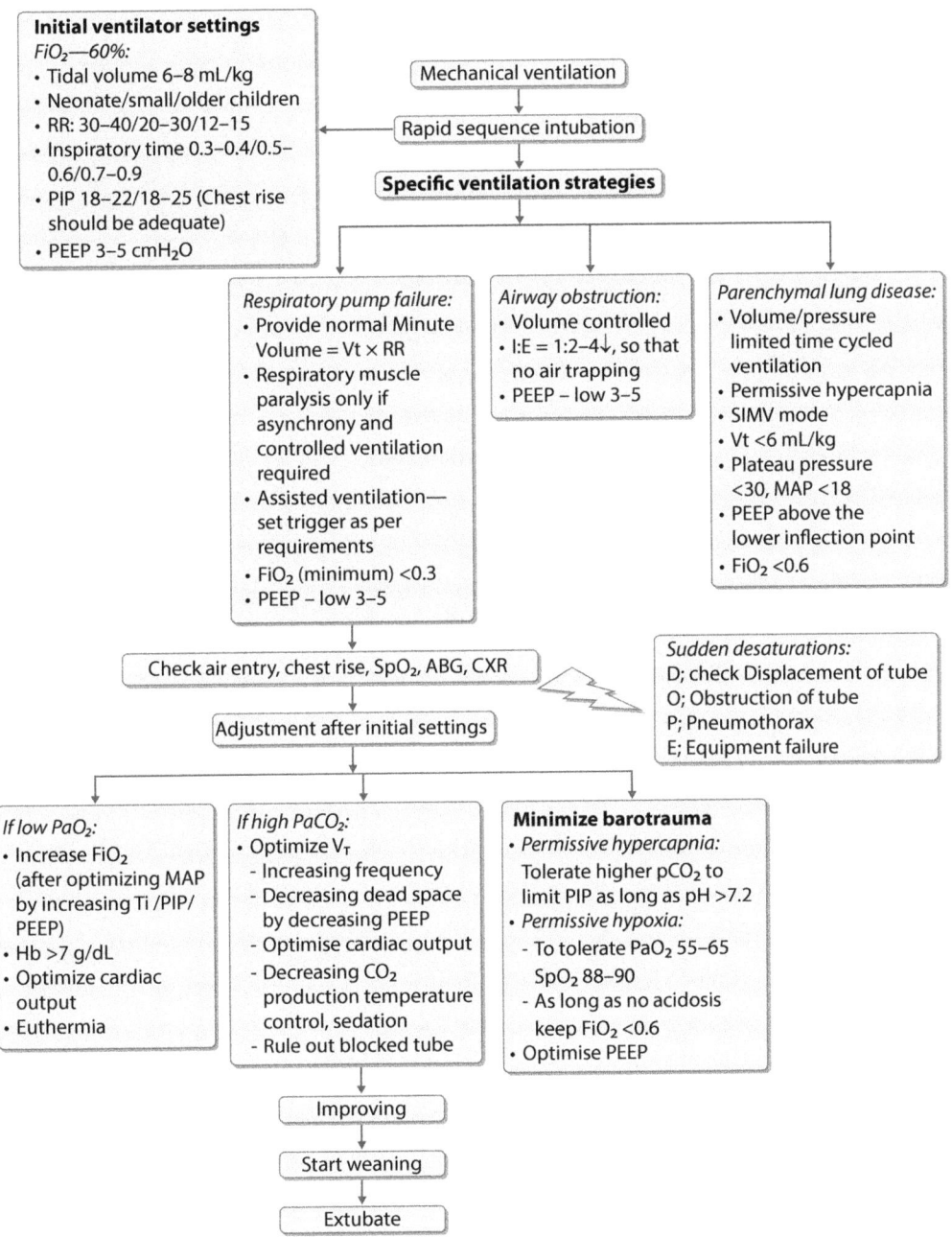

(ABG: arterial blood gas analysis; CXR: chest X-ray; MAP: mean airway pressure; PEEP: positive end expiratory pressure; PIP: peak inspiratory pressure)

SECTION 3

Cardiovascular Disorders

- **Approach to Cyanotic Infant**
  Arvind Mishra, Aradhana Dwivedi, Mukti Sharma

- **Cyanotic Spells or "Tet Spells"**
  Aradhana Dwivedi, Mukti Sharma, Arvind Mishra

- **Congestive Cardiac Failure**
  Mukti Sharma, Aradhana Dwivedi, Arvind Mishra

- **Hypertensive Emergencies in Children**
  Aradhana Dwivedi, Mukti Sharma, Arvind Mishra

CHAPTER 23

Approach to Cyanotic Infant

Arvind Mishra, Aradhana Dwivedi, Mukti Sharma

- Determine whether the cyanosis is *central* or *peripheral*.
  - Central cyanosis is a bluish discoloration of the skin, nail beds, mucus membranes, and tongue. Cyanosis is dependent on the absolute concentration of deoxygenated hemoglobin and is observed when it is >5 g/dL in capillary bed or >3 g/dL in arterial blood. Thus visible cyanosis is dependent on both the degree of desaturation as well as the hemoglobin concentration. In polycythemia, cyanosis is detectable at a higher value of arterial oxygen saturation (SaO_2) vis-à-vis anemia, where the reverse is true. This implies that cyanosis can be masked in severe anemia.
  - It is detected consistently at lips and oral mucosal membranes, tip of tongue, finger nails and conjunctiva. It is confirmed with a low hemoglobin oxygen saturation (SaO_2) and arterial partial pressure of oxygen (PaO_2) on arterial blood gas (ABG) analysis.
  - Peripheral cyanosis spares the mucus membranes and tongue. SaO_2 and PaO_2 are normal. It is often a normal finding in newborns where only the extremities are affected (acrocyanosis) due to vasoconstriction as a result of transient hypothermia. Other causes include sepsis, hypothermia, hypoglycemia, and low cardiac output state.
- Determine whether the cyanosis is of *cardiac or noncardiac origin* by analyzing the time of onset of respiratory distress and cyanosis.
  - There is usually effortless tachypnea without respiratory distress in cyanosis of cardiac origin.
  - Neonates who become symptomatic at birth are more likely to have respiratory conditions such as transient tachypnea of the newborn, hyaline membrane disease (HMD), pneumothorax, meconium aspiration syndrome, and congenital diaphragmatic hernia.
  - If the newborn develops respiratory distress and cyanosis several hours after birth, it is usually related to cyanotic congenital heart disease (CCHD), aspiration, or tracheoesophageal fistula.
  - *Consider neurological disorders:* Observe for apnea and periodic breathing, which may be related to immaturity of the nervous system. Seizures can also cause cyanosis.
  - *CCHD presenting with early cyanosis:* Transposition of great arteries (TGA), tricuspid atresia, pulmonary atresia–intact ventricular septum (PA-IVS)
  - Late-onset cyanosis is typically seen in patients with tetralogy of Fallot (TOF).
- Determine if the cyanosis is *uniform or differential.*
  - Peripheral oxygen saturation (SpO_2) in the right hand (preductal) and foot (postductal) helps identify differential cyanosis and a difference of >3% is significant.

- *Differential cyanosis* is seen in patent ductus arteriosus (PDA) with reversal of shunt or in the setting of persistent pulmonary hypertension of newborn (PPHN) or interrupted aortic arch.
- *Reverse differential cyanosis* is seen in the setting of TGA with PDA with reversal of shunt.
- *Typical symptoms of cyanosis with increased pulmonary blood flow (PBF):* Tachypnea, feeding difficulty, recurrent respiratory tract infections, and failure to thrive.
- *Typical symptoms of cyanosis with decreased PBF:* Cyanotic or "tet" spells, squatting in older children.
- *Check the vitals:*
  - Signs of respiratory distress such as tachypnea, retractions, nasal flaring, grunting or crepitations usually indicate a respiratory problem.
  - *Features suggestive of sepsis:* Peripheral cyanosis, increased heart rate (HR) and respiratory rate (RR), decreased blood pressure (BP), increased/decreased temperature
- *Identify right versus left ventricular apex:*
  - *Right ventricular apex (diffuse apex):* TOF, double-outlet right ventricle with ventricular septal defect (VSD) with pulmonary stenosis (PS), TGA with VSD with PS, atrioventricular septal defect with PS, congenitally corrected transposition of great arteries (CCTGA) with VSD with PS, hypoplastic left heart syndrome (HLHS), total anomalous pulmonary venous connection (TAPVC).
  - *Left ventricular apex (localized apex):* Tricuspid atresia, single ventricle (double-inlet left ventricle), PA-IVS with hypoplastic right ventricle
- *Heart sounds:* The focus should be on the second heart sound (S2), which is loud and single in patients with pulmonary arterial hypertension (PAH). In contrast, S2 is single with inaudible pulmonic component (P2) in cardiac lesions with reduced PBF.
- *Murmurs:* An ejection systolic murmur is audible in most forms of CCHD with decreased PBF. An absence of a murmur does not rule out CCHD as serious lesions such as TGA, TAPVC, and HLHS do not manifest with murmur.

Differential diagnosis: To determine the underlying cause of cyanosis, try to find the various mechanisms of cyanosis.
- *Decreased SaO_2:*
  - Decreased atmospheric pressure—high altitude
  - Impaired pulmonary function
    - *Alveolar hypoventilation:* Central nervous system (CNS) depression, airway obstruction, neuromuscular disease
    - V-Q mismatch: Airway disease, extrinsic compression of lungs
    - *Impaired oxygen diffusion:* Pulmonary edema
- *Anatomic shunts:*
  - Cyanotic congenital heart disease

- Pulmonary arteriovenous (AV) fistula
- Intrapulmonary shunts
■ *Abnormal hemoglobin*:
  - Methemoglobinemia
  - Sulfhemoglobinemia
■ *Peripheral cyanosis:* Sepsis, hypothermia, polycythemia, hypoglycemia, or low cardiac output state
■ *Hyperoxia test:*
  - Administer 100% oxygen for >10 minutes, obtain ABGs.
  - If PaO_2 >150 mm Hg then pulmonary disease likely; if PaO_2 >250 mm Hg then cardiac cause is virtually eliminated
  - If PaO_2 <100 mm Hg, rise by <30 mm Hg or SaO_2 unchanged: Cardiac cause (right to left shunt) likely.
  - Total anomalous pulmonary venous return (TAPVR) may respond positively to O_2 despite being a CCHD.
  - Pulmonary disease with a massive intrapulmonary shunt may not respond.
  - It is infrequently practiced nowadays given the easy availability of echocardiography.

Chest X-ray (CXR): To identify pulmonary causes of cyanosis: Pneumothorax, pulmonary hypoplasia, diaphragmatic hernia, pulmonary edema, pneumonia, HMD, etc.
■ Characteristic CXR findings may point to a particular cardiac diagnosis.
  - *TGA:* Egg-on-a-string sign (appears because of a narrow vascular pedicle due to typical anteroposterior relationship of great vessels in TGA)
  - *TOF:* Boot-shaped heart
  - *Obstructed TAPVC:* Ground-glass appearance suggestive of pulmonary venous hypertension, mimics HMD
  - *Supracardiac TAPVC:* Snowman, figure of 8; these features may not appear in early infancy.
■ *Electrocardiogram (ECG):* This must be done in all patients to identify certain characteristic findings.
  - Early R-to-S transition from V1 to V2—TOF
  - Left-axis deviation—tricuspid atresia, AVSD with PS, single ventricle with PS
  - Monomorphic QRS in V1–V6—single ventricle with PS
  - Complete heart block—CCTGA, AVSD with PS

Echocardiography: This is a diagnostic modality for almost all cardiac lesions.

Management of neonate with cyanosis is shown in **Flowchart 1**.

Flowchart 1: Management of neonate with cyanosis.

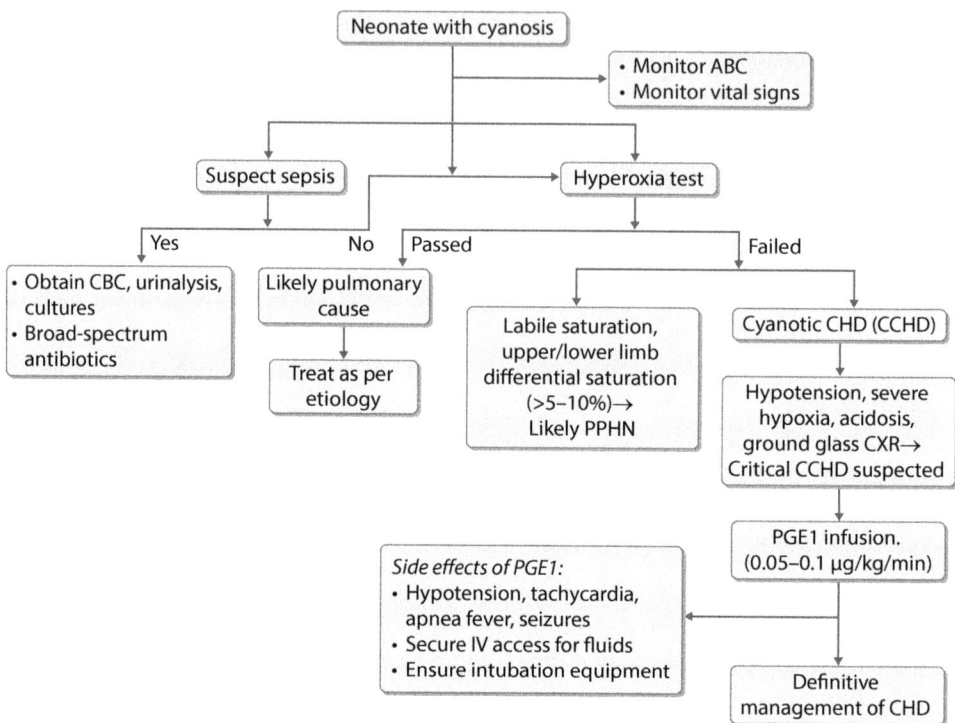

(ABC: airway, breathing, circulation; CBC: complete blood count; CHD: congenital heart disease; CXR: chest X-ray; IV: intravenous; PGE1: prostaglandin E1; PPHN: persistent pulmonary hypertension of newborn)

CHAPTER 24: Cyanotic Spells or "Tet Spells"

Aradhana Dwivedi, Mukti Sharma, Arvind Mishra

- *Definition:* A typical "tet" spell begins with a progressive increase in the rate and depth of breathing and culminates in paroxysmal hyperpnea, deepening cyanosis, limpness, syncope, and occasionally convulsions, cerebrovascular accidents, and death.
- Peak incidence is between the second and sixth month of life. Spells in infants are typically initiated by the stress of feeding, crying, or a bowel movement, particularly after awakening from a long deep sleep.
- It is commonly found in tetralogy of Fallot physiology.
- Any event such as sudden tachycardia, hypovolemia, crying, defecation, or increased physical activity that suddenly lowers the systemic vascular resistance (SVR) or produces a large, right-to-left ventricular shunt may initiate the spell and, if not corrected, establishes a vicious circle of hypoxic spells.
- Pathogenesis

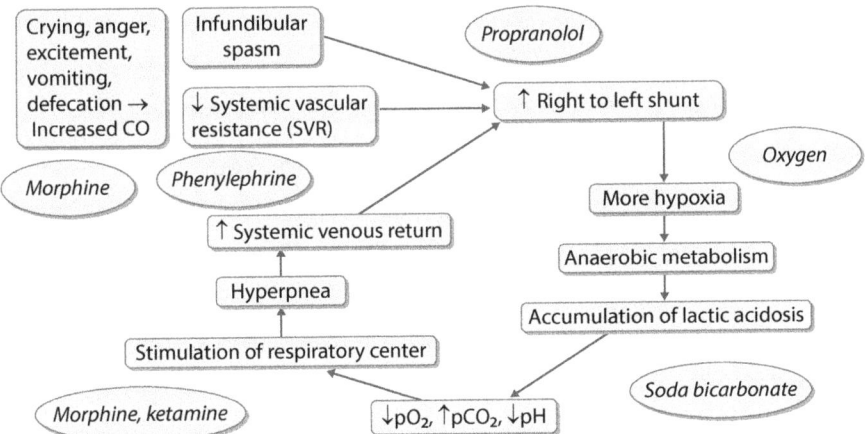

(CO: cardiac output; pO$_2$: partial pressure of oxygen; pCO$_2$: partial pressure of carbon dioxide)

- *Clinical features:*
  - *General:* Irritability, diaphoresis, inconsolable crying
  - *Skin:* Increased cyanosis
  - *Cardiovascular system (CVS):* Tachycardia, decrease in intensity or disappearance of murmur
  - *Respiration:* Tachypnea, grunting, hyperpnea, respiratory distress
  - *Central nervous system (CNS):* Seizures, coma
- Management of cyanotic spell is shown in **Flowchart 1**.

Flowchart 1: Management of cyanotic spell.

```
                    ┌──────────────────┐
                    │  Cyanotic spell  │────────► • Ensure ABC
                    └────────┬─────────┘          • Calm the child
                             ▼                    • Rule out breath-holding spell
              ┌────────────────────────────┐
              │ Knee-chest position        │
              │ Oxygen administration      │
              │ IVF: 10 mL/kg NS bolus     │
              │ 5 mL/kg PRBC if anemic     │
              └────────────┬───────────────┘
                           │ Ensure sedation
                           ▼
        ┌──────────────────────────────────────────────────┐
        │ Injection morphine 0.05–0.1 mg/kg SC or IV       │
        │ Alternatively intranasal or IV midazolam         │
        │   0.1 mg/kg OR                                   │
        │ Injection ketamine 0.5–1 mg/kg IV or 3–5 mg/kg IM│
        └──────────────────────────────────────────────────┘
                           │ Correct acidosis
                           ▼
              ┌────────────────────────────┐
              │ Injection NaHCO₃ 1–2 mEq/kg│
              │ IV stat (diluted 1:1 with DW)│
              └────────────┬───────────────┘
                           │ No relief
                           ▼
```

Correct underlying abnormalities:
- Anemia, hypovolemia,
- Tachyarrhythmias
- Hypoglycemia

Indicators of improved pulmonary blood flow:
- Decreased cyanosis
- Heart murmur becomes audible/louder

Injection propranolol 0.1 mg/kg/dose slow IV push
May repeat in 15 minutes × 1 [alternative metoprolol (0.1 mg/kg/dose)/esmolol 0.5 mg/kg/dose]

↓ No improvement

Injection phenylephrine 0.1 mg/kg/dose IM/SC or 0.01 mg/kg/dose IV

↓ No improvement

Intubation and mechanical ventilation

↓

Consider urgent BT shunt/RVOT stenting/PDA stenting/complete repair

↓

- *Prevention of spells:* Oral propranolol 1–4 mg/kg/day
- Iron supplementation
- Parental counseling for prevention of dehydration, knee-chest position
- Seek early medical attention

(ABC: airway, breathing, circulation; BT: Blalock–Taussig; DW: distilled water; IM: intramuscular; IV: intravenous; IVF: intravenous fluid; NS: normal saline; PDA: patent ductus arteriosus; PRBC: packed red blood cell; RVOT: right ventricular outflow tract; SC: subcutaneous)

CHAPTER 25: Congestive Cardiac Failure

Mukti Sharma, Aradhana Dwivedi, Arvind Mishra

- Heart failure (HF) in children is a clinical and pathophysiologic syndrome that results from ventricular dysfunction, volume, or pressure overload, alone or in combination. It leads to characteristic signs and symptoms, such as poor growth, feeding difficulties, respiratory distress, exercise intolerance, and fatigue, and is associated with circulatory, neurohormonal, and molecular abnormalities. Symptoms are related to a failing heart and venous congestion.
- In early congestive heart failure, increased cardiac contractility and other compensatory mechanisms maintain adequate cardiac output. When these compensatory mechanisms are exhausted, cardiogenic shock becomes manifest.
- Causes of heart failure in CHD based on age of onset of HF are given in **Table 1**.
- The age of onset of congestive cardiac failure (CCF) in other conditions is given in **Table 2**.

TABLE 1: Causes of heart failure (HF) in congenital heart disease (CHD) based on age of onset of HF.

Age at onset	Conditions
At birth	• HLHS • Volume overload lesions: – Severe TR—Ebstein's anomaly – Severe PR – Large systemic AV fistula, i.e., vein of Galen malformation
1st week	• TGA • PDA in small premature infants • HLHS (with more favorable anatomy) • TAPVR with pulmonary venous obstruction • Systemic AV fistula • Critical AS or PS
1–4 weeks	• COA with associated anomalies • Critical AS • Large L-R shunt lesions (VSD, PDA) in premature infants • All other lesions previously listed
4–6 weeks	• AVSD
6 weeks to 4 months	• Large VSD/PDA • Anomalous left coronary artery from pulmonary artery (ALCAPA)

(AS: aortic stenosis; AV: atrioventricular; AVSD: atrioventricular septal defect; COA: coarctation of the aorta; HLHS: hypoplastic left heart syndrome; L-R: left to right; PDA: patent ductus arteriosus; PR: pulmonary regurgitation; PS: pulmonary stenosis; TAPVR: total anomalous pulmonary venous return; TGA: transposition of the great arteries; TR: tricuspid regurgitation; VSD: ventricular septal defect)

TABLE 2: Age of onset of congestive cardiac failure (CCF) in other conditions.

Condition	Age of onset
Kawasaki disease	1–4 years
Viral myocarditis	Small children >1 year
Acute rheumatic carditis	School-age children
Duchenne muscular dystrophy (DMD) and Friedreich's ataxia	Older children and adolescents
Endocardial fibroelastosis	Infancy
Metabolic abnormalities (severe hypoxia, acidosis, hypoglycemia and hypocalcemia)	Newborns
Supraventricular tachycardia/complete heart block	Early infancy
Severe anemia/thyroid abnormalities	Any age
Bronchopulmonary dysplasia in preterm causing right heart failure	Early Infancy
Primary carnitine deficiency	2–4 years

- *Clinical manifestations*:
    - *History:* Recent infection, possible drug/toxin ingestion, family history, poor feeding, failure to thrive, increased sweating
    - *General exam:* Pallor, cyanosis, mottling, dependent edema especially sacral
    - *Cardiovascular system (CVS):* Tachycardia, gallop rhythm, decreased or unequal pulses, hypotension
    - *Respiratory:* Tachypnea, wheezing, crackles, dyspnea
    - *Gastrointestinal (GI):* Hepatomegaly
    - *Central nervous system (CNS):* Irritability, lethargy
- Check for acute decompensation

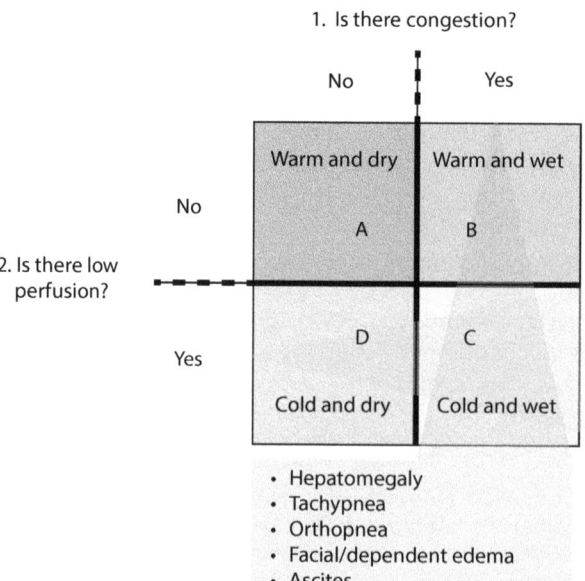

- *Investigations:*
  - *Blood:* Complete blood count (CBC), arterial blood gas (ABG), blood urea nitrogen (BUN), creatinine, electrolytes, glucose, aspartate aminotransferase (AST), alanine aminotransferase (ALT), C-reactive protein (CRP)
  - *Cardiac biomarkers:* Brain natriuretic peptide (BNP), N-terminal prohormone of brain natriuretic peptide (NT-pro BNP); Useful as an adjunctive marker to aid in diagnosis and establish prognosis or disease severity; serial measurement has prognostic value. Cardiac troponin I and T can be done if myocarditis is suspected.
  - *Urine:* Urinalysis, urine output
  - *Chest radiograph:* Look for cardiomegaly, pulmonary edema
  - *Electrocardiogram:* To rule out rhythm abnormalities, low-voltage complexes, chamber hypertrophy, ST-T changes
  - *Echocardiogram:* Detailed diagnosis, ventricular function (assessed by LV fractional shortening, normal value 28–42%, LV ejection fraction, normal value 55–65%)
  - *Cardiac magnetic resonance imaging (MRI):* For evaluation of myocarditis, right ventricular assessment and determine prognosis and timing of treatment in slowly progressive ventricular dysfunction such as Duchenne muscular dystrophy (DMD) or anthracycline-related cardiomyopathy (CM).
  - *Metabolic primary screening tests:* If indicated
- *Management of CCF:*
  - Stepwise goal-directed management
  - *The treatment of patients with CHF consists of:* (1) Elimination of the underlying causes; (2) treatment of the precipitating or contributing causes (e.g., infection, anemia, arrhythmias, fever); and (3) control of heart failure state.
  - Most of the drugs used in children with CCF have been extrapolated from adult studies. There are no randomized controlled trials (RCTs) for these drugs in pediatric population **(Table 3)**.

  Management of cardiogenic shock is shown in **Flowchart 1**.
  Management of CCF is shown in **Flowchart 2**.
  The stepwise introduction of medical therapy in HF is given in **Figure 1**.

TABLE 3: Drugs and dosage for management of CCF.

Drugs	Dosage
Digoxin	10 µg/kg/day in two divided doses (maintenance dose)
Furosemide	1–4 mg/kg/day (1–2 doses)
Spironolactone	1–3 mg/kg/day (2 doses)
Captopril	0.5–5 mg/kg/day in 3 divided doses
Enalapril	0.1–0.5 mg/kg/day
Losartan	0.5 mg/kg/day once daily
Metoprolol	0.1–0.2 mg/kg/day (2 doses, maximum 1 mg/kg/dose)
Carvedilol	0.1 mg/kg/day twice daily (increase gradually to 0.5–1 mg/kg/day)
Levocarnitine	50–100 mg/kg/day (2–3 doses)

SECTION 3: Cardiovascular Disorders

Flowchart 1: Management of cardiogenic shock.

Congestive cardiac failure (CCF)
- Ensure ABC
- Supplemental oxygen
- Pulse oximetry
- Monitor BP (four limbs)
- Cardiorespiratory monitoring

Assess compromise of end-organ perfusion: Decreased urinary output, altered mentation, hypotension

No → CCF → Stepwise management of CCF

Yes → Cardiogenic shock

Ongoing supportive measures:
- Normothermia
- Catheterize and monitor urine output
- CVP monitoring
- Support ventilation/oxygenation (avoid high PEEP)
- Antibiotics if indicated

- Manipulate preload
- Isotonic NS 5–10 mL/kg IV bolus if necessary
- Maintain PDA in duct-dependent lesion
- PGE1 infusion
- (0.05–0.1 µg/kg/min)
- Echocardiogram (if feasible)
- Shift to PICU

- Inotropic support (avoid in idiopathic hypertrophic subaortic stenosis)
- Dopamine 8–20 µg/kg/min IV infusion
  Or
- Epinephrine 0.05–1.5 µg/kg/min IV infusion Plus
- Dobutamine 5–10 µg/kg/min
- *Once stable, consider:* Milrinone 50–75 µg/kg/dose IV bolus followed by continuous infusion at 0.25–0.75 µg/kg/min

Flowchart 2: Management of congestive cardiac failure.

Congestive cardiac failure

Management goals:
- Control of congestive state
- Management of precipitating events
- Treatment of cause

Step 1
- Bed rest, propped up position, humidified oxygen, respiratory support
- Stop oral feeds if severe tachypnea
- Volume restriction if required
- Sodium restriction is generally not required; ensure good caloric intake

Step 2
Medical management:
- Loop diuretics (reduces pulmonary and systemic congestion)
- Mineralocorticoid receptor antagonists (MRA)—spironolactone
- ACE inhibitor/ARNI (reduces disproportionally elevated afterload)

Contd...

Contd...

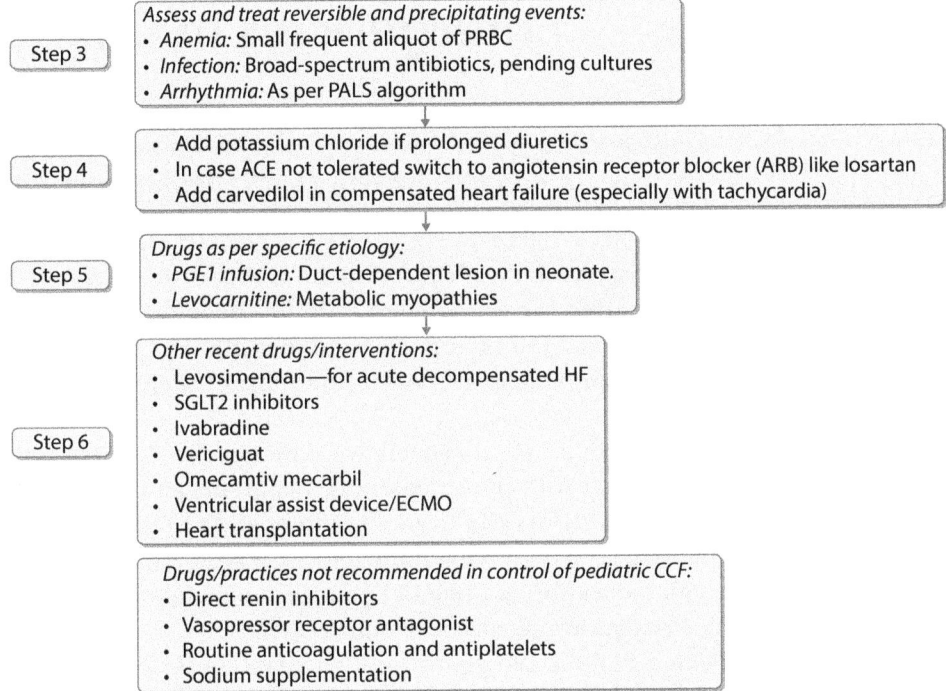

(ABC: airway, breathing, circulation; ACE: angiotensin-converting enzyme; ARNI: angiotensin receptor neprilysin inhibitor; BP: blood pressure; ECMO: extracorporeal membrane oxygenation; IV: intravenous; PALS: pediatric advanced life support; PDA: patent ductus arteriosus; PEEP: positive end-expiratory pressure; PGE1: prostaglandin E1; PRBC: packed red blood cell; SGLT2: sodium–glucose cotransporter 2)

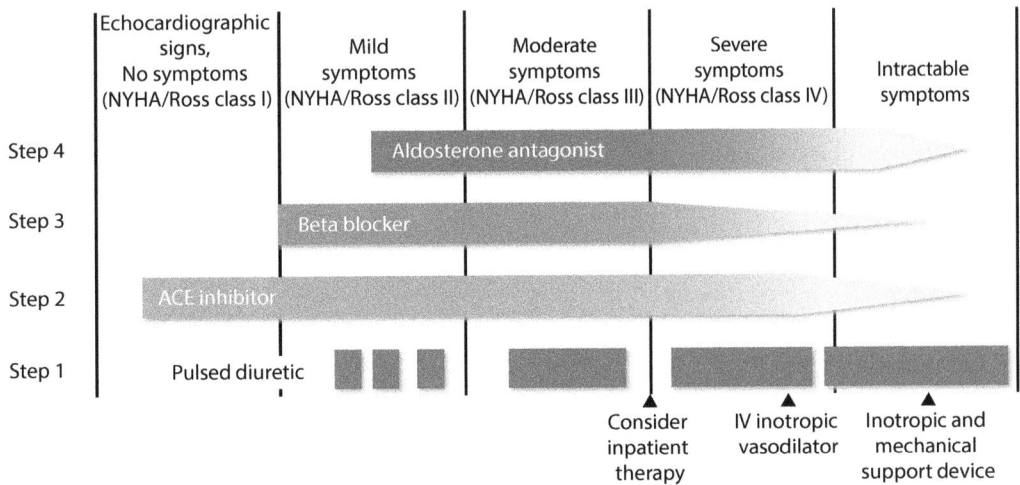

Fig. 1: Stepwise introduction of medical therapy in heart failure (HF). (ACE: angiotensin-converting enzyme; IV: intravenous; NYHA: New York Heart Association)

CHAPTER 26

Hypertensive Emergencies in Children

Aradhana Dwivedi, Mukti Sharma, Arvind Mishra

- *Definition*: Acute severe hypertension (HTN) can be defined as an acute blood pressure (BP) elevation that fulfills (and usually exceeds) the definition of stage 2 HTN (≥95th percentile + 12 mm Hg, or ≥140/90 mm Hg) and that is accompanied by severe symptoms. Physical examination and/or laboratory findings of accelerated HTN are frequently also present.
- Traditionally, it has been divided into hypertensive emergencies and hypertensive urgencies, the former associated with life-threatening symptoms and/or target-organ injury and the latter associated with less significant symptoms and no target organ injury.
- If the BP reading is at the stage 2 HTN level and the patient is symptomatic, or the BP is >30 mm Hg above the 95th percentile (or >180/120 mm Hg in an adolescent), refer to an emergency department or pediatric intensive care unit (PICU).
- Organs commonly affected include the central nervous system (CNS) (hypertensive encephalopathy, retinal vasculopathy-induced visual changes, cerebral infarction, and hemorrhage); the CVS (congestive heart failure, myocardial ischemia, aortic dissection); and the kidneys (proteinuria, hematuria, and acute renal insufficiency).
- *Symptoms*: Common CNS symptoms in acute severe HTN are headache, dizziness, nausea/vomiting, visual impairment, seizures, and altered mental state. The renal manifestations can be evidence of acute kidney injury (AKI), such as hematuria, albuminuria, and azotemia.
- The possible triggering event that precipitates the acute severe HTN in an underlying state of chronic HTN needs to be elucidated. This can be activation of sympathetic nervous system as in pain, anxiety, postoperative stress, any new drug intake, or any factor increasing systemic vascular resistance.
- *Common secondary causes of HTN in children:*
  - Renovascular
  - Coarctation of aorta
  - Renal parenchymal disease
  - Endocrine
  - Malignancy
  - Others
    - Child on steroids/calcineurin inhibitors
    - Guillain–Barré syndrome
    - Substance abuse (in adolescents)
    - Rebound HTN

CHAPTER 26: Hypertensive Emergencies in Children

- *Evaluation—history:*
  - *History suggestive of secondary causes of HTN, most commonly renal and cardiac disease:* Polyuria, recurrent urinary tract infection (UTI), hematuria, anasarca, failure to thrive, dyspnea
  - *History suggestive of target organ damage:* Breathlessness, palpitations, increased chest activity, headache, vomiting, lethargy, irritability, altered sensorium, seizures, visual disturbances, blindness
- *Examination:*
  - Heart rate—bradycardia can be a marker for raised intracranial pressure (ICP)
  - BP and pulse in all four limbs—to rule out coarctation of aorta
  - Anthropometry
  - *General examination:* Obesity, acne, striae, hirsutism, virilization, ambiguous genitalia
- *Systemic examination:*
  - *Cardiovascular system:* Look for features of congestive cardiac failure; auscultate over epigastrium, and flanks for renal artery bruit
  - *Abdominal examination:* Look for abdominal masses, palpable kidneys
  - *Neurological examination:* Features of encephalopathy raised ICPs
  - *Ocular examination:* Fundus
- *First-line investigations*:
  - Renal function tests (renal failure)
  - Electrolytes (hypokalemia/hyperkalemia)
  - Urinalysis (acute or chronic glomerulonephritis)
  - Complete blood counts/peripheral blood smear (PBS) [chronic renal failure, hemolytic uremic syndrome (HUS)]
  - Chest X-ray (cardiomegaly, pulmonary edema)
  - Electrocardiogram (ECG), echo [cardiomegaly, left ventricular hypertrophy (LVH)]
- *Special investigations:*
  - Neuroimaging (target organ damage: Brain)
  - *Ultrasonography (USG) abdomen and kidneys, ureters, and urinary bladder (KUB) including Doppler:* Renal etiology
  - MCU/DMSA
  - C3 levels, antinuclear antibody (ANA)
  - Levels of renin, aldosterone, cortisol, thyroid-stimulating hormone (TSH)
  - DSA
  - Catecholamine in 24 hours urine
  - I-123 MIBG (^{123}I-metaiodobenzylguanidine) scintigraphy
- *Management*:
  - Establish the distinction between hypertensive emergency and hypertensive urgency.
  - Maintain airway, breathing, circulation (ABC)
  - Admit in PICU, continuous arterial BP monitoring is preferred
  - *Goals of therapy:*
    - Reverse/prevent end organ damage
    - Restore normal BP
    - Identify and treat the underlying cause

- Mean arterial BP [one-third systolic blood pressure (SBP) + two-thirds diastolic blood pressure (DBP)]
- Treatment may be initiated with oral agents, if the patient can tolerate oral therapy and if life-threatening complications have not yet developed.
- Drug therapy aims to reduce BP in a controlled, predictable, and safe manner, which is best achieved with continuous infusion of pharmacologic agents that have rapid onset, short half-life, and ease of titration.
- Intravenous agents are indicated when oral therapy is not possible because of the patient's clinical status, or when a severe complication has developed (such as congestive heart failure) that warrants a more controlled BP reduction.
- *Target control of BP:* The BP should be reduced by no >25% of the planned reduction over the first 8 hours, with the remainder of the planned reduction over the next 12-24 hours. The ultimate short-term BP goal in such patients should generally be around the 95th percentile.
- Reduction is slow in order to preserve cerebral autoregulation.
- The long-term the treatment goal with nonpharmacologic and pharmacologic therapy should be a reduction in SBP and DBP to <90th percentile and <130/80 mm Hg in adolescents ≥13 years old.

- Antihypertensives prescribed are given in **Table 1**.

Management of hypertensive crisis is given in **Flowchart 1**.

TABLE 1: Dosing of antihypertensives.

Drug	Onset	Duration of effect	Route	Dose and remarks
Labetalol	5–10 minutes	3–6 hours	• IV infusion • IV bolus	• 0.25–3 mg/kg/h • 0.2–1 mg/kg/dose q 5–10 minutes (maximum 40 mg)
Sodium nitroprusside	2 minutes	<10 minutes	IV infusion	Starting 0.3–0.5 µg/kg/min (in 5% dextrose); titrate to effect; maximum dose 10 µg/kg/min; protect from light; cyanate and thiocyanate toxicity usually seen after 72 hours, follow levels of methemoglobin and thiocyanate
Nicardipine	1–10 minutes	3 hours	• IV infusion • IV bolus	• 0.5–4 µg/kg/min (maximum 5 mg/h) • 30 µg/kg (maximum 2 mg/dose) q 15 minutes
Esmolol	1 minutes	10–20 minutes	IV infusion	Loading with 100–500 µg/kg over 1–2 minutes; then maintain at 25–100 µg/kg/min
Sodium nitroglycerine	2–5 minutes	5–10 minutes	IV infusion	• Begin with 0.25–0.5 µg/kg/min • Usual dose 1–5 µg/kg/min • *Maximum dose:* 20 µg/kg/min
Phentolamine	10 minutes	30–60 minutes	IV bolus	0.1–0.2 mg/kg (maximum 5 mg) q 2–4 hours if required; can be used in pheochromocytoma

Contd...

Contd...

Drug	Onset	Duration of effect	Route	Dose and remarks
Fenoldopam	10 minutes	1 hour	IV infusion	• 0.2–0.5 mg/kg/min up to 0.8 mg/kg/min • Promotes natriuresis and improves urine output; develops tolerance in 48 hours
Diazoxide	3–5 minutes	2–12 hours	• IV infusion • IV bolus	• 0.3–5 µg/kg/min • 1–5 mg/kg q 5–30 minutes
Hydralazine	5–20 minutes	2–6 hours	• IV/IM • Oral	• 0.5 mg/kg q 4–6 hours • 0.25 mg/kg/dose (maximum 25 mg)
Nifedipine	10–30 minutes	1–4 hours	Oral	0.1–0.25 mg/kg (maximum 10 mg) q 4–6 hours
Clonidine	15–30 minutes	1.5–4 hours	Oral	2–5 µg/kg/dose, up to 10 µg/kg/dose given q 6–8 hours; can cause rebound hypertension
Minoxidil	30 minutes	2–5 days	Oral	0.1–0.2 mg/kg/dose (maximum 5 mg)
Isradipine	60 minutes	3–8 hours	Oral	• 0.05–0.1 mg/kg/dose • Up to 5 mg/dose

(IM: intramuscular; IV: intravenous)

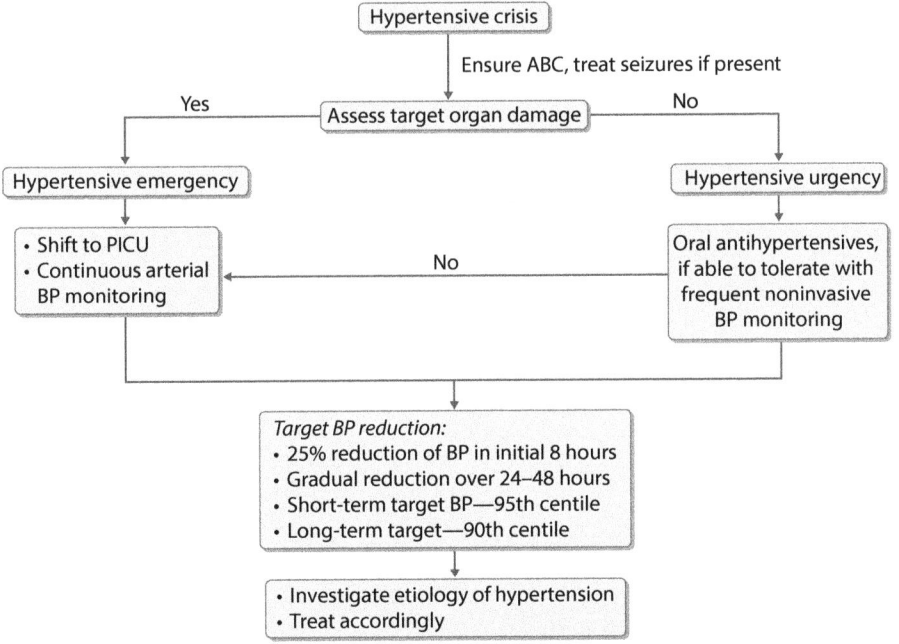

Flowchart 1: Management of hypertensive crisis.

(ABC: airway, breathing, circulation; BP: blood pressure; PICU: pediatric intensive care unit)

SECTION 4

Hematological and Oncological Disorders

- **Disseminated Intravascular Coagulation**
  Amit Devgan, Barnali Mitra
- **Febrile Neutropenia**
  Vishal Sondhi, Barnali Mitra
- **Tumor Lysis Syndrome**
  Barnali Mitra, Vishal Sondhi
- **Hemophilia Emergencies**
  Barnali Mitra, Amit Devgan
- **Acute Transfusion Reactions**
  Barnali Mitra, Vishal Sondhi
- **Acute Illness in a Child with Sickle Cell Disease**
  Barnali Mitra, Vishal Sondhi
- **Bleeding Disorders**
  Vishal Sondhi

CHAPTER 27: Disseminated Intravascular Coagulation

Amit Devgan, Barnali Mitra

- Disseminated intravascular coagulation (DIC) is a clinic-pathological syndrome characterized by activation of coagulation pathways and formation of fibrin clots leading to multiorgan dysfunction. Usually, bleeding is predominant problem, but 10% of DIC cases can present with exclusively thrombotic problem.
- Pathogenesis

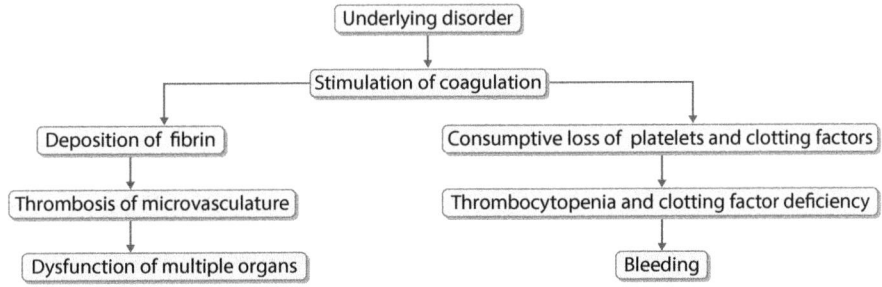

The causes, clinical features, and laboratory workup of DIC are given in **Table 1**.

Causes	Clinical features	Laboratory workup
<ul><li>Infection and sepsis</li><li>Polytrauma</li><li>Pancreatitis</li><li>*Malignancy:*<ul><li>Solid tumors</li><li>Leukemia</li></ul></li><li>*Obstetric:*<ul><li>Amniotic fluid embolism</li><li>Placental abruption</li><li>Preeclampsia</li></ul></li><li>Hemangiomas</li><li>Liver cell failure</li><li>*Toxins and immune insults:*<ul><li>Snake envenomation</li><li>Recreational drugs</li><li>ABO incompatibility</li><li>Graft rejection</li></ul></li><li>*Microangiopathic disorders:*<ul><li>HUS</li></ul></li><li>Kasabach–Merritt syndrome</li></ul>	<ul><li>Petechiae or purpura</li><li>Purpura fulminans</li><li>Ooze from venipuncture or surgical sites</li><li>Epistaxis or mucosal bleeding</li><li>Hematemesis, malena, hematochezia</li><li>Hemoptysis</li><li>Hematuria</li><li>Renal insufficiency</li><li>Intracranial bleed</li><li>Tachycardia</li><li>Hypotension</li></ul>	<ul><li>Decreased platelet count</li><li>Increased PT, aPTT, TT</li><li>*PBS:* Schistocytes on smear</li><li>*Fibrinogen:* Decreased</li><li>*D-dimer:* Increased</li><li>*FDP:* Increased</li><li>Factor VIII, V, II, antithrombin III, protein C, S: Decreased</li><li>*Other investigations to rule out multiorgan dysfunction:* RFT, LFT, electrolytes, blood culture, urinalysis, and culture, chest X-ray</li><li>Blood group and crossmatch</li></ul>

TABLE 1: Causes, clinical features, and laboratory workup of disseminated intravascular coagulation (DIC).

(aPTT: activated partial thromboplastin time; HUS: hemolytic–uremic syndrome; LFT: liver function test; PBS: peripheral blood smear; PT: prothrombin time; RFT: renal function test; TT: thrombin time)

Diagnosis and management of DIC is given in **Flowchart 1**.

Flowchart 1: Diagnosis and management of disseminated intravascular coagulation (DIC).

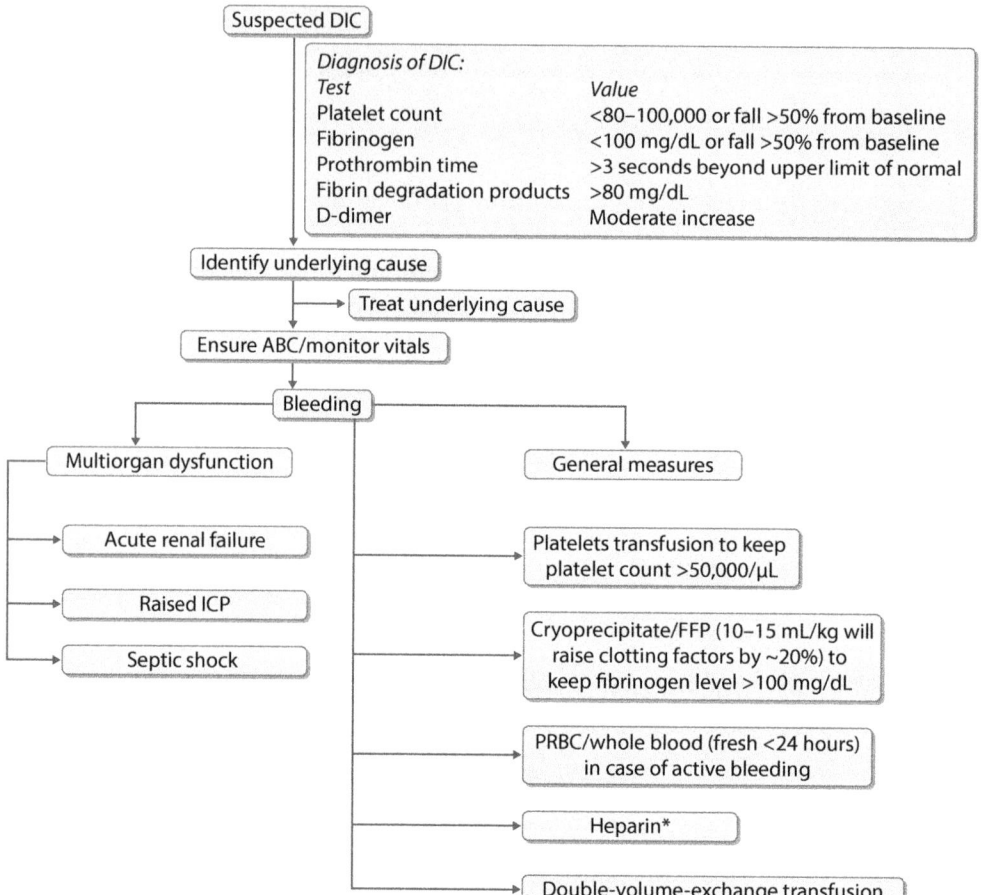

*Anticoagulation is not the primary treatment for pediatric DIC, but it may help manage it. Use anticoagulant therapy, like unfractionated heparin (UFH), only in patients with life-threatening or symptomatic thrombosis, e.g., acral ischemia, without clinically significant bleeding. Patients with recent severe traumatic brain injury or liver failure should not receive therapeutic heparin. IV UFH is preferred due to precise titration and quick cessation in case of bleeding. Start UFH infusion at 5–10 U/kg/h.
(ABC: airway, breathing, circulation; FFP: fresh frozen plasma; ICP: intracranial pressure; IV: intravenous; PRBC: packed red blood cell)

CHAPTER 28

Febrile Neutropenia

Vishal Sondhi, Barnali Mitra

- *Definition:*
  - *Neutropenia:* For the purposes of management of fever in children with cancer or hematopoietic cell transplant, neutropenia is defined as an absolute neutrophil count (ANC) <500 cells/μL or an ANC that is expected to decrease to <500 cells/μL during the next 48 hours. The ANC is calculated using the following formula = Total white blood cell count (cells/μL) × [percent polymorphonuclear (PMN) cells + percent bands] ÷ 100.
  - *Fever:* In neutropenic patients, fever is defined as a single oral temperature ≥38.3°C (101°F), a temperature ≥38°C (100.4°F) for longer than 1 hour, or two elevations >38°C (100.4°F) during a 12-hour period.
- *Evaluation:* History and thorough physical examination—focus in oropharynx/ gastrointestinal tract (GIT)/respiratory/central lines/skin and soft tissue/urinary tract; history of (H/o) recent invasive procedure; absence of toxic appearance does not hold significance
- *Assess:* Vitals
  - Oral intake, sensorium, any focal deficit
  - Classical signs of inflammation may be absent
- *Investigations:*
  - Complete blood count with ANC
  - *Blood cultures (urgent)* from peripheral and central line (both aerobic and anaerobic)
  - Urine culture/stool culture
  - Pus culture depending on the clinical presentation
  - Biochemistry—renal function test (RFT), liver function test (LFT), electrolytes
  - Chest radiograph—if signs/symptoms suggestive of lung involvement
  - *Other investigations:* Radiograph sinus, computed tomography (CT) chest/abdomen, throat swab culture, sputum for gram stain and culture based on clinical presentation
- *Management:*
  - Broad-spectrum intravenous (IV) antibiotics should be started at the earliest (must commence within 60 minutes of arrival) after obtaining all culture samples.
  - The first-line antibiotic should be based on the unit guidelines and may typically comprise piperacillin + tazobactam or cephalosporin (ceftazidime/cefoperazone + sulbactam) and aminoglycoside (amikacin). If there is an obvious cutaneous infection/ hemodynamically unstable/high prevalence of methicillin-resistant *Staphylococcus aureus* (MRSA) infection in center or suspected central line infection—staphylococcal cover (vancomycin) should be started upfront.
  - Daily physical examination to be done after starting antibiotics.
  - In case of radiograph chest suggestive of consolidation, cover for community-acquired pneumonia.

- No response to antibiotics in 36–48 hours or clinical worsening, vancomycin should be added. Further, change to carbapenems and vancomycin.
- With no improvement (persistent fever >96 hours)/worsening or child is at high risk of developing invasive fungal infection—antifungals (caspofungin/amphotericin) should be added; serum biomarker (galactomannan or D-glucan) not recommended for starting antifungal therapy.
- Trimethoprim and sulfamethoxazole prophylaxis is continued and fresh blood cultures sent at every antibiotic change.

Algorithm for management of febrile neutropenia is given in **Flowchart 1**.

Flowchart 1: Algorithm for management of febrile neutropenia.

```
Neutropenia and fever
        ↓
Strict isolation and immediate blood culture
Start antibiotics within 1 hour of admission
        ↓
H/E: Check vitals, sensorium, oral intake, focal deficit
INV: CBC, biochemistry, CXR, all cultures, special investigations
Monitor daily for fever response, neutropenia, focus of infection, secondary infection
        ↓
Start broad-spectrum antibiotics based
on unit protocol (piptaz/cefoperazone—
sulbactam and amikacin)
```

Low risk (all):
- ANC < 500 cells/μL expected to resolve within 7 days (i.e., neutrophil count increasing)
- Stable and adequate hepatic function
- Stable and adequate renal function
- No active comorbidities

High risk (1 or more):
- ANC <500 cells/μL anticipated to last for >7 days
- Evidence of hepatic insufficiency (aminotransferase levels >5 times normal values)
- Evidence of renal insufficiency (creatinine clearance <30 mL/min)
- Comorbid medical problems including, but not limited to:
  – Hemodynamic instability/oral or GI mucositis that interferes with swallowing or causes diarrhea/GI symptoms, including abdominal pain, nausea, vomiting, or diarrhea/new-onset neurologic or mental status changes/signs of intravascular catheter infection/new pulmonary infiltrate or hypoxemia or underlying chronic lung disease/new findings or symptoms associated with localized infection
  – Acute lymphoblastic leukemia in infant <12 months of age
  – Acute myeloid leukemia
  – Within 30 days of hematopoietic cell transplant

Does fever resolve within 72 hours?

Continue empiric antibiotics until:
- Afebrile for 48 hours, and
- ANC > 500 cells/μL and increasing

Yes ← / No →

- Evaluate for occult fungal infection
- Add vancomycin
- Consider adding broader coverage (carbapenems)
- Repeat cultures for bacteria and fungi
- *Further studies:* CBC, DIC profile, CRP, CXR, other imaging

Does fever resolve within 48 hours?

Yes / No

- Add amphotericin B/caspofungin
- If fever persists on amphotericin B consider increasing dose

(ANC: absolute neutrophil count; CBC: complete blood count; CRP: C-reactive protein; CXR: chest X-ray; DIC: disseminated intravascular coagulation; GI: gastrointestinal; H/E: histopathological examination; INV: investigation)

CHAPTER 29: Tumor Lysis Syndrome

Barnali Mitra, Vishal Sondhi

- Tumor lysis syndrome (TLS) is an oncological emergency due to death of tumor cells characterized by hyperuricemia, hyperphosphatemia, hyperkalemia, and hypocalcemia. If untreated, it can rapidly progress to acute renal failure **(Table 1)**.
  The classification of tumor risk groups is given in **Table 2**.

TABLE 1: Metabolic derangements and clinical features.

Metabolic cause	Signs and symptoms
Hypocalcemia	Vomiting, anorexia, tetany, carpopedal spasm, seizures, cardiac arrest
Hyperkalemia	Gastrointestinal (GI) symptoms, weakness, paralysis, arrhythmia
Hyperuricemia	Lethargy, nausea, vomiting, hypertension, altered sensorium
Renal failure	Flank pain, oliguria/anuria, dysuria, hematuria

TABLE 2: Classification of tumor risk groups.

High-risk group tumors (>5% risk)	Intermediate-risk group tumors (1–5% risk)	Low-risk group tumors (<1%)
Burkitt lymphoma	Stage III or IV anaplastic large-cell lymphoma with serum LDH level <2 times the ULN	AML with WBC count <25,000/µL and serum LDH level <2 times the ULN
ALL with WBC ≥100,000/µL and/or serum LDH level ≥2 times the ULN	Early-stage lymphoblastic lymphoma with serum LDH level <2 times the ULN	CLL with WBC ≤50,000/µL
AML with WBC ≥100,000/µL	CLL with WBC 10,000–50,000/µL	Other non-Hodgkin lymphomas that do not meet the criteria for high risk or intermediate risk, with serum LDH level within normal limits
Stage III or IV lymphoblastic lymphoma or early stage lymphoblastic lymphoma with serum LDH level ≥2 times the ULN	T-cell lymphoma/leukemia, diffuse large B-cell lymphoma, peripheral T-cell lymphoma, transformed lymphoma, or mantle cell lymphoma with serum LDH level above the ULN but *without* bulky disease	Other solid tumors
T-cell lymphoma and mantle cell lymphoma	Early stage Burkitt lymphoma with serum LDH level <2 times the ULN	

Contd...

Contd...

High-risk group tumors (>5% risk)	Intermediate-risk group tumors (1–5% risk)	Low-risk group tumors (<1%)
Stage III or IV diffuse large B-cell lymphoma	ALL with WBC <100,000/µL and serum LDH level <2 times the ULN	
Patients with intermediate-risk disease with renal dysfunction and/or renal involvement or uric acid, potassium, or phosphate levels above the ULN	AML with WBC 25,000–100,000/µL or AML with WBC <25,000/µL and LDH ≥2 times the ULN	
	Bulky solid tumors (neuroblastoma)	

(ALL: acute lymphoblastic leukemia; AML: acute myeloid leukemia; CLL: chronic lymphocytic leukemia; LDH: lactate dehydrogenase; ULN: upper limit of normal; WBC: white blood cell)

- High index of suspicion is required for TLS in children with cancer (Cairo-Bishop criteria).
- Cairo–Bishop definition of TLS and investigations

Laboratory TLS: Two or more of below-mentioned criteria within 3 days before to 7 days after initiation of therapy in the setting of adequate hydration (with or without alkalinization) and use of a hypouricemic agent:
- Uric acid ≥476 µmol/L (8 mg/dL) or 25% increase from baseline
- Potassium ≥6.0 mmol/L (or 6 mEq/L) or 25% increase from baseline
- Phosphorus ≥2.1 mmol/L (6.5 mg/dL) for children or 25% increase from baseline
- Calcium ≤1.75 mmol/L (7 mg/dL) or 25% decrease from baseline

Clinical TLS: Laboratory TLS plus any one or more of the following criteria:
- Creatinine 1.5 times upper limit of normal
- Cardiac arrhythmia/sudden death
- Seizure

Investigations:
- CBC
- Na, K, Cl, PO_4, HCO_3
- Calcium (ionic and serum albumin in serum calcium is low)
- Uric acid
- LDH
- Urea, creatinine, urine RE/ME (urate crystals)
- Chest X-ray
- ECG—hypocalcemia, hyperkalemia

(CBC: complete blood count; ECG: electrocardiogram; ME: microscopic examination; LDH: lactate dehydrogenase; RE: routine examination; TLS: tumor lysis syndrome)

- Tumor-related factors associated with a higher risk of TLS include:
  - High tumor cell proliferation rate
  - Chemosensitivity of the malignancy
  - Large tumor burden, as manifested by bulky disease >10 cm in diameter and/or a white blood cell count >50,000/µL

- Pretreatment serum lactate dehydrogenase (LDH) more than two times the upper normal
- Organ infiltration, or bone marrow involvement
- Clinical features that predispose to the development of TLS:
  - Pretreatment hyperuricemia (serum uric acid >7.5 mg/dL or hyperphosphatemia)
  - A preexisting nephropathy or exposure to nephrotoxins
  - Oliguria and/or acidic urine
  - Dehydration, volume depletion, or inadequate hydration during treatment
- *Management (Flowchart 1)*:
  - *Hydration:* Urine output maintained at >100 mL/m^2; specific gravity of urine should be <1.010; target urine pH between 7 and 7.5.

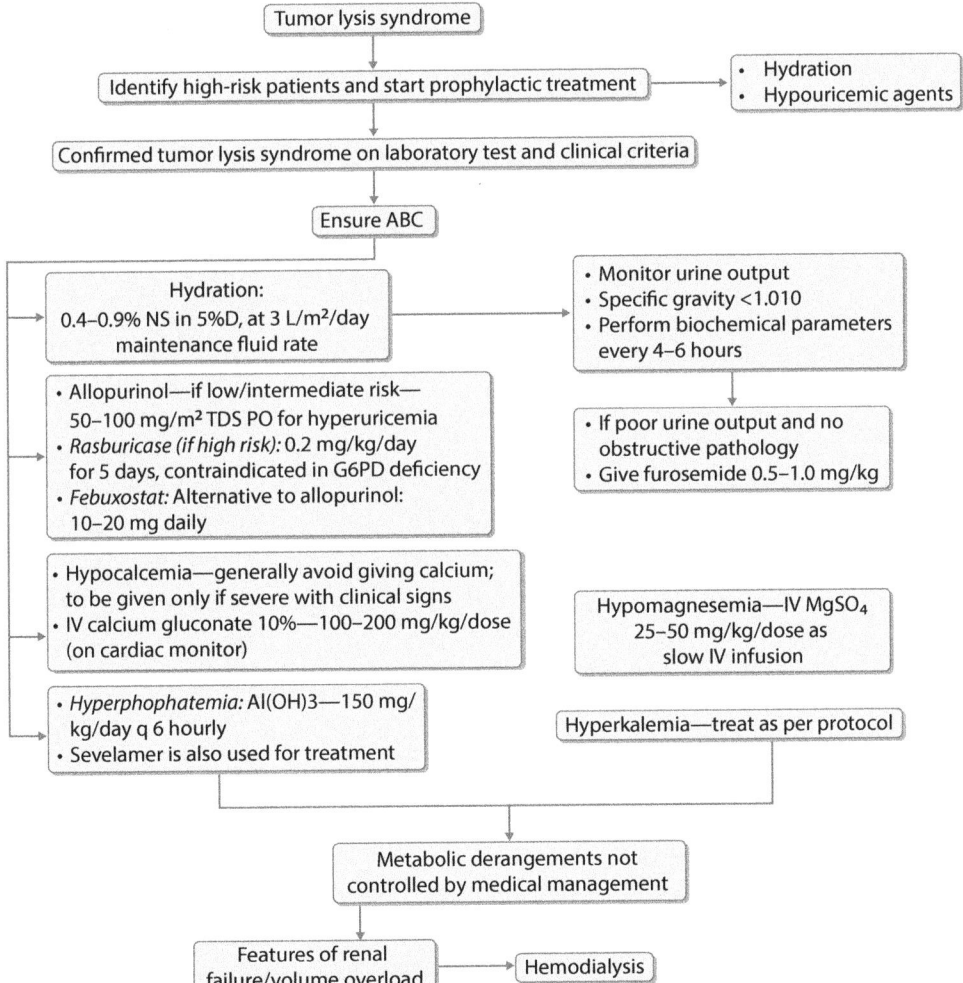

Flowchart 1: Management of tumor lysis syndrome.

(ABC: airway, breathing, circulation; 5%D: 5% dextrose; G6PD: glucose-6-phosphate dehydrogenase; IV: intravenous; NS: normal saline)

- *Intravenous (IV) fluid:* 3 L/m^2/day or 200 mL/kg/day if weight is <10 kg, maintenance fluid with 0.45–0.9% normal saline (NS) with 5% dextrose
- Diuretics given only if urine output is poor—give loop diuretics
- Hyperuricemia—managed with allopurinol (xanthine oxidase inhibitor)/rasburicase (recombinant urate oxidase)—urine alkalization not recommended
- Hyperphosphatemia treated with aluminum hydroxide
- Hypocalcemia should be treated only if symptomatic with seizures, tetany, and arrhythmia.
- When the calcium phosphate product exceeds 60 mg^2/dL^2, there is an increased risk of calcium phosphate precipitation in the renal tubules.
- The indications for renal replacement therapy in patients with TLS are:
  - Severe oliguria or anuria
  - Persistent hyperkalemia
  - Hyperphosphatemia-induced symptomatic hypocalcemia

CHAPTER 30: Hemophilia Emergencies

Barnali Mitra, Amit Devgan

- Assessment of severity

Severity	Clotting factor level% activity (IU/mL)	Bleeding episodes
Severe	1% (<0.01)	Spontaneous bleeding, predominantly in joints and muscles
Moderate	1–5% (0.01–0.05)	Occasional spontaneous bleeding; severe bleeding with minor trauma, surgery
Mild	5–40% (0.05–0.40)	Severe bleeding with major trauma or surgery

- Sites of bleeding:
  - *Serious:* Joints, muscle, soft tissue, mouth, gums, nose, hematuria
  - *Life threatening:* Central nervous system (CNS), gastrointestinal, neck, throat, severe trauma
- Clinical features:
  - *Acute hemarthrosis:* Pain, swelling, limitation of movements (target joint—a target joint is defined as a joint with ≥3 recurrent bleeding episodes in a 6-month period)
  - *Intracranial bleed:* Post-traumatic head injuries, significant headaches
  - *Intramuscular bleed:* H/o of trauma, deep-seated, may lead to atrophy, fibrosis, and contractures
  - *Iliopsoas bleed:* Pain in the lower abdomen, groin, and/or lower back and pain on extension, signs of femoral nerve compression; may progress to life-threatening retroperitoneal bleed.

Management of hemophilia emergencies is given in **Flowchart 1**.

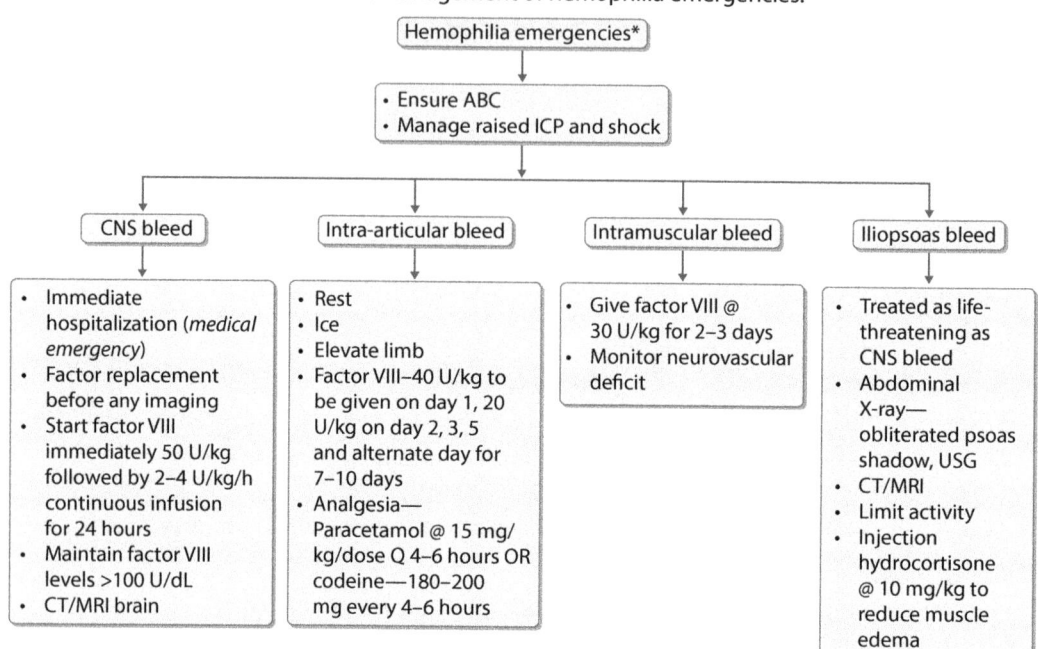

Flowchart 1: Management of hemophilia emergencies.

*For hemophilia B: For severe bleeding, give factor IX at *100–140 U/kg* as soon as possible to produce a factor IX level of 80–100%. For less-severe joint or muscle bleeding, a target factor IX level of 40–50% may be used, by giving a factor IX at a dose of 50–70 U/kg **(Table 1)**.
(ABC: airway, breathing, circulation; CNS: central nervous system; CT: computed tomography; ICP: intracranial pressure; MRI: magnetic resonance imaging)

	Site of hemorrhage	Desired factor level (%)	Hemophilia A/VIII	Hemophilia B/IX
Life-threatening	CNS	100	50–75	100–120
	Neck/retropharyngeal	100	50	100
	Abdominal/retroperitoneal	100	50	60–80
	GIT	60–100	30–60	60–100
Serious	Hemarthrosis	30–50	25	30–50
	Intramuscular	30–50	25	30–50
	Oral/epistaxis	30–50	25	30–50
	GU/renal	50	25	50

TABLE 1: Dose of factor replacement therapy (per kg).

(CNS: central nervous system; GIT: gastrointestinal tract; GU: genitourinary)

CHAPTER 31: Acute Transfusion Reactions

Barnali Mitra, Vishal Sondhi

- A transfusion is defined as an infusion of whole blood or any one of its components. Acute transfusion reactions (ATRs) present as adverse signs or symptoms during or within 24 hours of transfusion of blood/blood components. Immediate reactions by definition occur during transfusion or within 6 hours of end of transfusion. Rate of ATR is 0.5–3% of transfusions. Platelet is the component with highest number of reaction among all blood components.
- The acute reactions are classified as immunological and non-immunological reactions **(Boxes 1 and 2)**.

BOX 1: Immunological reactions.

- *Mild reactions:*
  - Mild hypersensitivity
  - Allergic/urticarial reaction
- *Moderately severe reactions:*
  - Moderate-to-severe urticarial reaction
  - Febrile nonhemolytic transfusion reactions (FNHTR)
  - Possible bacterial contamination
- *Life-threatening reactions:*
  - Acute intravascular hemolysis
  - Bacterial contamination and septic shock
  - Anaphylactic reactions
  - Transfusion-related acute lung injury (TRALI)

BOX 2: Nonimmunological reactions.

CCF: Transfusion-associated circulatory overload (TACO)
Marked fever with shock: Bacterial contamination
Hypothermia: Rapid infusion of cold blood
Hemolysis: Physical/chemical destruction of blood
Air embolus: Air infusion in line
Hyperkalemia: Rapid and multiple transfusion of stored WBC/PRBC
Hypocalcemia: Massive transfusion, citrated

(CCF: congestive cardiac failure; PRBC: packed red blood cell; WBC: white blood cell)

- Clinical features of ATR are given as follows:
    - Urticaria, rash
    - Anxiety, pruritus, palpitations, dyspnea, headache, hypoxia, wheezing, stridor
    - Burning and pain along infusion site
    - Fever with chills, sweating, feeling of impending doom
    - Back (lumbar) pain
    - Tachycardia, tachypnea, hypotension
    - Hemoglobinuria, oliguria, anuria, acute renal failure
    - Oozing from IV site, features of DIC

    (DIC: disseminated intravascular coagulation; IV: intravenous)

- The laboratory tests to be performed are given as follows:
    - Repeat grouping and crossmatching
    - DCT, ICT
    - PT, aPTT
    - Donor and recipient Gram stain and culture
    - Tests for DIC if suspected
    - Urine for hemoglobin and myoglobin

    In case of reaction, blood administered along with tubing should be preserved for analysis by blood bank.

    (aPTT: activated partial thromboplastin time; DCT: direct Coombs test; DIC: disseminated intravascular coagulation; ICT: indirect Coombs test; PT: prothrombin time)

The management of suspected transfusion reaction is given in **Flowchart 1**.

CHAPTER 31: Acute Transfusion Reactions

Flowchart 1: Management of suspected transfusion reaction.

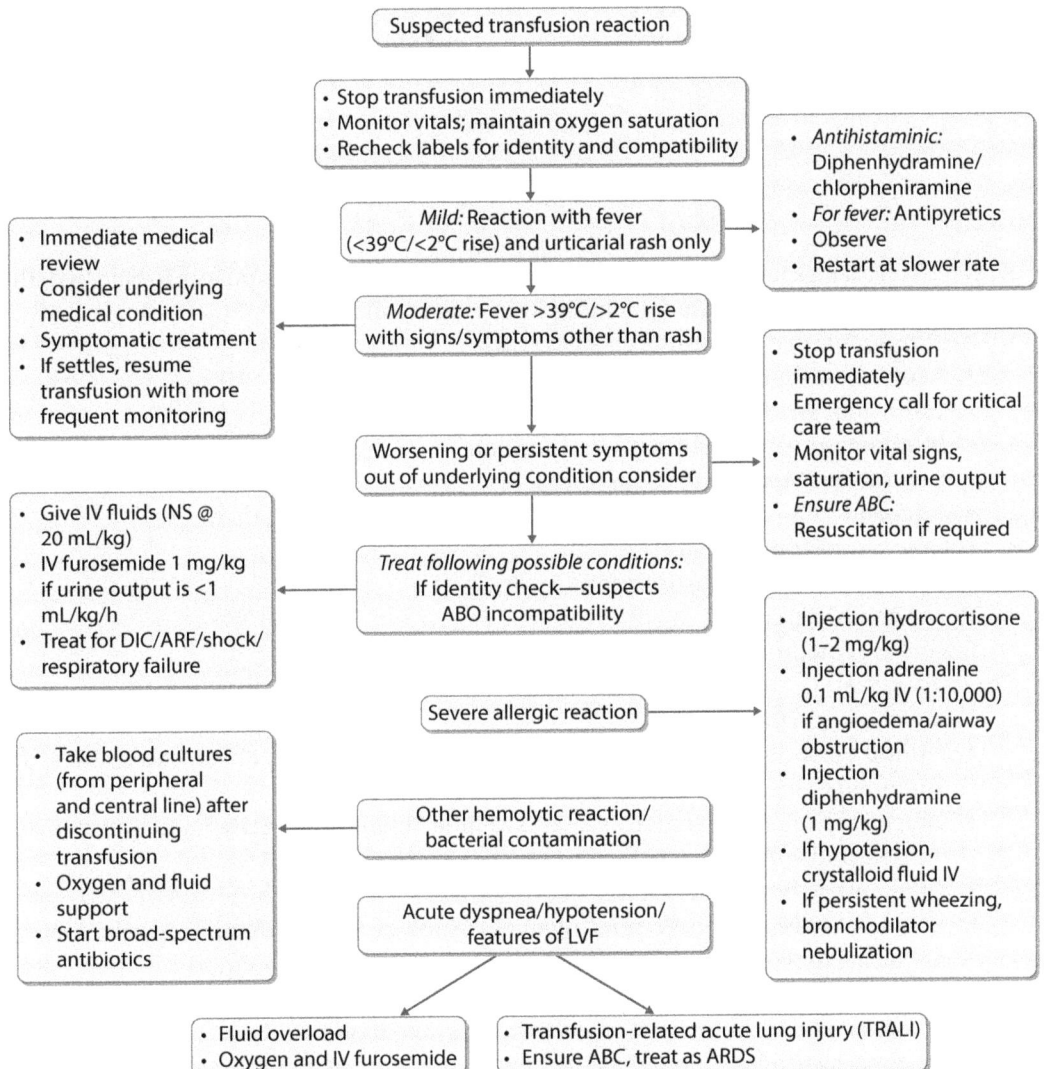

(ABC: airway, breathing, circulation; ARDS: acute respiratory distress syndrome; ARF: acute respiratory; DIC: disseminated intravascular coagulation; IV: intravenous; NS: normal saline)

CHAPTER 32

Acute Illness in a Child with Sickle Cell Disease

Barnali Mitra, Vishal Sondhi

- *Sickle cell crisis:* Risk factors for sickling are hypoxia, dehydration, exposure to cold/whether changes, stress, and infection. It includes following conditions:
  - *Acute painful episode (vaso-occlusive crisis):*
    - Acute chest syndrome
    - Hand–foot syndrome (dactylitis)
    - Intrahepatic vaso-occlusive sequestration
    - Central nervous system (CNS) crisis
    - Priapism
  - Splenic sequestration crisis
  - Erythroblastopenic (aplastic) crisis
  - Hyper hemolytic crisis
  - Infection—pneumococcal infection is most common
- *Clinical features:*
  - *Vaso-occlusive crisis:*
    - Painful episodes can involve any part of body, with back, chest, extremities, and abdomen being most commonly involved
    - Objective clinical signs such as fever, swelling, tenderness, tachypnea, hypertension, nausea, and vomiting
    - Differentiate bone pains from osteomyelitis
    - Rule out underlying precipitating events (dehydration, infection, stress, menses, nocturnal hypoxemia, especially obstructive sleep apnea)
  - *CNS crisis:* Presenting as focal neurological deficits, motor disabilities (e.g., hemiparesis, gait dysfunction, focal seizures, speech defects, and deficit in IQ
  - *Acute chest syndrome:* Defined as the new appearance of an infiltrate with pulmonary symptoms in a patient with sickle cell anemia; presents with fever, chest pain, cough, and hypoxia; rule out infection (cultures), pulmonary infarction (angiography), and pulmonary fat embolism [ventilation–perfusion (VQ) mismatch]; this is responsible for almost 25% deaths are due to sickle cell disease (SCD).
  - *Splenic sequestration:* Present with sudden splenomegaly with acute fall in hemoglobin (Hb), and pallor, lethargy, abdominal fullness, and cardiovascular collapse
  - *Aplastic crisis:* Present with acute fall in Hb, marked decrease in reticulocyte count without splenomegaly
  - *Infection:* The most common with pneumococcal sp. followed by *Haemophilus influenzae* type B, and *Salmonella* sp. (consider immunization if not already done)
- Course of treatment of acute illness in a child with sickle cell disease is shown in **Flowchart 1**.

CHAPTER 32: Acute Illness in a Child with Sickle Cell Disease

Flowchart 1: Course of treatment of acute illness in a child with sickle cell disease.

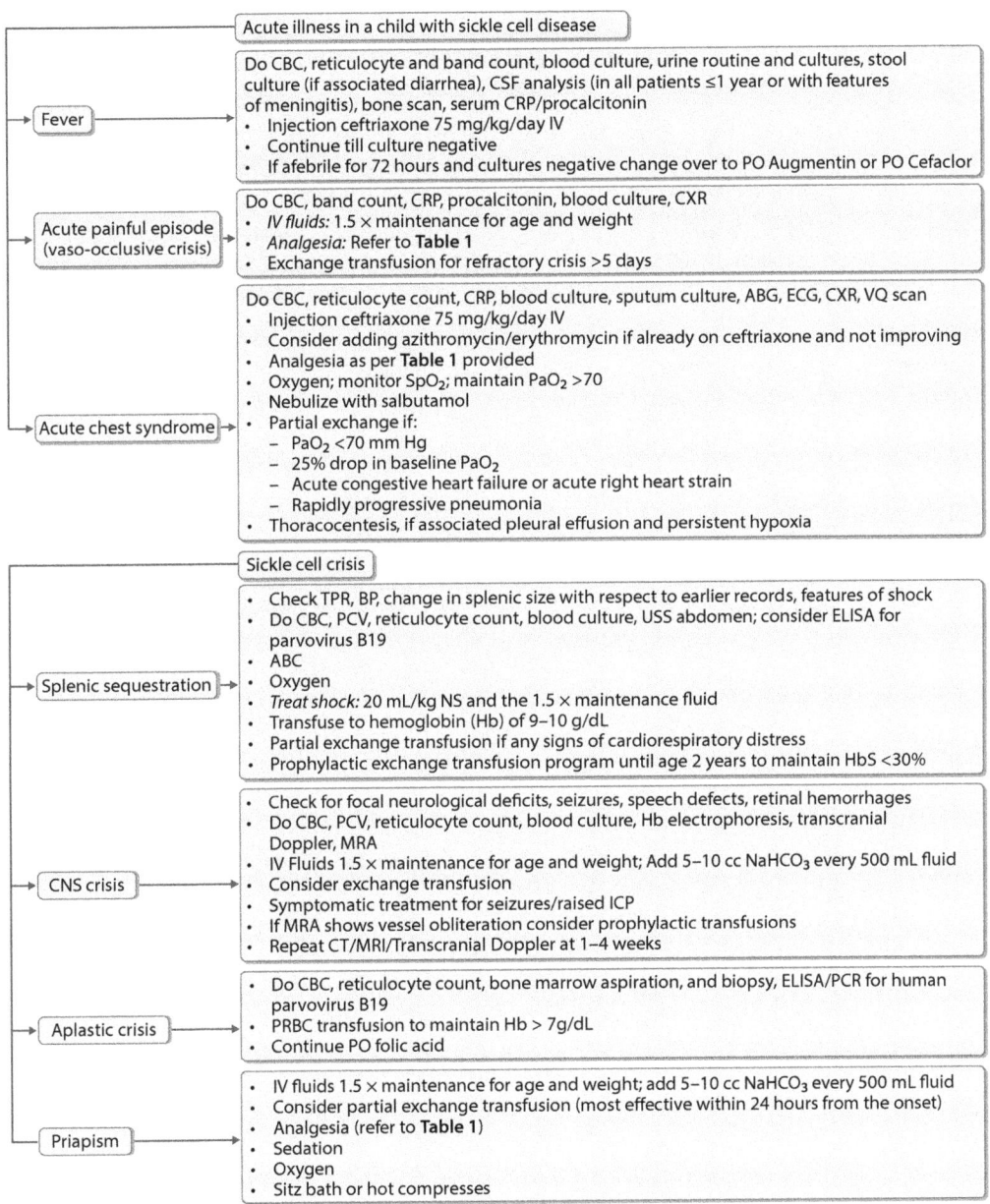

(ABC: airway, breathing, circulation; ABG: arterial blood gas; BP: blood pressure; CBC: complete blood count; CRP: C-reactive protein; CSF: cerebrospinal fluid; CXR: chest X-ray; ECG: electrocardiogram; ELISA: enzyme-linked immunosorbent assay; HbS: hemoglobin S; MRA: magnetic resonance angiography; NS: normal saline; PaO_2: partial pressure of arterial oxygen; PCV: packed cell volume; PRBC: packed red blood cell; packed SpO_2: peripheral oxygen saturation; TPR: temperature, pulse rate, respiration; USS: ultrasound scan; VQ: ventilation–perfusion)

The analgesics for sickle cell crisis are given in **Table 1**.

TABLE 1: Analgesics for sickle cell crisis.

	Maximum dose	Route	Interval	Comments
Severe pain				
Morphine	0.15 mg/kg/dose (maximum 10 mg)	SC, IM	Q 3 hours	Drug of choice
Meperidine	1.5 mg/kg/dose (maximum 100 mg)	IM	Q 3 hours	Increased incidence of seizures; avoid in patients with renal or neurologic disease
Moderate pain				
Oxycodone	5–10 mg/dose	PO	Q 4 hours	For children >5 years
Methadone	0.15 mg/kg/dose	PO	Q 6 hours	Effective in patients usually requiring parenteral narcotics; NOT FOR ROUTINE USE
Mild pain				
Codeine	0.75 mg/kg/dose	PO	Q 4 hours	May be effective up to 6 hours
Acetaminophen	1.5 g/m^2/day divided into 6 doses	PO	Q 4 hours	May be given with a narcotic for added analgesia

CHAPTER 33: Bleeding Disorders

Vishal Sondhi

- Bleeding disorders are often confronted in day-to-day practice. When evaluating a patient with bleeding, the first step is to take a detailed history. This should include the age of the child, as inherited disorders may be a factor. Additionally, sex is important to note as hemophilia is more common in males. The clinical presentation of the bleed, whether it is mucocutaneous or deep-seated, should also be considered. Any past history of blood or blood component transfusion should be taken into account, as well as any family history of inherited disorders. Obtain a complete medication history, including herbal remedies. Pay special attention to the use of aspirin and other nonsteroidal anti-inflammatory drugs.
- During the history-taking process, it is important to pay attention to the specific type of bleeding that is present and to differentiate between disorders of coagulation from disorders of platelets and blood vessels (**Table 1**).
- The common bleeding disorders are given in **Table 2**.

TABLE 1: Differentiation between disorders of coagulation and disorders of platelets and blood vessels.

Clinical findings	Disorders of coagulation	Disorders of platelets and blood vessels (including von Willebrand disease)
Petechiae	Usually not seen	Characteristic
Ecchymoses	Common; large, one or more	Characteristic—small or many scattered
Soft-tissue bleed	Characteristic	Rare
Joint bleed	Characteristic feature of disease	Usually not seen
Prolonged bleeding	Common	Rare
Bleeding from minor superficial skin injuries	Uncommon	Common and recurrent

TABLE 2: Common bleeding disorders.

Congenital disorders	Acquired disorders

• *Disorders of platelet number/function*: Thrombocytopenia—Due to disease of bone marrow or defective megakaryocyte maturation
• *Disorders of platelet function*: Bernard–Soulier syndrome, Glanzmann thrombasthenia, storage pool diseases
  – Factor VIII deficiency
  – Factor IX deficiency
  – von Willebrand disease
	• *Disseminated intravascular coagulation*: Will have prolonged PT and aPTT, decreased fibrinogen and platelets, increased fibrin degradation products, and increased D-dimer
	• *Liver disease*: The liver is the predominant site of factors V, VII, IX, X, XI, XII, XIII, prothrombin, plasminogen, fibrinogen, protein C and S, and ATIII synthesis
	• *Vitamin K deficiency*: Factors II, VII, IX, X, protein C, and protein S are vitamin K-dependent; early vitamin K deficiency may present with isolated prolonged PT, because factor VII has the shortest half-life; fibrinogen would be normal
	• *Hemolytic–uremic syndrome/thrombotic thrombocytopenic purpura (HUS/TTP)*: Has triad of microangiopathic hemolytic anemia, uremia, and thrombocytopenia

(aPTT: activated partial thromboplastin time; ATIII: antithrombin III; PT: prothrombin time)

Flowchart 1 shows approach to a child with bleeding.

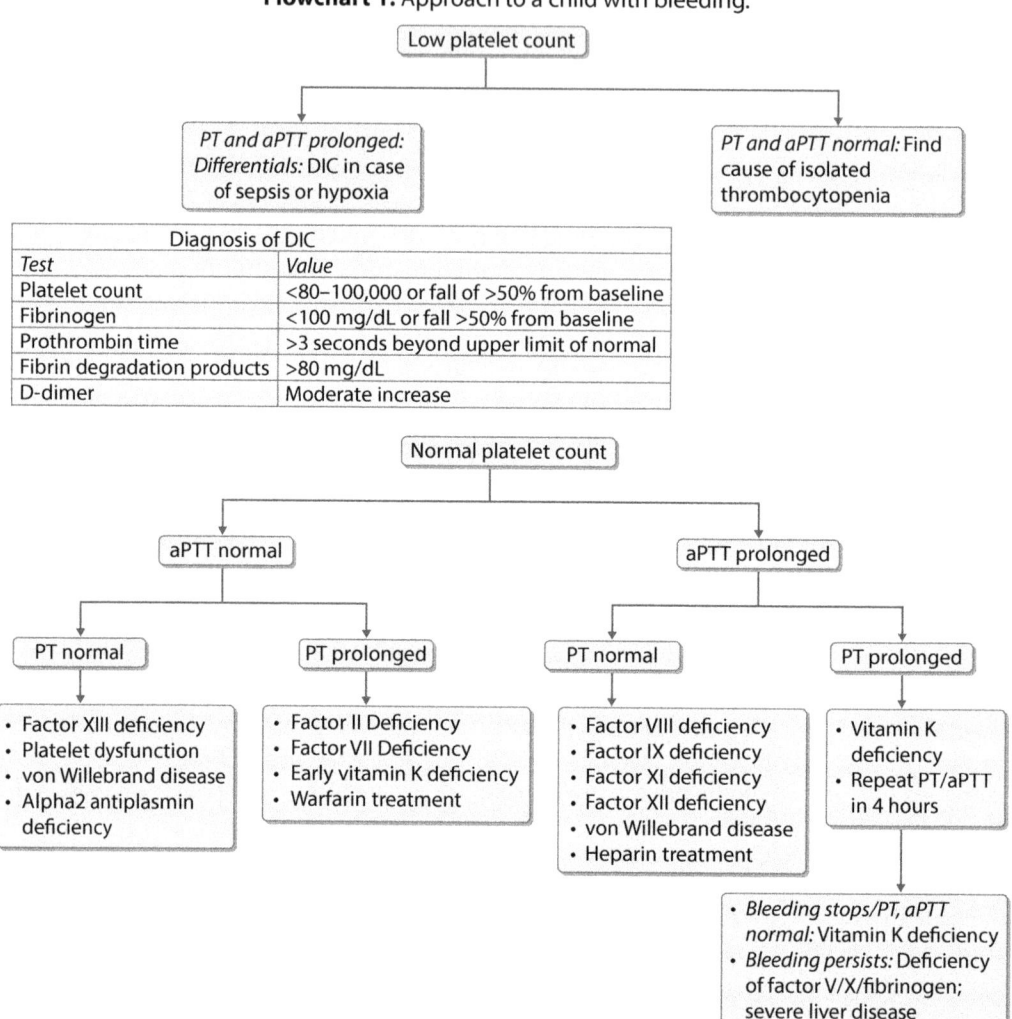

Flowchart 1: Approach to a child with bleeding.

(aPTT: activated partial thromboplastin time; DIC: disseminated intravascular coagulation; PT: prothrombin time)

SECTION 5

Endocrine Disorders

- **Diabetic Ketoacidosis**
  Bikash Shreshta, V Venkateshwar, Biju M John

- **Hypoglycemia**
  Bikash Shreshta, V Venkateshwar

- **Syndrome of Inappropriate Antidiuretic Hormone Secretion**
  V Venkateshwar, Bikash Shreshta

- **Adrenal Crisis**
  Bikash Shreshta, V Venkateshwar

- **Diabetes Insipidus**
  Bikash Shreshta, V Venkateshwar

CHAPTER 34

Diabetic Ketoacidosis

Bikash Shreshta, V Venkateshwar, Biju M John

- Diabetic ketoacidosis is the triad of hyperglycemia (>200 mg/dL), metabolic acidosis (venous pH <7.3 and bicarbonate <15 mEq/L) and ketonemia.
- A total of 20–40% of new-onset diabetes may present as diabetic ketoacidosis.
- Clinical features of diabetic ketoacidosis may be extremely variable and it requires a high degree of suspicion.
- Fluid therapy is the backbone of the diabetic ketoacidosis management. It includes the deficit correction (maximum 10% dehydration = 100 mL/kg), maintenance therapy as well as ongoing losses. The choice of fluid is dependent upon the corrected sodium level. Generally, it is NS at first for rapid expansion of the volume and may be changed to N/2 or ringer lactate or balanced salt solution depending upon the corrected sodium level.
- Dextrose should be added to maintenance fluid as per the blood glucose level. The range of dextrose in maintenance fluid can range from 0 to 12.5%. Dextrose level should be adjusted accordingly to aim for a blood sugar level fall between 50 and 100 mg/dL every hour and maintain between 200 and 300 mg/dL 6 hours after initiating fluid therapy.
- Insulin therapy has to be started only after 1 hour of starting fluid therapy. The dose of insulin is 0.1 U/kg/h. The additional dextrose level can be changed (0–12.5%) to maintain blood sugar fall and level as desired. If the required fall and level of blood sugar is not achieved despite change in dextrose level, then change in insulin level may be done accordingly (0.05–0.2 U/kg/h).
- Despite the adjustment in dextrose as well as insulin therapy, if the blood sugar level is not controlled, then a fault in insulin preparation, sepsis, insulin resistance, inadequate hydration, lactic acidosis, or electrolytes disturbance should be suspected.
- The insulin has to be continued till acidosis is corrected. Once acidosis is corrected (pH >7.3 and HCO_3^- >15 mEq/L), and the patient is able to take orally, then insulin infusion should be switched to subcutaneous insulin. The insulin infusion must be continued for 30–60 minutes after the first subcutaneous dose is administered to allow for delayed onset of action of the injected insulin.
- Generally, ongoing losses are taken care of by maintenance fluids. However, gastric losses by emesis/diarrhea should be replaced. Urinary losses should not be added to maintenance fluids.
- Bicarbonate therapy is contraindicated. Bicarbonate therapy may be used in condition where arterial pH <6.9 and there is impaired cardiac contractility and vascular tone as in cases with hypotensive shock undergoing active resuscitation with vasopressors.

- Start potassium therapy with administration of insulin. Starting concentration in fluid should be 40 mEq/L as a combination of potassium acetate and potassium phosphate. If the patient is hypokalemic (<3.5 mEq/L), a higher concentration of potassium, 60–80 mEq/L, may be necessary. Administer high concentrations of potassium only with electrocardiographic monitoring. If hyperkalemic (>6 mEq/L) at the outset, give only 0–20 mEq/L of potassium.
- Antibiotics are used if clinical or laboratory features of infection are present.
- Blood glucose to be measured 1 hourly till the levels are stabilized and electrolytes and blood gas analysis should be done 2–4 hourly till acidosis is corrected.
- *Mild diabetic ketoacidosis (DKA):* pH 7.2–7.29 or bicarbonate <15 mEq/L, we could assume 5% dehydration.
  Moderate DKA: pH 7.1–7.19 or bicarbonate <10 mEq/L, we could assume 7% dehydration.
  Severe DKA: pH <7.1 or bicarbonate <5 mEq/L, we could assume 10% dehydration.
- **Usually we correct 10 mL/kg for 1% dehydration.**
  Pre-illness weight could be an accurate way to analyze level of dehydration.
- **Insulin infusion could be started at 0.05 U/kg/h for mild cases.**
- Most of the cases shall recover and get re-hydrated in 12–18 hours.
- In case blood gas does not improve, pay attention to the non-gap acidosis, which could be due to extra chloride getting in from too much normal saline. In this situation, plasmalyte or balance salt solutions with lower chloride may be a better choice.
  Details of diabetic ketoacidosis are given in **Flowchart 1**.
  (Can try the two-bag system of infusing glucose and saline)

CHAPTER 34: Diabetic Ketoacidosis

Flowchart 1: Diabetic ketoacidosis.

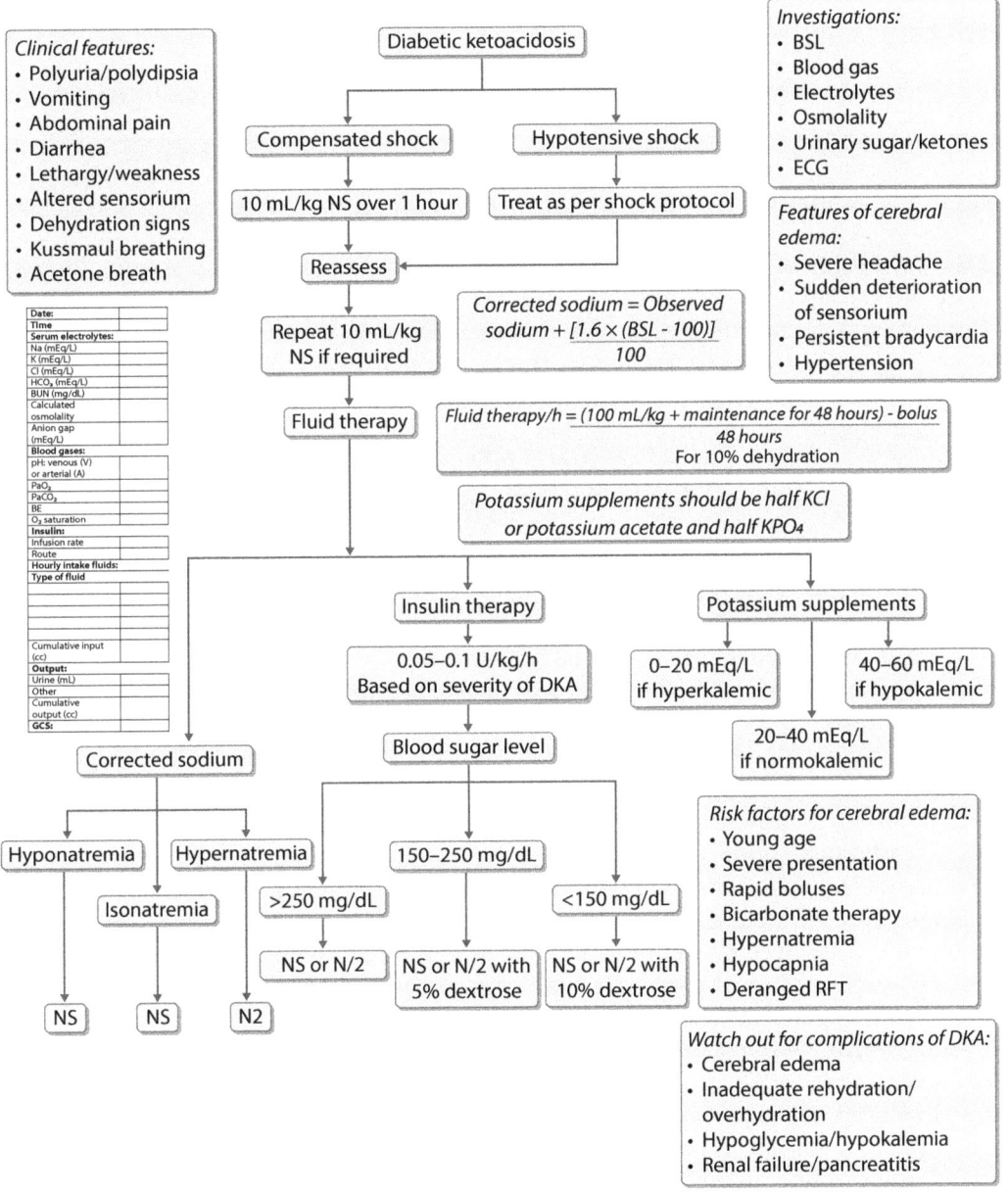

CHAPTER 35

Hypoglycemia

Bikash Shreshta, V Venkateshwar

- The definition of hypoglycemia is controversial. A glucose level <40 mg/dL is generally accepted to represent severe hypoglycemia. However, counter-regulatory hormones response start occurring before this level—insulin hormone secretion at 80–85 mg/dL and counter regulatory hormones [cortisol, glucagon, epinephrine, and growth hormone (GH)] get released as level reaches to 65 mg/dL of plasma glucose level. The operational cut-off similar to the level that elicits counter-regulatory hormones response, seems appropriate to prevent complication (60–65 mg/dL).
- According to operational threshold (Cornblath et al.), the indications for action in neonates are:
  - *Healthy term neonates:* 30–35 mg/dL (<24 hours) and 45–50 mg/dL (>24 hours)
  - *Symptomatic neonates:* 45 mg/dL
  - *Asymptomatic neonates with risk factors:* 36 mg/dL
- The symptoms of hypoglycemia can be classified as:
  - *Autonomic features:* Weakness, hunger, sweating, anxiety, palpitations, pallor, nausea, and emesis
  - *Neuroglycopenic symptoms:* Headache, confusion, seizures, personality changes, visual disturbances, lethargy, ataxia, stroke, and coma
- It is important to draw samples for diagnostic testing during hypoglycemia, ideally before glucose administration.
- The immediate management of symptomatic hypoglycemia is intravenous glucose bolus, followed by continuous glucose infusion.
- Refractory hypoglycemia requires investigations, which include the urine for ketones, serum insulin level, cortisol level, growth hormone levels, blood ammonia level, lactic acid levels, reducing substances, and urinary aminoacidogram.
- Refractory hypoglycemia may respond to glucagon, diazoxide, or hydrocortisone.
- Some hints to the etiology of hypoglycemia are:
  - Hypoglycemia with low insulin levels and elevated ketone levels suggests ketotic hypoglycemia, a common cause of hypoglycemia in childhood.
  - Absence of ketones points to hyperinsulinemia or fatty acid oxidation defect.
  - If the requirement of glucose infusion exceeds 10 mg/kg/min, hyperinsulinemic state is likely.
  - Hypoglycemia occurring 2–4 hours after a meal is seen in defects of glycogenolysis and ketonuria is present.
  - Fasting hypoglycemia occurring 6–12 hours after a meal suggests disorder of neoglucogenesis.

Management of hypoglycemia is given in **Flowchart 1**.

CHAPTER 35: Hypoglycemia

Flowchart 1: Hypoglycemia.

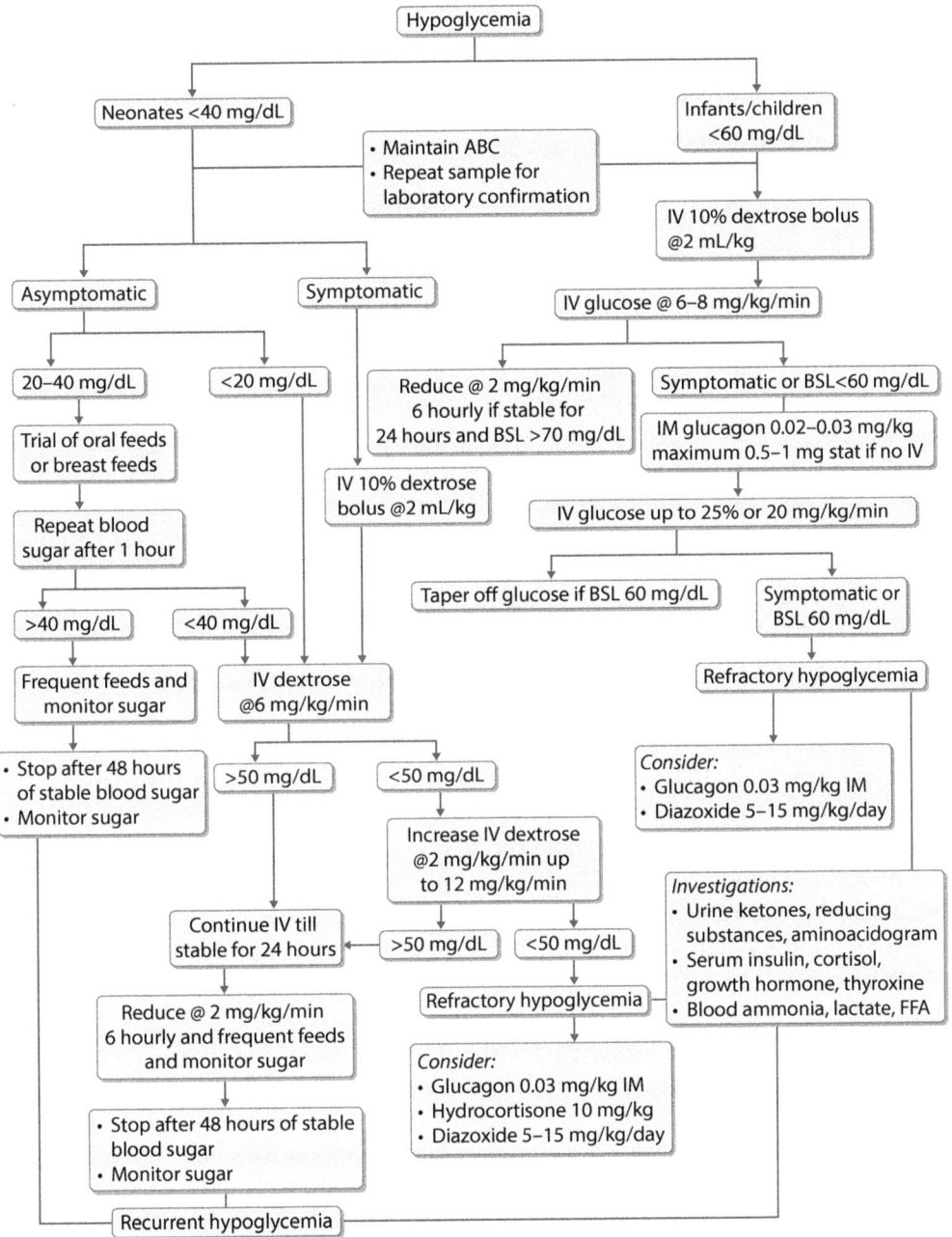

CHAPTER 36

Syndrome of Inappropriate Antidiuretic Hormone Secretion

V Venkateshwar, Bikash Shreshta

- SIADH or syndrome of inappropriate secretion of antidiuretic hormone is a non-physiologic condition of AVP excess. Excessive secretion of antidiuretic hormone (ADH) accompanying normal or low plasma osmolality or [Na^+] is inappropriate because it further depresses the plasma osmolality and [Na^+].
- *Types of SIADH:* Type A—due to random hypersecretion of ADH, typically seen in lung carcinoma. Type B—elevated basal level of ADH. Type C—abnormal reset of osmostat causing ADH secretion to low thresh hold. Type D—due to activation mutation of V_2 receptor/production of antidiuretic principle other than AVP.
- The conditions associated with SIADH include central nervous system (CNS) disorders (meningitis, encephalitis, trauma, tumors, abscess, surgery, and excessive stress), pulmonary disorders (pneumonia, bronchiolitis, pneumothorax, asthma, and positive pressure ventilation), tumors (lymphoma, thymoma, bronchogenic carcinoma, etc.) and drugs (ADH analogs, vincristine, cyclophosphamide, haloperidol, chlorpropamide, carbamazepine, barbiturates, etc.).
- The diagnostic criteria of SIADH include the following:
  - Hyponatremia (<135 mEq/L), reduced serum osmolality (<275 mOsm/kg)
  - Urine osmolality inappropriately elevated (>100 mOsm/kg)
  - Urinary sodium concentration >30 mEq/L
  - Absence of hypovolemia, CCF, nephritic syndrome, cirrhosis, or diuretic drugs
  - Normal renal, adrenal, and thyroid function
- The other findings supportive of SIADH are low serum uric acid and blood urea nitrogen (BUN) levels.
- Generally, the patient remains asymptomatic till serum sodium is <125 mEq/L. Common manifestations include lethargy, apathy, nausea, vomiting, confusion, irritability, weakness, muscle cramps, seizures, sluggish deep tendon reflexes, pseudobulbar palsy, Cheyne-Stokes respiration, etc.
- Treatment involves identifying the underlying pathology and correcting it if feasible. Symptomatic treatment is aimed at correcting hyponatremia.
- Acute cases of hyponatremia may be corrected rapidly if there are neurological features such as seizures whereas in chronic cases of hyponatremia (duration >48 hours), the correction of sodium should not be >12 mEq/L/day to prevent central pontine myelinolysis. If seizures occur, anticonvulsants should be added along with sodium correction.
- Certain drugs are effective in established SIADH not responding to fluid restriction. Frusemide increases water excretion but requires simultaneous saline or salt

administration to counter sodium loss. Demeclocycline inhibits the renal response to ADH. Newer drugs such as conivaptan/tolvaptan inhibit the binding of ADH to renal receptors and cause aquaresis.

Management of SIADH is given in **Flowchart 1**.

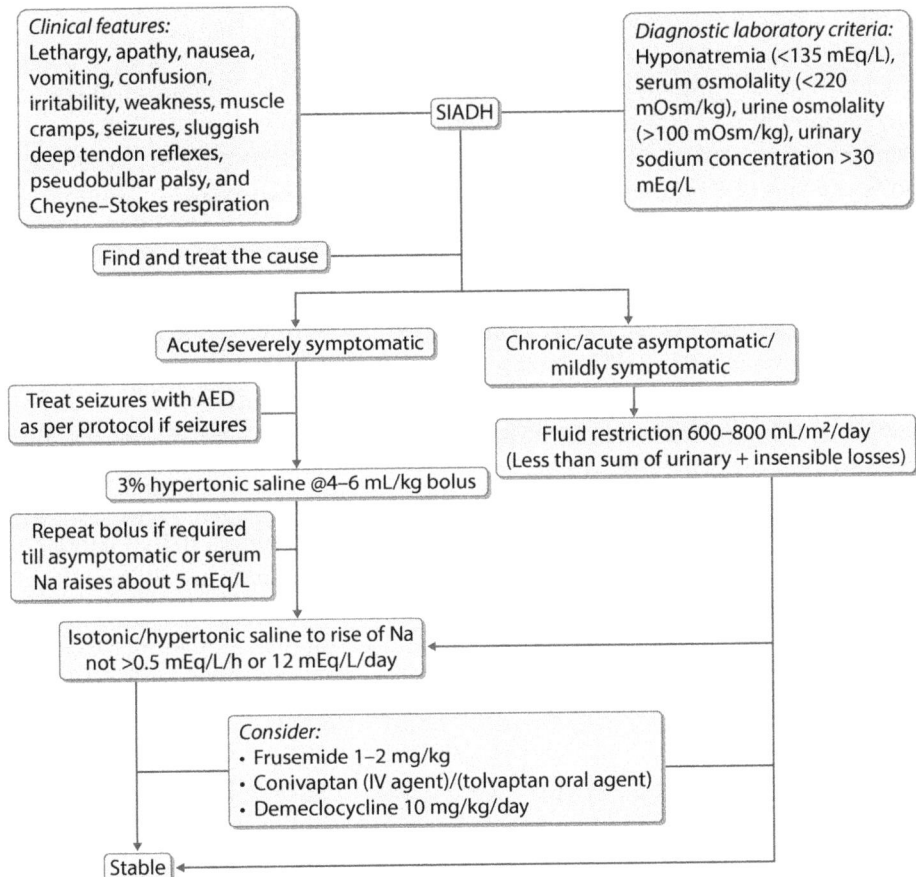

Flowchart 1: Syndrome of inappropriate antidiuretic hormone (SIADH).

CHAPTER 37

Adrenal Crisis

Bikash Shreshta, V Venkateshwar

- Adrenal crisis is the impaired secretion of adrenocorticoid steroid hormone as a result of adrenal dysfunction or lack of adrenocorticotropic hormone.
- It is either primary or secondary. Primary adrenal insufficiency is caused when the adrenal gland is the site of dysfunction (e.g., Addison disease), whereas in secondary adrenal insufficiency, there is defect in the hypothalamic-pituitary-adrenal (HPA) axis resulting in low or no adrenocorticotropic hormone (ACTH) production.
- Important causes of primary adrenal insufficiency in children include congenital adrenal hyperplasia, adrenal hemorrhage, adrenoleukodystrophy, Wolman disease, familial unresponsiveness to ACTH, infections, and autoimmune conditions.
- Secondary adrenal insufficiency occurs in a setting of neurosurgical procedures, head injury, central nervous system (CNS) disorders and chronic diseases with prolonged steroid use (on steroid withdrawal).
- Primary adrenal insufficiency has a gradual onset with symptoms of generalized malaise, fatigue, weight loss, salt craving, anorexia, and chronic pigmentation. In secondary adrenal insufficiency, salt wasting is not present and CNS manifestations are apparent.
- A rapid decompensation in the face of metabolic stress is an important indicator of adrenal insufficiency. Symptoms to be associated with intensive care unit (ICU) admission are sudden hypovolemic shock, hyperkalemia, vomiting, diarrhea, abdominal pain, and coma.
- Serum cortisol level (morning) <3 µg/dL along with normal or elevated ACTH level is indicative of adrenal insufficiency, whereas a level >18 µg/dL can reasonably exclude the condition. ACTH stimulation test should be used in new onset cases and where the diagnosis is in doubt.
- Treatment must be immediate and vigorous. Normal saline bolus is the first line of therapy, along with steroids.
- Periodic monitoring of serum electrolytes and glucose is important during management. Intravenous fluids must not contain potassium till serum potassium is in the normal range. Specific treatment of hyperkalemia is not required unless there are cardiac arrhythmias. Management of adrenal crisis is shown in **Flowchart 1**.

Flowchart 1: Adrenal crisis.

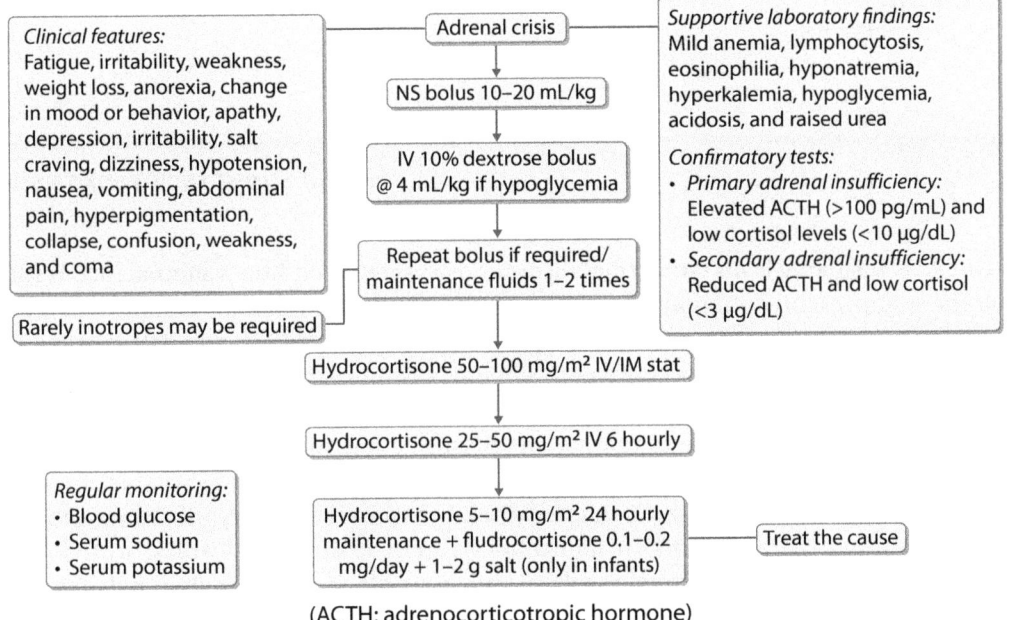

(ACTH: adrenocorticotropic hormone)

CHAPTER 38

Diabetes Insipidus

Bikash Shreshta, V Venkateshwar

- Diabetes insipidus is an endocrine disorder of dysregulated free water balance resulting from vasopressin deficiency or insensitivity of the kidneys to vasopressin action, characterized by polyuria, polydipsia, dilute urine, hypernatremia, and dehydration.
- Diabetes insipidus can be of two types—central (vasopressin deficiency) and nephrogenic (renal insensitivity to anti-diuretic action of vasopressin). Central diabetes insipidus can be genetic or acquired due to trauma, neoplasms, congenital malformations, infiltrative disorders, autoimmune disorders, infections, or drugs. Nephrogenic diabetes insipidus can be genetic or acquired due to kidney disease, hypercalcemia, hypokalemia, or drugs.
- The basic pathology results in failure of water reabsorption leading to hypertonic dehydration if the normal thirst mechanism is not able to maintain fluid balance, due to lack of access to water or inability to drink (emesis, immaturity, neurological impairment, anorexia etc.).
- The clinical suspicion of diabetes insipidus is based on symptoms of polyuria and polydipsia. The other manifestations are weight loss, irritability, features of dehydration, and fever.
- The diagnostic criteria for diabetes insipidus are elevated serum osmolality >300 mOsm/L, urine osmolality <300 mOsm/kg and hypernatremia >145 mEq/L. The other findings are low urine specific gravity <1.005. Serum osmolality is usually not <270 mOsm/kg, and urinary osmolality is not >600 mOsm/kg in diabetes insipidus. If serum osmolality is 270–300 mOsm/kg, a water deprivation test is performed to confirm the diagnosis and differentiation of central and nephrogenic diabetes insipidus. Following water deprivation, desmopressin challenge test is done by administering intranasal desmopressin 5–20 µg and then urinary and serum osmolalities are measured after 1 hour to diagnose central/nephrogenic DI. Serum vasopressin level is not routinely measured in clinical practice.
- The emergency management is based on immediate correction of dehydration and meticulous fluid balance.
  Management of DI is given in **Flowchart 1**.
- Central diabetes insipidus can be treated with vasopressin or vasopressin analogs such as desmopressin (DDAVP). Treatment of nephrogenic diabetes insipidus consists of thiazide and indomethacin and typically depends upon reversal of the underlying cause.

CHAPTER 38: Diabetes Insipidus

Flowchart 1: Management of DI.

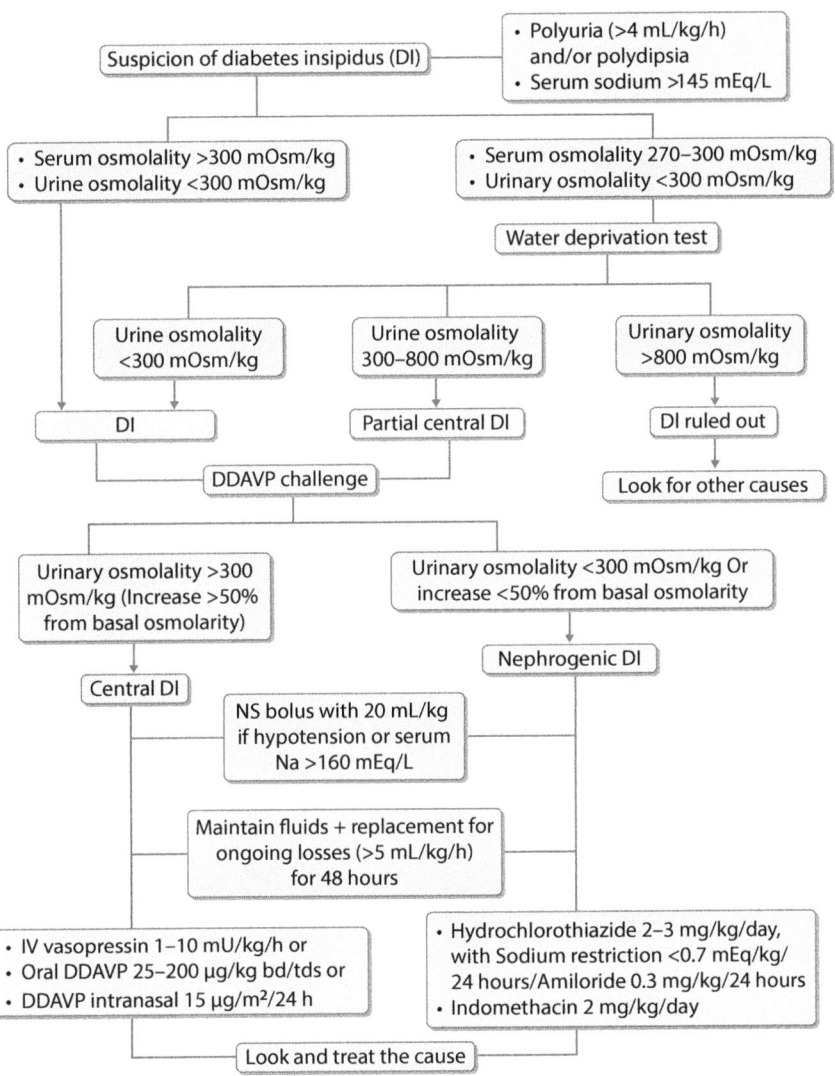

SECTION 6

Renal Disorders

- **Acute Kidney Injury**
  V Venkateshwar, Bikash Shreshta, Suprita Kalra

- **Hemolytic Uremic Syndrome**
  Bikash Shreshta, V Venkateshwar, Suprita Kalra

- **Renal Replacement Therapy**
  Bikash Shreshta, V Venkateshwar, Suprita Kalra

CHAPTER 39: Acute Kidney Injury

V Venkateshwar, Bikash Shreshta, Suprita Kalra

- Acute kidney injury (AKI) is defined as a rapid deterioration of renal function resulting in retention of nitrogenous waste and inability of kidney to regulate fluid and electrolyte homeostasis.
- It is recommended to use Kidney Disease: Improving Global Outcomes (KDIGO) 2012 classification for an early diagnosis of AKI so that measures are taken to prevent the progression of the condition **(Table 1)**.
- 30–40% of children in pediatric intensive care unit (PICU) manifest AKI, which is independently associated with higher mortality (40–50%).
- The common causes of AKI differ between resource-limited and resource-sufficient regions and for community-acquired and hospital-acquired AKI and include primary renal causes such as acute glomerulonephritis (GN), hemolytic uremic syndrome (HUS) etc. and those with secondary kidney injury due to dehydration, shock or multi organ dysfunction syndrome. Poststreptococcal glomerulonephritis (GN) typical HUS were common causes earlier, but their incidence has declined in India.
- The causes of AKI and their salient clinical features are given in **Table 2**.
  The evaluation of acute kidney injury is given in **Table 3**.
- Look for features of underlying chronic kidney disease such as growth retardation, rickets, anemia etc.

TABLE 1: Classification of acute kidney injury (KDIGO classification).

AKI severity	Serum creatinine criteria	Urine output criteria
Stage I	1.5–1.9 times baseline Or ≥0.3 mg/dL increase	<0.5 mL/kg/hour for 6–12 hours
Stage II	Increase ≥2–2.9 times baseline	<0.5 mL/kg/hour for ≥12 hours
Stage III	3.0 times baseline Or Increase in serum creatinine to ≥4.0 mg/dL Or Initiation of renal replacement therapy Or In patients <18 years, decrease in eGFR to <35 mL/minute per 1.73 m^2	<0.3 mL/kg/hour for 24 hours or anuria for 12 hours

(AKI: acute kidney injury; eGFR: estimated glomerular filtration rate; KDIGO: Kidney Disease: Improving Global Outcomes)

- Presentation of AKI may be with complications such as altered sensorium, acidotic breathing, pulmonary edema.
- Furosemide stress test (urine output of >2 mL/kg over 2 hours after 1 mg/kg IV furosemide is a test of renal tubular integrity and has been shown to be a reliable predictive marker of progression to stage III AKI in children though larger prospective studies are still required for validation.
- *Renal Angina Index (RAI):* A product of the risk and injury score calculated 8–12 hours after PICU admission in critically ill children. Score of >8 predicts day 3 severe AKI and need for kidney replacement therapy (KRT) with high sensitivity and specificity.
- Urinary and serum neutrophil gelatinase-associated lipocalin (NGAL) alone or along with other biomarkers may help predict AKI but not easily available and validated so far.

TABLE 2: Causes of acute kidney injury (AKI) and their salient clinical features.

Prerenal		*Salient clinical features*
	Acute diarrhea with dehydration, shock, hemorrhage, CCF, burns, sepsis, massive ascites, angiotensin-converting enzyme (ACE) inhibitors	• History of underlying disorder • Signs of hypoperfusion • Oliguria present
Renal		
Acute tubular necrosis	• Sustained prerenal causes • Drug /toxin mediated • Envenomation (Viper) • Falciparum malaria • Leptospirosis • G6PD deficiency	• Setting of prolonged pre-renal causes (as above) • Occurrence in respective endemic area of malaria/leptospirosis • History of nephrotoxic drug intake • Oligo-anuria present
Acute glomerulonephritis	• Post-streptococcal • Other bacterial/viral and rarely fungal or protozoal infections	• Age 5–10 years, history of preceding skin/throat infection, cola colored urine, oliguria, hypertension, edema • Features of GN may start with ongoing severe infections and referred to as infection related GN (IRGN)
Vascular	Hemolytic uremic syndrome	Age <5 years, preceding diarrhea, followed by pallor, oliguria, hypertension, petechia, drowsiness
	Renal vein thrombosis	Dehydration/hypercoagulability as in nephrotic syndrome
Tubulo-interstitial nephritis	*Hypersensitivity to drugs:* Ampicillin, cephalosporins, sulfonamides, non-steroidal anti-inflammatory drug (NSAID), quinolones	• Drug history • Usually no oliguria
Postrenal		
	Bladder outlet obstruction due to posterior urethral valves in males, bilateral pelviureteric junction (PUJ)/ureteral obstruction	Distended bladder if outflow obstruction, poor urinary stream, and recurrent urinary tract infections (UTIs)

- *Treatment*
  - Treatment is basically supportive which includes delicate fluid balance, hemodynamic stability, avoidance of nephrotoxic drugs along with appropriate drug dose modification as per stage of AKI, prevention, and management of complications and treatment of the underlying cause if possible.
  - Antibiotics are considered if signs of infection are present.
  - Diuretic may be used for management of fluid overload but have no impact on development or progression of AKI.
  - Dopamine used to be popular for hemodynamic stability but has not been shown to be of significance in terms of prognosis and outcome.

TABLE 3: Evaluation of acute kidney injury.

Test	Prerenal	Intrinsic renal	Postrenal
BUN/Cr ratio	>20	10-20	10-20
Urine specific gravity	>1.020	~1.010	<1.010
Urine osmolality	>350	~300	~300
Urine sodium	<20	>30	>40
Fractional excretion of sodium (FE_{Na})	<1%	>2%	>3%
Urine Cr/plasma Cr	>40	<20	<20
Urine microscopy	Normal Hyaline casts	• *ATN:* Dark granular casts, renal epithelial cells/casts • *GN:* RBCs, RBC casts, WBCs, proteinuria • *Acute interstitial nephritis (AIN):* Urine eosinophilia, WBCs, hyaline casts	Normal Hyaline casts
Ultrasound kidney, ureter, and bladder (KUB)	Essentially normal	Increased echogenicity and poor corticomedullary differentiation, may identify focal lesions such as calculi/cysts etc., which indicate acute on chronic or chronic kidney disease	Hydroureteronephrosis and/or distended bladder may be seen in obstructive causes
Kidney biopsy	\multicolumn{3}{l}{Small shrunken kidneys indicate chronic kidney disease (CKD)}	
	\multicolumn{3}{l}{Indicated in suspected rapidly progressive glomerulonephritis (RPGN)/unexplained AKI primarily renal in origin}	
Additional investigations as per clinical setting for underlying cause	\multicolumn{3}{l}{• Peripheral smear examination, platelet, and reticulocyte count, complement C3, and lactate dehydrogenase (LDH) levels for suspected hemolytic uremic syndrome (HUS) • Malarial parasite; serologies for leptospirosis, typhoid, rickettsial infection, dengue hemorrhagic fever for underlying infections as cause • Blood ASO, C3, ANA, antineutrophil cytoplasmic antibody (cANCA), and Perinuclear antineutrophil cytoplasmic antibody (pANCA) in acute or rapidly progressive GN • Doppler ultrasonography (suspected arterial or venous thrombosis) • Noncontrast computerized tomography (NCCT) for obstructing calculi.}	

- CVP measurement is useful for assessment of fluid status and deciding about fluid replacement.
- Packet red blood cell (PRBC) transfusion and other blood component therapy as per standard guidelines to maintain tissue oxygenation and prevent/treat bleeding diathesis.
- Hyponatremia may require fluid restriction or if central nervous system (CNS) symptoms predominate, then 3% NS can be used.
- Hypocalcemia may need oral or IV calcium correction.
- Metabolic acidosis, if refractory, might require IV soda bicarbonate.
- Hyperphosphatemia may require phosphate restricted diet or phosphate binders.
- Hyperkalemia is life-threatening complication and needs to be addressed vigorously but systematically.
- Hypertension (HTN) or HTN encephalopathy may require IV antihypertensives.
- Administer IV calcium before sodium bicarbonate therapy in metabolic acidosis.

- *Kidney replacement therapy or dialysis*
  - In a PICU patient, estimation of cumulative fluid overload by the following formula is helpful in deciding requirement of renal support: (Fluid input in liter)—(fluid output in liter)/PICU admission weight in kilogram. If >10%—evaluate for renal support; if >20%—strongly consider renal support.
  - Peritoneal dialysis is easier to perform, more gradual and requires minimal infrastructure and expertise. It can be employed even in hemodynamically unstable children.
  - Intermittent hemodialysis may not be tolerated well by children with shock or hemodynamic instability where sustained low efficiency dialysis (SLED) or CRRT (continuous renal replacement therapy) are better suited but require expertise and are more expensive. They are preferred in hypercatabolic states such as sepsis, multiorgan failure, tumor lysis syndrome, etc.

- *Prognosis*
  - It is not favorable in severe crescentic glomerulonephritis, atypical HUS, sepsis, multiorgan failure, etc., especially if diagnosis is delayed and complications have set in.
  - Acute tubular necrosis (ATN) due to hypoperfusion, intravascular hemolysis, D+HUS, acute interstitial nephritis, drug, and toxin related AKI usually show complete recovery with timely appropriate management.

The indications for dialysis are given in **Box 1**.

Algorithm of suspected acute kidney injury is given in **Flowchart 1**.

BOX 1: Indications for dialysis.

- Fluid overload (>15%) not responding to diuretics or causing congestive cardiac failure or hypertension
- Severe unresponsive metabolic acidosis (pH <7.2)
- Hyperkalemia despite of medical management (Serum K >6.0 mEq/L)
- *Uremic symptoms:* Altered sensorium/seizures/urea >160–200 mg/dL
- Hyponatremia unresponsive to treatment (Serum Na <120 mEq/L)
- Create space for more fluid (blood product, drugs nutrition)
- Removal of dialyzable toxins (salicylate/phenobarbitone)

Flowchart 1: Management of suspected AKI.

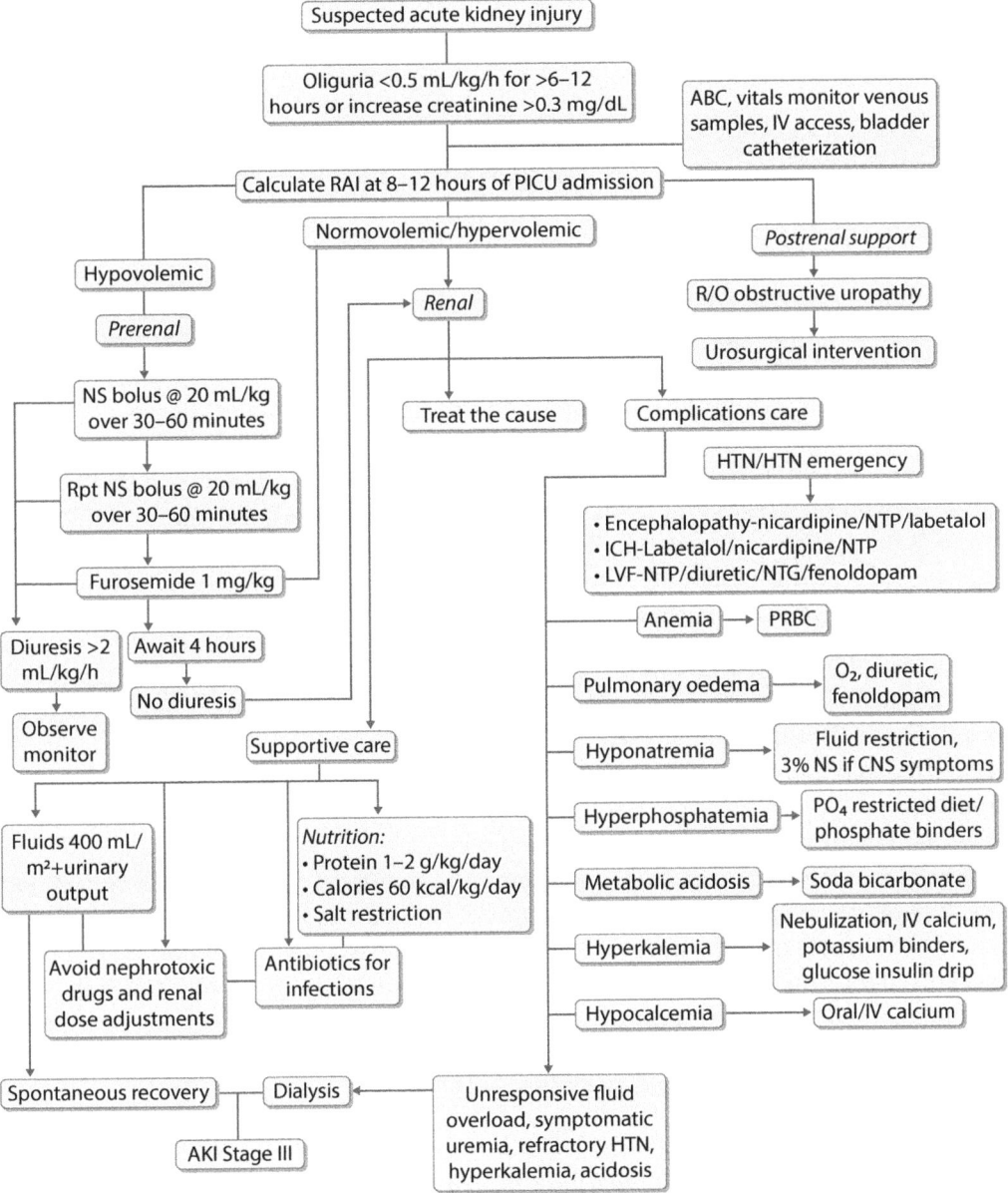

(AKI: acute kidney injury; CNS: central nervous system; HTN: hypertension; PICU: pediatric intensive care unit; PRBC: packet red blood cell)

CHAPTER 40

Hemolytic Uremic Syndrome

Bikash Shreshta, V Venkateshwar, Suprita Kalra

- Hemolytic uremic syndrome (HUS) is characterized by triad of microangiopathic hemolytic anemia (Hb <10 gm%, schistocytes >2%. High lactate dehydrogenase (LDH) >450 IU/L or undetectable haptoglobin), thrombocytopenia (platelet <150,000/mm^3) and acute kidney injury (AKI) (>50% rise of creatinine from base line).
- Hemolytic uremic syndrome is an important cause of severe AKI in children.
- Most cases of HUS occur following gastrointestinal infection with Shiga toxin-producing organisms, chiefly *Escherichia coli* or *Shigella* which is seen predominantly in children between 6 months and 5 years of age (previously referred to as D+HUS).
- Hemolytic uremic syndrome might be associated with systemic illnesses, malignancy, pregnancy, various drugs, etc. (secondary HUS), and with disorders of complement regulation referred to as atypical HUS (previously referred to as D-HUS).

Typical hemolytic uremic syndrome:
- The clinical manifestation of typical HUS is pallor, oliguria, and lassitude following a prodrome of dysentery or diarrhea.
- Hypertension, hematuria, features of fluid overload, petechia and purpura are usually present.
- The child may manifest all complications of AKI.
- Therapy is supportive with fluid resuscitation to maintain euvolemia and control of BP. Renal replacement therapy with few sessions of dialysis may be required in some children.
- Antibiotics have controversial role as none have shown to reduce either the duration or severity of the symptoms but still recommended in children with bloody diarrhea.
- Maintenance of nutrition is critical.
- A total of 80% of typical HUS show complete recovery with about 5% mortality and rare recurrence and progression into end-stage renal disease (ESRD).

Atypical hemolytic uremic syndrome:
- Encompasses HUS due to complement dysregulation due to anti-factor H antibodies, genetic mutations in various regulatory proteins or factors of the alternative complement pathway and rarely due to recessive mutations in diacylglycerol kinase epsilon (DGKE) gene (usually presents in infancy).
- Hemolytic uremic syndrome has to be differentiated from thrombotic thrombocytopenic purpura (TTP), which presents in a similar clinical pattern except for the fact that fever

and neurological symptoms are more characteristic in TTP and most children have severe thrombocytopenia with only mild AKI.
- Evaluation and exclusion of disseminated intravascular coagulation (DIC) and common infections that can mimic or trigger HUS, e.g., malaria, leptospirosis, and dengue.
- The broad management principles of HUS include early establishment of diagnosis based on clinical and laboratory criteria, initiation of therapy for renal management and stabilization of hematological status along with evaluation of underlying cause for specific management (anti-factor H antibody responds to immunosuppression) and prognostication.
- In children presenting with severe AKI and oliguria along with other features suggestive of atypical hemolytic uremic syndrome (aHUS), after sending relevant investigations (mentioned in algorithm below) placement of double lumen hemodialysis catheter in internal jugular vein (IJV) (or femoral vein in very sick children) and urgently initiate double volume plasma exchange (PEX) (with fresh frozen plasma as replacement fluid) and hemodialysis sessions for AKI.
- Anti-FH antibody related aHUS is the commonest cause of aHUS in Indian subcontinent accounting for almost half of all cases of aHUS in pediatric age group.
- Start immunosuppressive therapy with oral prednisolone (1 mg/kg/day; for 4 weeks followed by 1 mg/kg alternate day tapered slowly over next 12–18 months) and either intravenous cyclophosphamide (500 mg/m^2 3-weekly for six doses) or intravenous rituximab (375 mg/m^2 weekly for two doses) followed by mycophenolate mofetil 750–1,000 mg/kg/day for 18–24 months only after labor confirmation of presence of anti-FH antibodies (available at AIIMS New Delhi and KEM, Pune).
- Further treatment plan would be: Alternate day 1.5 times volume plasma exchanges (60 mL/kg body weight) for four sessions followed by twice weekly 1.5 times volume plasma exchanges (60 mL/kg body weight) for six sessions.
- The plasma exchanges are stopped at this point in case of anti-factor H antibody disease. The exchanges or plasma infusions (once AKI and fluid overload has resolved) may however have to be continued for prolonged periods once or twice a week to maintain hematological remission in children with aHUS due to other genetic abnormalities in the complement pathway.
- Therapy with eculizumab is recommended in Western protocols but difficult in resource constrained setting due to prohibitive costs and difficulty in procurement.
- (i) Eculizumab is, therefore, recommended in lack of remission despite 7–10 PEX; (ii) life-threatening complications (seizures, cardiac dysfunction); (iii) complications due to PEX or vascular access; and (iv) inherited defect in complement regulation.
- Renal biopsy is not mandatory for establishing the diagnosis and cannot be performed in the acute stage due to thrombocytopenia. It is indicated if the diagnosis is in doubt, or in recurrent or severe disease. The pathognomic finding of thrombotic microangiopathy (TMA) is seen in all types.
Algorithm of hemolytic uremic syndrome is given in **Flowchart 1**.

SECTION 6: Renal Disorders

Flowchart 1: Hemolytic uremic syndrome.

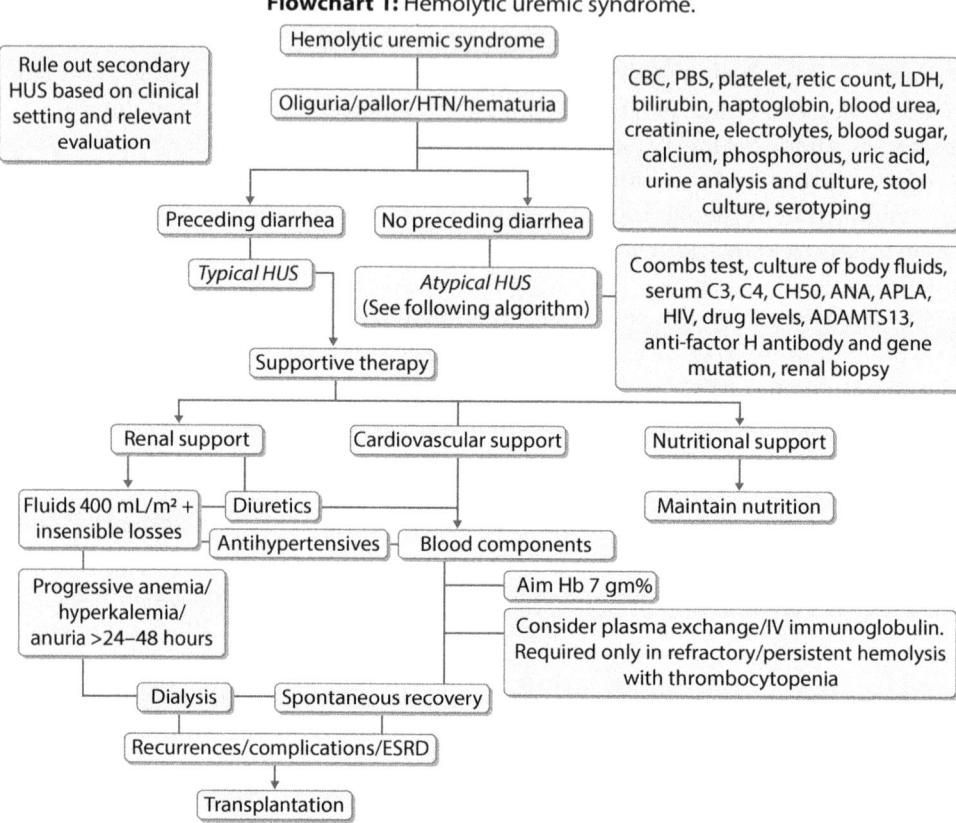

(ANA: antinuclear antibody; APLA: antiphospholipid antibody; CBC: complete blood count; ESRD: end-stage renal disease; HIV: human immunodeficiency virus; HTN: hypertension; LDH: lactate dehydrogenase; PBS: peripheral blood smear)

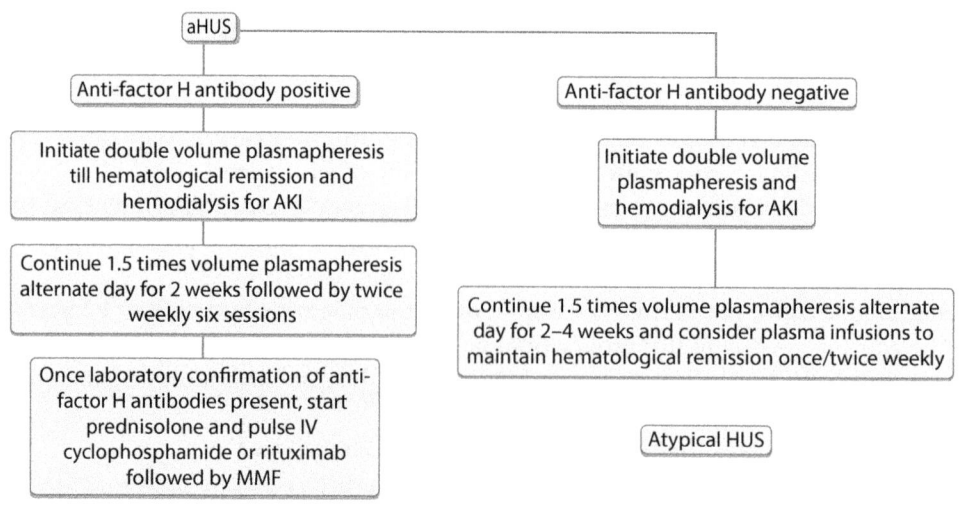

(AKI: acute kidney disease; MMF: mycophenolate mofetil)

CHAPTER 41

Renal Replacement Therapy

Bikash Shreshta, V Venkateshwar, Suprita Kalra

- Renal replacement therapy (RRT) means various life supporting treatments for renal failure, including dialysis, and renal transplantation.
- RRT is indicated both in cases of acute kidney injury (AKI) and in chronic kidney disease (CKD).
- The indications for RRT in AKI are as follows:

> **Indications for dialysis**
> - Fluid overload not responding to diuretics or causing congestive cardiac failure or hypertension
> - Severe unresponsive metabolic acidosis (pH <7.2)
> - Hyperkalemia (serum K >6.0 mEq/L)
> - *Uremic symptoms:* Altered sensorium/seizures
> - Hyponatremia unresponsive to treatment (serum Na <120 mEq/L)
> - Hypercatabolic state
> - Create space for more fluid (blood product, drugs nutrition)
> - Removal of dialyzable toxins (salicylate/phenobarbitone)
> *No single value of urea and/or creatinine by itself forms indication for RRT*

- In cases of CKD, RRT may be used as a bridge therapy before transplantation or in due to CKD V, i.e., glomerular filtration rate (GFR) <15 mL/min/1.73 m^2 with or without medically uncontrolled complications such as HTN/fluid overload, failure to thrive, gross electrolyte abnormalities.
- *Acute peritoneal dialysis:*
  - Acute peritoneal dialysis is the preferred choice in neonates/young infants with acute presentation of AKI because it is inexpensive, and requires minimum equipment and expertise. This is especially true in centers where continuous renal replacement therapy (CRRT) is not available or feasible due to financial constraints. Also, vascular access in neonates and infants is difficult to secure and appropriate size catheters and dialyzers are not readily available making peritoneal dialysis the most resorted to modality in this subset of patients.
  - It is based on blood purification by ultrafiltration, diffusion, and convection methods. In children with urgent need of fluid removal, rapid clearance of toxin or severe hyperkalemia, CRRT is preferred method because of low efficiency of peritoneal dialysis (PD).
  - Peritoneal dialysis catheters:
    - Stiff non-cuffed peritoneal dialysis catheter can be placed under local anesthesia at the bedside in a critically ill child.
    - The soft Tenckhoff peel-away PD catheters with introducer kit are available as peel away catheters with introducer kit for insertion at the patient's bedside under local

anesthesia and sedation using the Seldinger technique. These catheters are available both as single or double cuffs made of Dacron which help to anchor the catheter to the peritoneum and the skin thereby preventing displacement and infection. When a single cuff catheter is used, the cuff is usually left in the subcutaneous tissue under the skin while in double cuff catheters, one cuff is placed deeper just over the peritoneum and the second one is left superficially under the skin.

The advantage of these soft-cuffed silicon Tenckhoff catheters include less risk of leakage and infection which makes the catheter last longer.

- Peritoneal dialysis prescription depends upon the clinical condition of the child including estimated fluid overload, severity of hyperkalemia, metabolic acidosis, and underlying etiology.
- Peritoneal dialysis prescription:
    - *Duration of each cycle:* It includes 5–10 minutes for fill phase, dwell time of 30–45 minutes (shorter dwell time of 15–20 minutes recommended for severe hyperkalemia) and 5–10 minutes for drain time.
    - The dwell volume should be 30–40 mL/kg (800–1,100 mL/m^2) except if initiating PD soon after surgical catheter placement, when smaller (10–15 mL/kg) dwells are preferred to avoid leakage.
    - Number of cycles of exchanges per day depends on condition of child but 16–20 per day is the standard norm with shorter more rapid cycles for hyperkalemia as mentioned above. The standard fluid used for acute PD is commercially available dextrose-based dialysate fluid (1.5–1.7%).

In absence of PD fluid, the same may be prepared by mixing:
  - Solution A—440 mL 5% dextrose + 60 mL of HCO$_3$
  - Solution B—500 mL of NS
  (The mixture of the 250 mL solution A and 500 mL of solution B gives dialysate fluid with composition 140 mEq/L, bicarbonate 40 mEq/L and dextrose 1.5 g/dL. Dialysis may be done manually or by a machine).

- Dextrose is correlated with ultrafiltration and its concentration is increased when there is significant fluid overload.
- Bicarbonate-based solutions are preferred to lactate-containing solutions in patients with hepatic dysfunction, hemodynamic instability, and worsening metabolic acidosis.
    - To prevent catheter-related clotting and infection, injection heparin 500–1,000 units/L of dialysate fluid and prophylactic antibiotic should be added in fluid. Addition of potassium also may be required in dialysate fluid in children with continuous PD.
    - *One should be watchful for PD related complications:* Increased abdominal pressure, catheter block, catheter insertion site infection, and peritonitis.
        Method for stiff PD catheter insertion: Stiff PD catheter insertion is like *Bag and Mask* for the kidneys, its simple but lifesaving.

Steps of the procedure:
- Take written informed consent.
- Prepare a peritoneal dialysis prescription as above.

- Keep PD monitoring chart ready to record inputs and outflow and ultrafiltrate.
- Check the PD fluid, the peritoneal dialysis catheter, inflow and outflow lines, medications for sedation and multipara monitor for monitoring the child during the procedure.
- Catheterize the urinary bladder if not done so already.
- Under strict asepsis, hang two PD fluid bottles on an IV stand and keep them ready for connection to PD catheter inflow track using tubings with Y connector. Hang a urobag with urometer for connection to the outflow tract of the PD catheter.
- Keep child nil per orally (NPO) for minimum 4 hours prior to the procedure.
- Sedate the child with appropriate dose of midazolam or Ketamine or as per institutional policy.
- Clean and drape the child maintaining strict asepsis.

For stiff peritoneal dialysis catheter insertion:
- Place the patient in supine position.
- Clean and drape the child's abdomen.
- Insert a 16 G cannula 1–1.5 cm below the umbilicus in the midline to create ascites using 20–30 mL/kg of 1.5 or 1.7% PD fluid such that the flanks are full on palpation. This can be avoided if patient already has ascites.
- Put a small stab wound using a sterile blade at the same puncture site and push a stiff PD catheter with the trocar through it till a feeling of give is palpable.
- Once the give is felt, remove the trocar, and advance the catheter into the right Iliac fossa enough to insert all the side holes intraperitoneally.
- Connect the catheter through a connector provided using a three way to the inflow and outflow tract kept ready.
- Open the inflow to fill the abdomen with 30 mL/kg or 1,000–1,200 mL/m^2 of PD fluid. Critically ill children especially those on ventilator may have worsening respiratory distress when PD fluid is put in the peritoneum so PD can be started with smaller volumes and the fill volume can be increased gradually.
- Check outflow and then create a reservoir with 20–30 mL/kg or 1,000–1,200 mL/m^2 of PD fluid and start the first cycle of PD.
- Suture the catheter and secure with sterile dressing.
- Intermittent hemodialysis (IHD) is used when there is profound volume, electrolyte disturbance in critically ill children. Blood is filtered through semipermeable membrane of the dialyzer filter to remove small waste product potassium, urea, and creatinine by diffusion method. This modality requires placement of hemodialysis catheter in a large vein which may be technically challenging in small children. Also, at the initiation of therapy, blood is pumped into the circuit equivalent to the volume of the tubings and dialyzer which may further destabilize a sick child. This can, however, be prevented by priming the circuit with blood or albumin. Sustained low efficiency dialysis (SLED) is another alternative which uses same equipment as IHD but the dialysis sessions are prolonged to 8–12 hours with gradual ultrafiltrate removal.
- Continuous renal replacement therapy is a form of renal replacement which is of long term, may be days or weeks. It is used in critically ill patients who are hemodynamically unstable, post operation, in multiple organ dysfunction syndrome (MODS), tumor lysis syndrome

or in metabolic disorders, etc. It is of three types—continuous venovenous hemofiltration (CVVH) and continuous venovenous hemodialysis (CVVHD), and continuous venovenous hemodiafiltration (CVVHDF). The standard prescription for CRRT is 2,000 mL/1.73 m² but this may required to be increased in conditions such as hyperammonemia **(Table 1)**.
- Ultimate treatment of renal failure is renal replacement therapy when temporary measures are insufficient or not feasible.

Types of renal replacement therapy is given in **Flowchart 1**.

TABLE 1: Continuous renal replacement therapy (CRRT) prescription.

Parameter	Description
Dialyzer type	CVVH, CVVHD, CVVHDF
Priming	In children <15 lbs, prime with PRBC rather than saline for hemodynamically stability
Blood flow rate	Access dependent, range 3–10 mL/kg/min
Dialysate flow rate	35–40 mL/kg/min or 2.5–3 L/1.7 m²
UF (ultrafiltration)	Start with zero then gradually increased to 10–29 mL/kg/min till fluid balance is achieved
Anticoagulant	• Heparin but risk of bleeding and thrombocytopenia • Citrate-based anticoagulant—less risk of bleeding
Dosage	Effluent volume of 20–25 mL/kg/h
Thermal control	Temperature maintained by machine and external warming device

(CVVH: continuous venovenous hemofiltration; CVVHD: continuous venovenous hemodialysis; CVVHDF: continuous venovenous hemodiafiltration; PRBC: packed red blood cell)

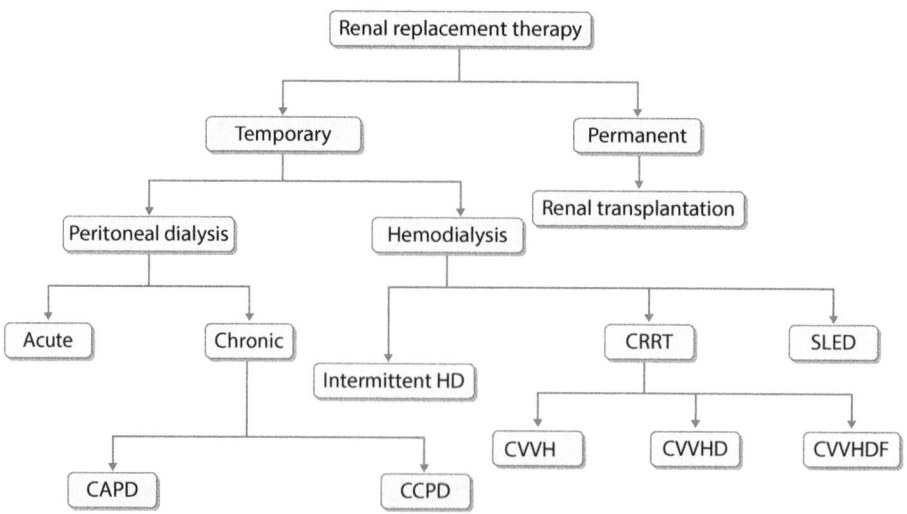

Flowchart 1: Renal replacement therapy.

(CAPD: continuous ambulatory peritoneal dialysis; CCPD: continuous cyclic peritoneal dialysis; CRRT: continuous renal replacement therapy; CVVH: continuous venovenous hemofiltration; CVVHD: continuous venovenous hemodialysis; CVVHDF: continuous venovenous hemodiafiltration; SLED: sustained low efficiency dialysis)

SECTION 7

Gastrointestinal Tract and Liver Disorders

- **Acute Abdomen**
  Vinod Dagar, Amit Devgan

- **Gastrointestinal Bleed**
  Vinod Dagar, Amit Devgan

- **Intestinal Obstruction**
  Vinod Dagar, Amit Devgan

- **Button Battery Ingestion**
  Sarvesh Kohli

- **Approach to Acute Liver Failure**
  Vinod Dagar, Amit Devgan

CHAPTER 42: Acute Abdomen

Vinod Dagar, Amit Devgan

- The term acute abdomen has been used loosely to include a variety of illnesses that may cause acute abdominal pain from ischemia, infection, or inflammation, requiring prompt decision-making and often emergent surgery.
- Common causes of abdominal pain are listed in **Table 1**.
- *Evaluation:*
  - History:
    - Age

Neonate	Infants	Older children
• NEC, meconium ileus, intestinal atresia, intestinal atresia • *Ask history of* polyhydramnios (high intestinal atresia), maternal DM (small left colon syndrome) and birth trauma	Intussusception	Appendicitis, peptic ulcer disease, cholecystitis

(DM: diabetes mellitus; NEC: necrotizing enterocolitis)

  - Pain
    - Character of pain:
      - *Sharp, severe, and constant:* Peritonitis
      - *Crescendo-decrescendo:* Bowel distention
    - Timing of the pain:
      - *Sudden onset pain:* Acute event such as a perforated viscus from an ulcer or trauma

TABLE 1: Common causes of abdominal pain.

Primary abdominal cause	Complications in critical ill patient	Systemic diseases
Mechanical obstruction	Gastrointestinal tract (GIT) hemorrhage	Diabetic ketoacidosis
Acute intestinal ischemia	Ileus	Acute intermittent porphyria
Infection/inflammation	Acute pancreatitis	Henoch–Schönlein purpura
Hollow viscera perforation	Acute cholecystitis	Kawasaki disease
Abdominal trauma	Enteritis	Sickle cell crisis
Reproductive organ-related disorders	Toxic megacolon	
	Abdominal compartment syndrome	

- *Insidious onset pain (nagging and vague):* Gastritis, inflammatory bowel disease, irritable bowel syndrome, or early appendicitis
- *Writhing in pain with intervening periods of lethargy:* Intussusception
- *Antecedent trauma:* Liver or spleen lacerations
- Location of pain

Epigastrium	Hypogastrium	Lower abdomen
Upper GIT, pancreas, gallbladder, biliary tree	Large intestine	In females consider ruptured ovarian cyst, ectopic pregnancy or PID

(GIT: gastrointestinal tract; PID: pelvic inflammatory disease)

- Change of pain over time in location and character—shift from epigastric or periumbilical region to the right lower quadrant (appendicitis)
- Radiation of the pain

Epigastrium to right shoulder	Epigastrium to back	Loin to groin
Acute cholecystitis	Acute pancreatitis	Ureteric colic

- Aggravating or relieving factors

Improvement with food intake	Worsening with food intake
Gastritis and peptic ulcer disease	Biliary colic, cholecystitis, pancreatitis

- *Vomiting:* Bile suggests a problem distal to the ampulla of Vater.
- Bowel habits

Diarrhea	Neonate with bloody stools	Infant with currant jelly stools	Rectal bleed
IBD, enteritis, intra-abdominal abscess	Suspect NEC	Intussusception	IBD

(IBD: inflammatory bowel disease; NEC: necrotizing enterocolitis)

- Menstruation—ruptured follicular or corpus luteum cyst in relation to menses
- Comorbid conditions

Postoperation adhesions	Infectious mononucleosis (prone to trauma)	Hereditary spherocytosis (cholelithiasis)
Sickle cell disease (auto-infarctions)	Portal hypertension with ascites (spontaneous bacterial peritonitis)	Neutropenia (typhlitis)
Vasopressors/hypotension (mesenteric ischemia)	Drugs (pancreatitis—asparaginase)	

- *Red flag signs:* Bilious vomiting, hematochezia, hematemesis, nighttime waking with pain, hemodynamic instability, and weight loss
- Physical examination:
  - General appearance
  - Vital signs
  - *Chest examination:* Look for signs of pneumonia, pneumothorax, hemothorax or features suggestive of diaphragmatic hernia.

- Abdominal examination
  - Look for abdominal wall motion, any discoloration, hernias of abdominal wall and groin
  - Involuntary guarding and rigidity, intra-abdominal masses, bowel sounds, and features suggestive of ascites
- Findings on physical examination for common differential diagnoses

Distinguishing features of acute gastrointestinal tract pain in children are given in **Table 2**.

- *Management:*
  - *Investigations:*
    - *Blood:* Complete blood count (CBC), electrolytes, arterial blood gas (ABG) analysis, blood urea nitrogen (BUN), creatinine, glucose, culture, liver function test (LFT), serum amylase
    - *Urine:* Urine analysis and culture
    - *Imaging: Three* views abdominal radiograph, chest radiograph (to rule out pneumonia), ultrasound, upper gastrointestinal (GI) series, barium enema, computed tomography (CT) scan
    - *Others:* Stool culture, vaginal culture [pelvic inflammatory disease (PID)], peritoneal fluid for analysis and culture
  - *Treatment:*
    - *Immediate:*
      - Nil per oral, rehydration
      - Nasogastric decompression

TABLE 2: Distinguishing features of acute gastrointestinal tract pain in children.

Disease	Onset	Location	Referral	Quality	Comments
Pancreatitis	Acute	Epigastric, left upper quadrant	Back	Constant, sharp, boring	Nausea, emesis, tenderness
Intestinal obstruction	Acute or gradual	Periumbilical–lower abdomen	Back	Alternating cramping (colic) and painless periods	Distention, obstipation, emesis, increased bowel sounds
Appendicitis	Acute	Periumbilical, then localized to lower right quadrant; generalized with peritonitis	Back or pelvis if retrocecal	Sharp, steady	Anorexia, nausea, emesis, local tenderness, fever with peritonitis
Intussusception	Acute	Periumbilical—lower abdomen	None	Cramping with painless periods	Hematochezia, knees in pulled-up position
Urolithiasis	Acute, sudden	Back (unilateral)	Groin	Sharp, intermittent, cramping	Hematuria
Urinary tract infection	Acute, sudden	Back	Bladder	Dull to sharp	Fever, costochondral tenderness, dysuria, urinary frequency

- Serial abdominal examination
- Surgical/gynecological/GI evaluation
- Pain control and antibiotics as indicated
- *Definitive:*
  - Surgical or endoscopic exploration as warranted

Management of acute abdominal pain is given in **Flowchart 1**.

Flowchart 1: Management of acute abdominal pain.

```
                              Trauma?
                    Yes ─────────────── No
                     │                   │
        • Perforated viscus    Distension or previous abdominal surgery
        • Hemorrhage            Yes ─────────────── No
        • Hematoma               │                   │
        • Contusion           Obstruction?      Peritoneal signs?
                            Yes ──── Yes ──── Yes ─── No
                             │       │         │      │
```

Yes (Obstruction):
- Volvulus (neonates)
- Intussusception (<2 years)
- Hirschsprung's disease (<2 years)

Yes (second):
- Necrotizing enterocolitis (neonates)
- Appendicitis
- Spontaneous bacterial peritonitis
- Meckel's diverticulum
- Perforated ulcer
- Cholecystitis (>5 years)
- Pancreatitis

Peritoneal signs Yes:
- Testicular torsion
- Incarcerated hernia
- Myocarditis
- Henoch–Schönlein purpura (HSP)
- Lower lobe pneumonia
- UTI

Extra-abdominal findings?
- Yes → (above)
- No → Palpable mass?
  - No → Focal tenderness?
  - Yes:
    - Intussusception
    - Constipation
    - Abdominal abscess

Colicky pain?
- No → Fever?
  - Yes:
    - Appendicitis
    - Gastroenteritis
    - UTI
    - Viral illness
    - Pneumonia
    - Intra-abdominal abscess
    - Hepatitis
  - No → Chronic recurrent pattern
    - **+**
      - Colic
      - Dietary protein allergy
      - Malabsorption
      - Toxins
      - Constipation
      - Sickle cell pain crisis
      - IBD
      - Peptic ulcer disease
      - Functional pain
    - **−**
      - Viral illness
      - Diabetic ketoacidosis
      - Intussusception
      - Hemolytic uremic syndrome
      - HSP
      - Pancreatitis
      - Urolithiasis
      - Toxins (iron)
      - Hepatitis
- Yes:
  - Urolithiasis
  - Constipation
  - Intussusception
  - Gastroenteritis

Focal tenderness Yes:
- Appendicitis
- cholecystitis
- Pancreatitis
- Urolithiasis
- Ovarian torsion
- Intussusception with perforation (2 months to 2 years)

(IBD: inflammatory bowel disease; UTI: urinary tract infection)

CHAPTER 43

Gastrointestinal Bleed

Vinod Dagar, Amit Devgan

- *Definitions:*
  - *Melena:* Passage of black tarry stools
  - *Hematochezia:* Passage of bright or dark red blood per rectum
  - *Hematemesis:* Passage of vomitus that is black or contains frank blood

Age category	Etiological factors
Newborn	Swallowed maternal blood, hemorrhagic disease of newborn, gastritis, vascular malformations, neonatal sepsis, idiopathic
Infants	Gastritis, esophagitis, stress ulcers, Mallory Weiss tear, vascular malformations, anal fissure, gastrointestinal duplication, milk protein allergy, gastroenteritis, intussusception
1–12 years	Esophageal varices, peptic ulcer disease, gastritis, gastroenteritis, hemorrhoids, anal fissure, volvulus, Meckel's diverticulum, Henoch–Schönlein purpura (HSP), polyp, colitis, inflammatory bowel disease, vascular malformations

- *Initial assessment:*
  - *Historical information:*
    - *Present illness:* Source of bleeding, magnitude of bleeding, duration of bleeding, associated gastrointestinal (GI) symptoms (vomiting, diarrhea, pain) and associated systemic symptoms (fever, rash, joint pains)
    - *Review of systems:* Gastrointestinal tract (GIT) disorders, liver disease, bleeding diathesis, medications [nonsteroidal anti-inflammatory drugs (NSAIDs), warfarin, hepatotoxic drugs, and prolonged antibiotic therapy]
    - *Family history:* GIT disorders (polyp, ulcer, colitis), liver disease, bleeding diathesis
  - Food/additives/drugs that color vomitus/stools

Red	Beet, laxative, phenytoin, rifampicin, candies
Black	Bismuth, charcoal, iron, spinach, blueberry, licorice

  - Physical examination

Skin	Pallor, jaundice, ecchymosis, abnormal blood vessels, hydration, rash, jaundice, purpura
Head, ear, nose throat, eyes	Epistaxis, gum bleed, oral thrush, conjunctival hemorrhage, jaundice, iritis
Cardiovascular	Heart rate and pulse pressure (lying, sitting, upright), gallop rhythm, capillary refill
Abdomen	Tenderness, organomegaly, ascites
Perineum and rectum	Fissures, fistula, rash, hemorrhoids, vascular lesion, evidence of bleed, tenderness

- *Investigations:*
  - *Laboratory assessment:*
    - Complete blood count (CBC), erythrocyte sedimentation rate (ESR), prothrombin time (PT), partial thromboplastin time (PTT), guaiac stool test, emesis, aspartate aminotransferase (AST), alanine transaminase (ALT), gamma-glutamyl transferase (GGT), blood typing and crossmatching, blood urea nitrogen (BUN), creatinine, total protein, albumin, stool culture
    - Blood urea nitrogen/creatinine ratio >30 (98% sensitive, 68% specific)—upper gastrointestinal (UGI) bleed
  - *Alkali denaturation test (Apt) test:* This is used to differentiate maternal from fetal blood in case of a neonatal UGI bleed. Mix one part vomitus/stool with five parts water. Centrifuge for 2 minutes and mix five parts of the supernatant with one part of 0.1% NaOH. Fetal hemoglobin resists alkali denaturation and remains pink, while the maternal hemoglobin turns yellowish brown.
  - Imaging studies

Test	Indication
Barium meal, barium enema	Dysphagia, odynophagia, drooling, stricture found at colonoscopy, suspected intussusception
Abdominal USG including Doppler	Suspected portal hypertension, intussusception
Meckel's scan	Meckel's diverticulum
Sulphur colloid scan, labeled RBC scan	Obscure GI bleeding
Angiography	Obscure or refractory GI bleeding, suspected AV malformation

    (AV: arteriovenous; GI: gastrointestinal; RBC: red blood cell; USG: ultrasonography)

  - Endoscopy

Test	Indication
Esophagogastroduodenoscopy	Hematemesis, melena, hematochezia
Flexible sigmoidoscopy, colonoscopy	Hematochezia
Endoscopy, video capsule endoscopy	Obscure gastrointestinal (GI) bleeding

- Therapy

Supportive care	• IV fluids (normal saline, Ringer lactate) • Blood products • Nasogastric tube • Vasopressors • Airway protection with ETT if altered sensorium with poor GCS score
Specific care	• Barrier agents (sucralfate) • H$_2$ antagonists (cimetidine, ranitidine, famotidine, nizatidine) • Proton-pump inhibitors (omeprazole, lansoprazole, pantoprazole) • Somatostatin analog

Endoscopic therapy	• Injection (sclerosant, epinephrine, normal saline, hypertonic saline) • Coagulation (bipolar coagulation, heater probe, laser, argon, plasma coagulator • Variceal injection or ligation • Band ligation • Polypectomy
Etiological treatment	Treat sepsis, liver failure; laparoscopy, surgery, treat complications of excessive bleed like hepatic encephalopathy

(ETT: endotracheal tube; GCS: Glasgow Coma Scale; IV: intravenous)

- Pharmacotherapy

Drugs	Indication	Dosage
Ranitidine	Control of bleeding or prevention of rebleed	Continuous infusion, 1 mg/kg followed by infusion of 2–4 mg/kg/day; bolus infusion, 3–5 mg/kg/day divided 8 hourly
Pantoprazole	Control of active bleed	• <40 kg—0.5 mg/kg/day IV OD • >40 kg—20–40 mg IV OD
Octreotide	Control of bleeding	• 1 µg/kg IV bolus (maximum 50 µg) followed by 1 µg/kg/h, may increase to 4 µg every 8 hours (maximum 250 µg per 8 hours) • When bleeding controlled—taper 50% every 12 hours; stop when at 25% of starting dose
Somatostatin	Control of active bleed	250 µg IV bolus followed by 250 µg/h continuous infusion; monitor for hyperglycemia 6 hourly
Terlipressin	Control of active bleed	2 mg every 4 hours till bleeding free interval of 24–48 hours
Vasopressin	Control of active bleed	0.002–0.005 U/kg/min × 12 hours, then taper over 24–48 hours (maximum 0.2 U/min)
Sucralfate	Coating of ulcerated mucosa	40–80 mg/kg/day in 4 divided doses
Propranolol	Prevention of variceal bleed	1 mg/kg/day in 2–4 divided doses; increase every 3–7 days to maximum of 8 mg/kg/day to achieve 25% reduction from baseline pulse rate

- Common causes of lower GI bleed

Anal fissure	Blood-streaked stool or blood passed following defecation, history of constipation
Allergic	Formula-fed infant
Intussusception	• Intermittent colicky abdominal pain; vomiting • Sausage-shaped mass in RUQ while RLQ feels empty, currant jelly stools
Meckel's diverticulum	Painless voluminous bleeding
Polyp	Painless bright-red blood, mucocutaneous lesions

Midgut volvulus	• Bright-red or maroon bleeding in infant or toddler • Possible bilious vomiting and abdominal mass
Infectious	Abdominal pain, tenesmus, fever
Inflammatory	Fever, weight loss, poor growth, extraintestinal symptoms
Coagulopathy	Petechiae, purpura, other bleeding sites
Hemorrhoids	Teens with constipation, portal hypertension
Henoch–Schönlein purpura	• Colicky abdominal pain, arthralgias, hematuria • Symmetric purpuric rash on lower extremities, buttocks

(RLQ: right lower quadrant; RUQ: right upper quadrant)

Evaluation of UGI bleed is given in **Flowchart 1**.

Flowchart 2 shows the approach to evaluation of a patient with lower GI bleed.

Flowchart 1: Evaluation of upper gastrointestinal (GI) bleed.

- All patients are admitted
- Frequent vital signs monitoring
- Large-bore IV cannula inserted
- Type and crossmatch for blood, CBC, PT/PTTK

Melena/hematemesis → Patient hemodynamically stable?

Yes → Bleeding with nasogastric (NG) lavage?
- Yes → Urgent upper endoscopy? Consider treatment with octreotide or vasopressin
  - Ulcer, gastritis, Mallory–Weiss tear → Acid suppression; *Helicobacter pylori* therapy
  - Ulcer with visible vessel → Endoscopic hemostasis
  - Esophageal varices → Sclerotherapy or variceal banding
- No → Treat with H₂ blockers or proton-pump inhibitors; Nonurgent upper endoscopy

No → Patient stable after intravenous fluids and blood products?
- No → NG lavage
- Consider:
  - Octreotide or vasopressin
  - Sengstaken–Blakemore tube emergent upper GI endoscopy
  - Angiography
  - TIPS procedure
  - Exploratory laparotomy

(CBC: complete blood count; IV: intravenous; PT: prothrombin time; PTTK: partial thromboplastin time with kaolin; TIPS: transjugular intrahepatic portosystemic shunt)

Flowchart 2: Approach to evaluation of a patient with lower gastrointestinal (GI) bleed.

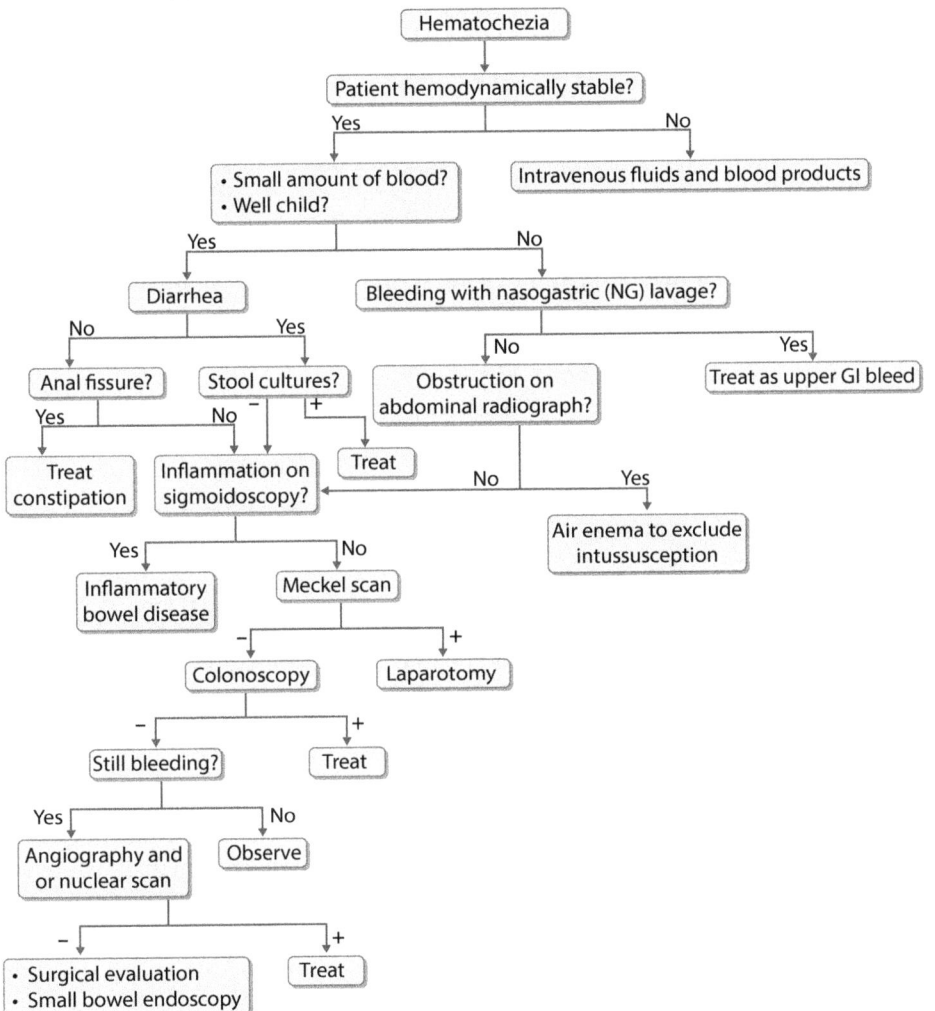

CHAPTER 44

Intestinal Obstruction

Vinod Dagar, Amit Devgan

- Bowel obstruction is a mechanical blockade to the transit of the intestinal contents that may be either intrinsic (Intraluminal or intramural) or due to extrinsic compression (extramural).
- *Etiology*:
  - Mechanical obstruction/dynamic obstruction

Intraluminal	Intramural	Extramural
Impaction	Stricture	Bands/adhesions
Foreign bodies	Malignancy	Hernia
Bezoars	Worms	Volvulus
Gallstones		Intussusception

  - *Adynamic obstruction:* Paralytic ileus (postoperative, infection, reflex ileus, and metabolic), mesenteric vascular occlusion, pseudo-obstruction
- *Clinical presentation*:
  - Features of obstruction:
    - *High small bowel obstruction:* Vomiting early and profuse with rapid dehydration, distension minimal with little evidence of fluid levels on abdominal radiography
    - *Low small bowel obstruction:* Pain is predominant with central distension; vomiting is delayed and multiple central fluid levels seen on radiography
    - *Large bowel obstruction:* Distension early and pronounced; pain is mild and vomiting and dehydration are late; proximal colon and cecum are distended on abdominal radiography
  - *General features:* Abdominal pain, bilious vomiting, diarrhea or constipation, increased nasogastric tube output, features of shock, absent bowel sounds, any evidence of previous surgery on abdominal wall, look for intra-abdominal masses or hernias.
- *Investigations*:
  - *Plain abdominal X-rays:* Air fluid levels in the small bowel, dilated small bowel or colon loops as well as edema or minimal intestinal gas distal to the obstruction (upright or lateral exposures)

    Radiological features of obstruction are given in **Table 1**.
  - *Abdominal ultrasound:* Diagnosis of intussusception and presence of free fluid, probe tenderness
  - Abdominal computed tomography (CT) scan
  - Complete hemogram, packed cell volume (PCV), serum electrolytes, kidney function tests

TABLE 1: Radiological features of obstruction.

Small bowel	Jejunum	Ileum	Cecum	Large bowel except cecum
Straight segments that are central and lie transversely; no gas in colon	Valvulae conniventes (across width of bowel, regularly spaced, ladder effect)	Featureless	Rounded gas shadow in right iliac fossa when distended	Haustral folds (spaced irregularly, do not cross whole diameter of the bowel)

TABLE 2: Common causes of intestinal obstruction.

Cause	Salient features	Investigations	Management
Intussusception	• Peak between 5 and 9 months of age • Triad of (severe paroxysmal colicky pain, normal or red jelly stools, sausage-shaped mass palpable)	Ultrasound (tubular mass in the longitudinal view and doughnut sign in transverse views)	• Nonsurgical reduction (air or saline solution enema with ultrasound or fluoroscopic guidance); contraindicated in symptoms >48 hours, peritoneal irritation, perforation, pneumatosis, presence of lead point • Surgical reduction or resection
Peritoneal adhesions	Following abdominal surgery or abdominal trauma	• X-ray abdomen • USG • CT scan	NG tube placement, hydration, presurgical antibiotic therapy effective against gram-negative aerobic and anaerobic bacteria and enterococci
Incarcerated hernia	Sudden attack of irritability and refusal to eat, irreducible mass protruding from the inguinal canal	Ultrasound with color Doppler flow	Urgent surgery
Meckel's diverticulum	• Lead point in intussusceptions, hernias, loop volvulus • Abdominal pain, bilious vomiting	• X-ray abdomen • Meckel's scan	Excision/surgery
Volvulus	Sudden pain abdomen with abdominal distension	• X-ray abdomen • USG abdomen	• Air enema • Surgery if required

(CT: computed tomography; NG: nasogastric; USG: ultrasonography)

- *Management:*
  - Nil per oral
  - Hydration and electrolyte balance
  - Placement of nasogastric tube—free drainage with 4 hourly aspiration
  - Evaluation of surgical resolution—indications for early surgical intervention (obstructed or strangulated external hernia, internal intestinal strangulation, acute obstruction)
- Common causes of intestinal obstruction are given in **Table 2**.
  Management of suspected gastrointestinal (GI) obstruction is given in **Flowchart 1**.

SECTION 7: Gastrointestinal Tract and Liver Disorders

Flowchart 1: Management of suspected gastrointestinal (GI) obstruction.

```
Suspected GI obstruction
           │
           ▼
┌─────────────────────────────┐
│ Fluid resuscitation:        │
│ NS or RL @ 20 mL/kg,        │
│ followed by maintenance     │
│ Correct metabolic acidosis  │
└─────────────────────────────┘
           │
           ▼
┌─────────────────────────────┐
│ Insert OG/NG tube to assess │
│ patency/allow decompression │
└─────────────────────────────┘
     │                 │
     ▼                 ▼
Difficulty in      Tube passes easily
passing tube             │
     │                   ▼
     ▼              NG aspirate
Chest radiograph:      │        │
Tube coiled in      Nonbilious  Bilious
chest—TEF/              │        │
esophageal       ┌──────┴──┐   ┌─┴────────┐
atresia/stricture│         │   │          │
              Abdomen   Nondis- Abdomen  Distended
              distended tended  nondistended
                 │        │        │
                 ▼        │        ▼
          Abdominal       │   Imaging:
          radiograph:     │   • Abnormal: Duodenal atresia,
          May show early  │     malrotation, jejunal atresia, ileal
          obstruction?    │     atresia, adhesion/band
              │           │   • Normal: Nonsurgical ileus/sepsis
     ┌────────┴────┐      │
     ▼             ▼      │
Nonprojectile  Projectile emesis:
emesis:        Palpable "olive"—
GERD           idiopathic hypertrophic
               pyloric stenosis
                      │
                      ▼
        Contrast enema: Intussusception, Hirschsprung's disease,
        meconium plug/ileus, small left colon, NEC, stricture

                                    Imperforate anus/
                                    obstructed or
                                    incarcerated hernia
```

(GERD: gastroesophageal reflux disease; OG: orogastric; NEC: necrotizing enterocolitis; NG: nasogastric; NS: normal saline; RL: Ringer's lactate; TEF: tracheoesophageal fistula)

CHAPTER 45: Button Battery Ingestion

Sarvesh Kohli

- Foreign body ingestion poses significant health risks and is associated with severe morbidity among children <6 years. Button batteries comprise 7–25% of these ingestions.
- *High risk of complications:*
  - Age >6 years
  - Battery >20 mm in diameter
- *Mechanisms of injury:*
  - Electrolysis
  - Pressure necrosis
  - Corrosive tissue injury (battery contents)
  - Heavy metal toxicity
- Complications may be life-threatening and can manifest from anywhere between hours to weeks.

Immediate/short-term (hours)	Delayed/long-term (weeks)
Mucosal damage	Esophageal strictures
Gastrointestinal perforation	Spondylodiscitis
Aortoesophageal fistula (bleeding)	Recurrent laryngeal nerve injury

- Symptoms are shown in **Figures 1A and B**.

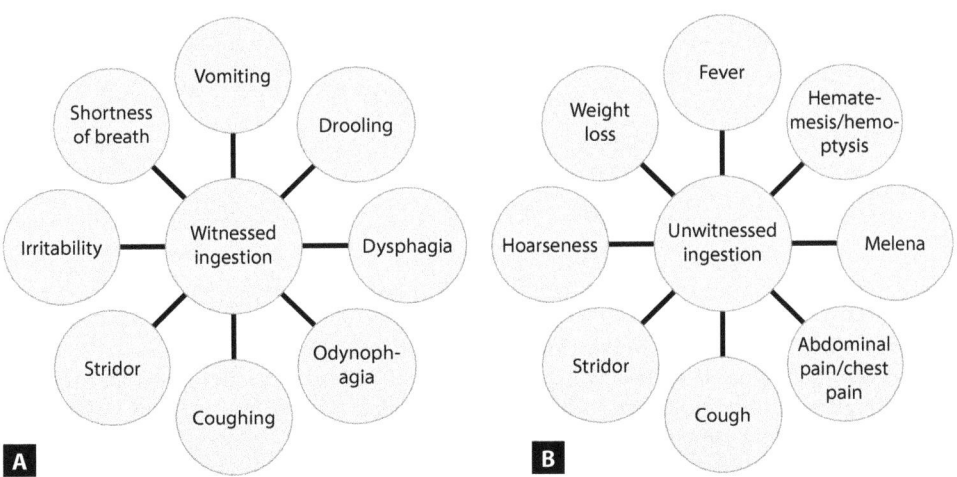

Figs. 1A and B: (A) Symptoms in witnessed ingestion; (B) Symptoms in unwitnessed ingestion.

SECTION 7: Gastrointestinal Tract and Liver Disorders

- *Investigations:*
    - Radiograph—neck, chest and abdomen (anteroposterior and lateral)
    - Contrast studies [computed tomography (CT) or magnetic resonance imaging (MRI)] after removal to identify complications
        - Severe symptoms at presentation/mucosal injury on endoscopy/delayed diagnosis of esophageal impaction—serial CT/MRIs of chest and neck **(Flowchart 1)**

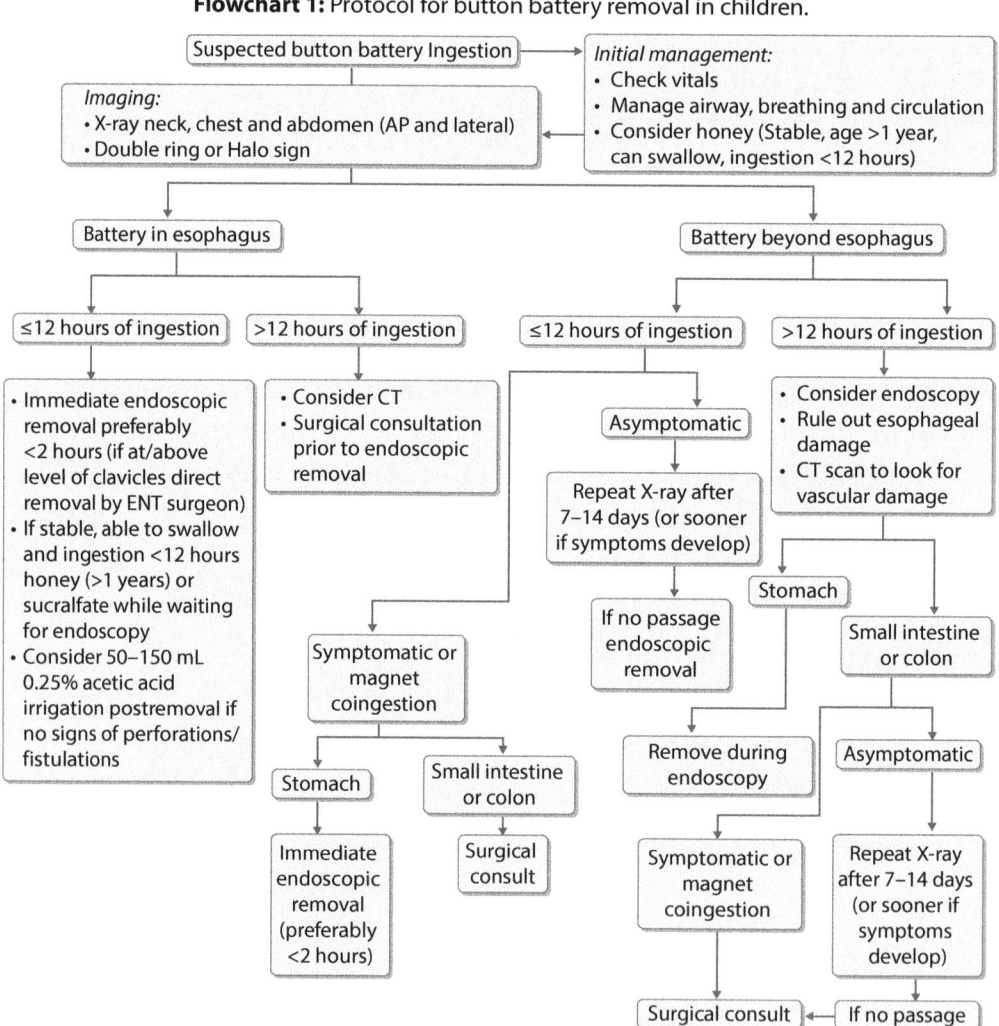

Flowchart 1: Protocol for button battery removal in children.

(AP: anteroposterior; ENT: ear, nose, and throat; CT: computed tomography)
Source: Mubarak A, Benninga MA, Broekaert I, Dolinsek J, Homan M, Mas E, et al. Diagnosis, Management, and Prevention of Button Battery Ingestion in Childhood: A European Society for Paediatric Gastroenterology Hepatology and Nutrition Position Paper. J Pediatr Gastroenterol Nutr. 2021;73(1):129-36.

CHAPTER 46

Approach to Acute Liver Failure

Vinod Dagar, Amit Devgan

- *Definition:*
  - Children with no known evidence of (e/o) chronic liver disease
  - Biochemical evidence of acute liver injury (usually <8 weeks)
  - *Hepatic-based coagulopathy not corrected by vitamin K, defined as:*
    - Prothrombin time (PT) ≥15 seconds or international normalized ratio (INR) ≥1.5 in the presence of hepatic encephalopathy (HE)
    - PT ≥20 seconds or INR ≥2.0 ± clinical HE
- Causes of acute hepatic failure in children are mentioned in **Table 1**.
- History-taking and examination is given in **Table 2**.

TABLE 1: Causes of acute hepatic failure in children.

Younger than 1 year		1 year and older	
Metabolic (mitochondrial, urea cycle defects, tyrosinemia, galactosemia, fructose intolerance)	42%	Unknown	47%
Neonatal hemochromatosis	16%	*Viral hepatitis:*	
		• Non-A, non-B hepatitis	27%
		• Hepatitis A	10%
		• Hepatitis B	4%
Undetermined	16%	Drug induced	10%
Viral hepatitis	15%	Others	2%
Others	10%		

TABLE 2: History-taking and examination.

For etiology	For course and severity	Clinical features
Fever	Jaundice	Signs of chronic liver disease
Blood transfusions	Mental status changes	Rapid decrease in liver size
Drugs	Alteration of sleep rhythm, personality changes	Liver span, splenomegaly, ascites, and complete neurological examination
Consanguinity	Evidences of coagulation disturbances	Infants—irritability, poor feeding, and change in sleep rhythm
Early infantile death	Nausea, vomiting, abdominal discomfort—nonspecific	Asterixis in older children
Developmental delay or seizures		
History suggestive of underlying chronic liver disease		

SECTION 7: Gastrointestinal Tract and Liver Disorders

- Stages of HE are mentioned in **Table 3**.
- *Immediate management:* This is shown in **Table 4**.
- *First-line investigations:* Complete hemogram, serum electrolytes, arterial blood gas (ABG), liver function test (LFT), renal function test (RFT), glucose, cholesterol, prothrombin time; blood ammonia and lactate, viral markers: Hepatitis B surface antigen (HBsAg), anti-HCV (hepatitis C virus), hepatitis A immunoglobulin M (HAV IgM), hepatitis E immunoglobulin M (HEV IgM); autoimmune markers—antinuclear antibodies (ANA)/smooth muscle antibodies (SMA)/liver-kidney microsome (LKM), ultrasonography (USG) abdomen, Wilson's disease workup—serum ceruloplasmin, eye examination [Kayser-Fleischer (KF)

TABLE 3: Stages of hepatic encephalopathy.

	Stages			
	1	2	3	4
Symptoms	Periods of lethargy, euphoria, reversal of sleep pattern, may be alert	Drowsiness, inappropriate behavior, agitation, wide mood swings, disorientation	Stupor but arousable, confused, incoherent speech	• Coma • 4A—responds to noxious stimulus • 4B—no response
Signs	Trouble drawing figures, performing mental tasks	Asterixis, fetor hepaticus, incontinence	Asterixis, hyperreflexia, extensor reflexes, rigidity	Areflexia, no asterixis, flaccidity
Electroencephalography (EEG)	Normal	Generalized slowing, theta waves	Markedly abnormal, triphasic waves	Markedly abnormal bilateral slowing, delta waves, electric cortical silence

TABLE 4: Immediate management of acute liver failure.

PICU care	Quiet environment
Central venous line	CVP, fluids, drugs, and samples
IV fluids	Start at three-fourths maintenance
GIR	6–8 mg/kg/min
Vasopressors	If clinically indicated
NG tube	For feeding or drainage
Strict input–output charting	
Nursing care	Care of bowel, back, bladder, skin, and eyes
Mechanical ventilation	Grade 3 or 4 encephalopathy or with hypoxia
Sedation	Only for invasive procedures, short acting

(CVP: central venous pressure; GIR: glucose infusion rate; IV: intravenous; NG: nasogastric; PICU: pediatric intensive care unit)

ring], 24-hour urinary copper excretion, special investigations for neonates and infants—urinary succinylacetone, alpha-fetoprotein, serum ferritin, and fructose challenge
- Fluids and metabolic complications and their management are given in **Table 5**.
  In case of any sudden change in mental status, evaluate for hypoglycemia, infections, and intracranial hemorrhage.
  - *Management of intracranial hypertension:* 70-80% of patients with grade 3-4 HE develop intracranial tension (ICT). It is the most common cause of death in them. Refer to chapter on management of raised intracranial pressure (ICP).
  - Management of coagulopathy is given in **Table 6**.
  - Management of hepatic encephalopathy (HE) is given in **Table 7**.

TABLE 5: Fluids and metabolic complications and their management.

Abnormality	Actions
Hypotension	• Resuscitate with NS, RL, plasma, or blood • Avoid fluid overload • If shock does not improve—vasopressors (norepinephrine, low-dose vasopressin)
Metabolic acidosis	• Suspect fluid deficit and correct • Look for sepsis
Hypokalemia	KCl infusion (per 100 mL IV fluids) K >3 3 mEq K 2.5–3 4 mEq K 2–2.5 5 mEq K <2 6 mEq
Metabolic alkalosis	Give KCl at the next higher level as above-mentioned
Respiratory alkalosis	Most common–acid-base disorder
Hyponatremia	Restrict fluids to two-thirds to three-fourths maintenance
Hypoglycemia	• Increase the GIR • Maintain blood sugar between 90 and 120 mg%

(GIR: glucose infusion rate; IV: intravenous; NS: normal saline; RL: Ringer's lactate)

TABLE 6: Management of coagulopathy.

Agent	Comment
Vitamin K	2–10 mg IV
FFP	Given in hemorrhage or in preparation for invasive procedures or if coagulopathy is severe (PT >60 sec)
Platelets	If platelets fall <50,000/mm^3
Prophylaxis of GI bleed	Proton-pump inhibitors (pantoprazole—20–40 mg/day or ranitidine—3–5 mg/kg/day)

(FFP: fresh frozen plasma; GI: gastrointestinal; PT: prothrombin time)

TABLE 7: Management of hepatic encephalopathy.

Bowel washes	With acidic fluids 6–8 hourly
Lactulose	• Oral/nasogastric (NG) tube 0.5 mL/kg/dose • Up to qid maximum of 30 mL/dose • 2–4 loose acidic stools/day
Enteral feeding	No restrictions in grade 1–2 encephalopathy, vegetable proteins preferred
Anticonvulsants	Phenytoin or phenobarbitone

TABLE 8: Etiology-specific management of underlying acute liver failure (ALF).

Etiology	Management
Hepatitis B	Lamivudine 4 mg/kg/day OD
Herpes simplex virus (HSV)	Acyclovir 10 mg/kg tds
Acetaminophen	N-acetylcysteine (NAC)
Amanita poisoning	Penicillin G 1 g/kg IV (intravenous), silibinin 15–30 mg/kg/day and NAC for acetaminophen poisoning
Autoimmune hepatitis	Methyl prednisolone 60 mg/kg IV
Galactosemia	Galactose- and lactose-free diets
Tyrosinemia	Nitisinone, a diet low in phenylalanine and tyrosine
Neonatal hemochromatosis	Antioxidants

- *Hepatorenal syndrome:* Most common cause of renal insufficiency in acute liver failure (ALF) secondary to intense vasoconstriction.
    - *Type 1:* Rapidly progressive reduction of renal function (doubling of the initial serum creatinine to >2.5 mg% or a 50% reduction of the initial 24 hours creatinine clearance to a level <20 mL/min in <2 weeks
    - *Type 2:* Slow progression
    - *Treatment:* Decreasing splanchnic circulation with drugs (vasoconstrictors) or through transjugular intrahepatic portosystemic shunt (TIPS) procedure
    - *Terlipressin:* 5–20 µg/kg/dose every 4 hours as IV bolus
    - *Norepinephrine:* Starting at 0.2 µg/kg/min, then titrate with blood pressure (BP)
- Etiology-specific management of underlying ALF is given in **Table 8**.
- Indications of liver transplantation are shown in **Table 9**.
- *Prognosis:*
    - *Overall mortality with supportive care alone:* 70%
    - *Mortality:* Raised ICP, infections, and multiorgan failure
    - 60–65% 1-year survival in transplantation for ALF
    - *Factors associated with (a/w) poor prognosis:*
    - Liver necrosis, multiorgan failure, age <1 year, stage 4 HE, and need for dialysis before transplantation
    The management of acute liver failure is given in **Flowchart 1**.

TABLE 9: King's college criteria for liver transplantation.

For acetaminophen poisoning	For other causes
Arterial pH <7.3	Prothrombin time (PT) >100 seconds
Or the following three factors:	*Or any three of the following:*
• PT >50 seconds	• PT >50 seconds
• Creatinine >3.5 mg%	• Bilirubin >17.5 mg%
• Grade 3 or 4 encephalopathy	• Age <10 years
	• Cryptogenic or drug-induced
	• Grade 3 or 4 encephalopathy

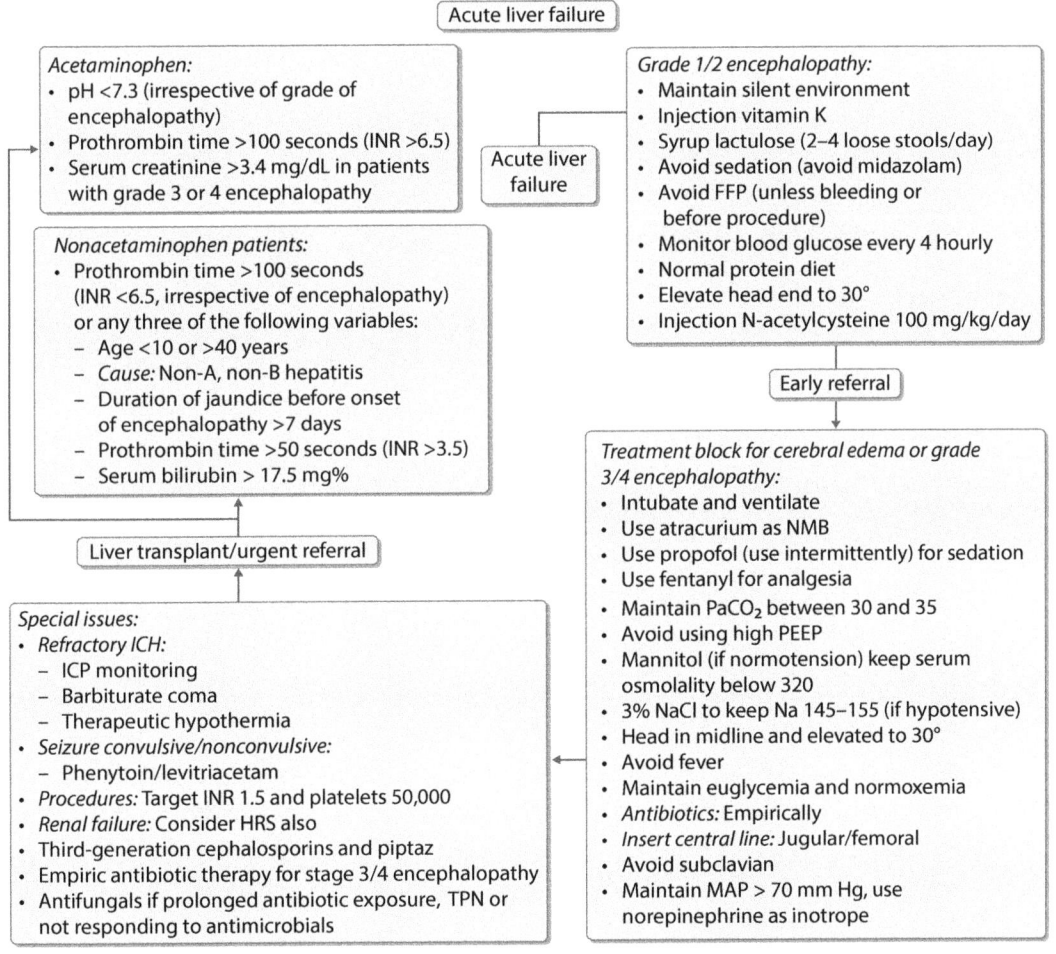

Flowchart 1: Management of acute liver failure.

(FFP: fresh frozen plasma; HRS: hepatorenal syndrome; ICH: intracranial hypertension; ICP: intracranial pressure; INR: international normalized ratio; MAP: mean arterial pressure; NMB: neuromuscular blocker; PaCO₂: partial pressure of arterial carbon dioxide; PEEP: positive end-expiratory pressure; TPN: total parenteral nutrition)

SECTION 8

Neurological Disorders

- **Approach to Coma**
  Arvind Mishra, KS Rana
- **Status Epilepticus**
  Vishal Sondhi
- **Increased Intracranial Pressure**
  Arvind Mishra, KS Rana
- **Head Injury in Children**
  Arvind Mishra, KS Rana
- **Acute Flaccid Paralysis**
  H Ravi Ramamurthy, KS Rana
- **Febrile Encephalopathy**
  Vishal Sondhi
- **Autoimmune and Demyelinating Disorders**
  Ruchika Jha, Vishal Sondhi

CHAPTER 47

Approach to Coma

Arvind Mishra, KS Rana

- *Definition:* Coma implies a total absence of arousal and awareness of surroundings, which is pathologic in origin. It is a state of medical and neurological emergency and requires urgent attention, preferably in an intensive care setting. 90% of pediatric trauma cases are traumatic and the most common cause of nontraumatic trauma is infection.

Term	Definition
Lethargy	Reduced wakefulness with attention deficits
Obtundation	Blunted alertness and diminished interaction with the environment
Stupor	Responsive only to pain
Coma	Unresponsive to pain

- *Causes of coma:*

Coma with focal signs	Generalized coma

• Intracranial hemorrhage
• *Stroke:* Ischemic or thrombotic
• Tumors
• Focal infections—brain abscess
• *Postseizure state:* Todd's paralysis
	• *Infections:* Sepsis, meningitis, toxic shock syndrome, enteric encephalopathy, cerebral malaria
	• *Hypoxia-ischemia:* Cardiovascular or respiratory failure
	• Metabolic disorders/Inborn errors of metabolism
	  – Hypoglycemia
	  – Acidosis [e.g., organic acidemias and diabetic ketoacidosis (DKA)]
	  – Hyperammonemia (hepatic encephalopathy, urea cycle disorders, valproic acid, fatty acid oxidation defects, and Reye syndrome)
	  – Uremia
	• Fluid and electrolyte disturbances
	• Acute disseminated encephalomyelitis
	• Postimmunization encephalopathy
	• Drugs and toxins
	• Hypertensive encephalopathy
	• Todd's paralysis
	• Nonconvulsive status epilepticus
	• Postmigraine

- Signs of trauma should be sought after an initial assessment of the comatose patient. Cervical immobilization should be maintained until trauma has been excluded or the cervical spine has been evaluated through radiographic and physical examinations.

- The clues to locate the site of abnormality are state of consciousness, pattern of breathing, pupillary size and reactivity, eye movements, and motor responses. The absence of the pupillary reflex in a comatose patient indicates a structural abnormality. Unequal pupillary size is a sign of uncal herniation.
- Papilledema is a late sign of increased intracranial pressure (ICP), and its absence does not rule out raised ICP.
- The oculocephalic responses (doll's eye reflex and the caloric responses) are specific maneuvers used for comatose children. Positive or normal oculocephalic responses indicate that the brainstem is intact.
- Basic principles of management:
  - Rapid assessment and stabilization.
  - Focused clinical evaluation to assess depth of coma and localization of lesion in the central nervous system.
  - Simultaneous etiologic evaluation for identification of cause.
  - Treatment—general and definitive therapy.
- *Airway management* is the most important step in the management of coma in children as their protective reflexes are obtunded and they are more prone to aspiration.
- Electroencephalography (EEG) is essential to diagnose nonconvulsive status epilepticus.
- Hypertension with bradycardia and a change in breathing pattern (Cushing triad) is an ominous sign of impending brain herniation.
- Decorticate posturing (flexion of the arms and extension of the legs) indicates supratentorial dysfunction and decerebrate posturing (extension and internal rotation of the arms and legs) indicates brainstem dysfunction.

The approach to coma is depicted in **Flowchart 1**.

CHAPTER 47: Approach to Coma

Flowchart 1: Approach to coma.

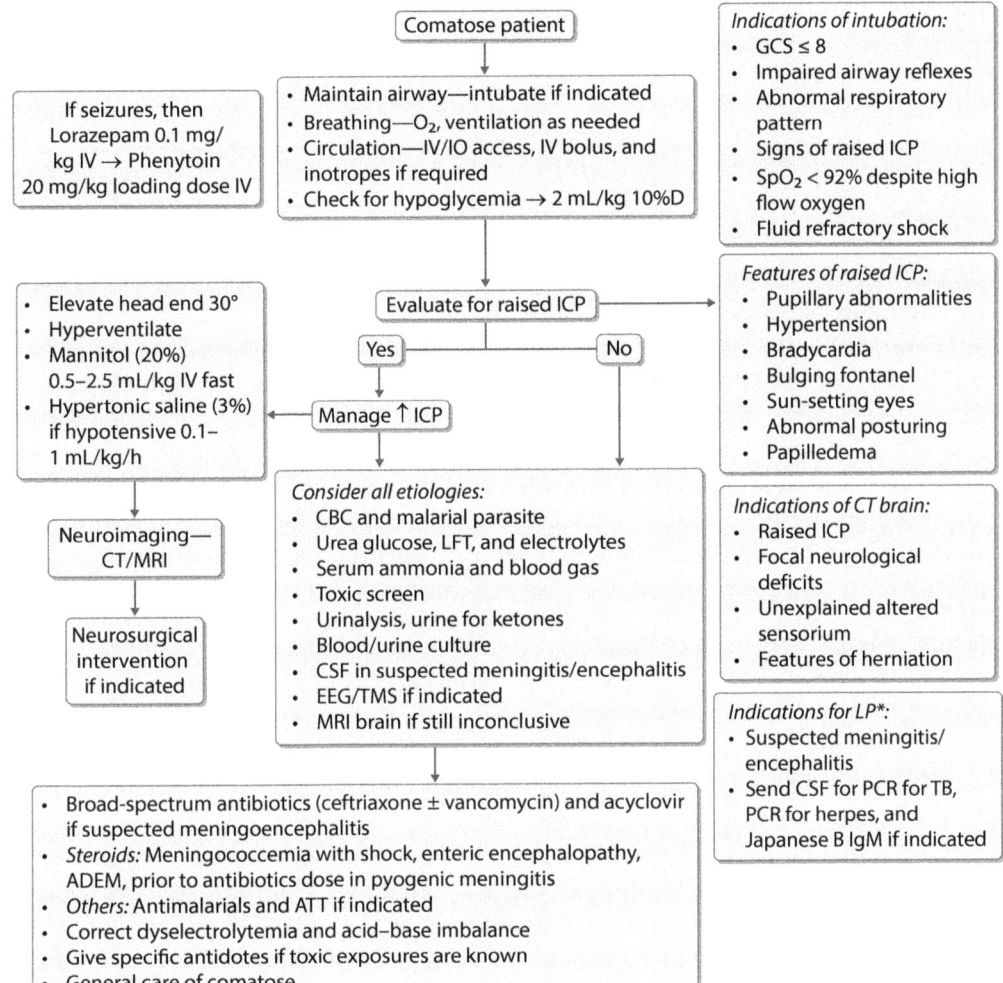

*LP should be preceded by neuroimaging

(ADEM: acute disseminated encephalomyelitis; ATT: antitubercular treatment; CBC: complete blood count; CSF: cerebrospinal fluid; CT: computed tomography; 10%D: 10% dextrose; EEG: electroencephalogram; GCS: Glasgow Coma Scale; ICP: intracranial pressure; LP: lumbar puncture; MRI: magnetic resonance imaging ; PCR: polymerase chain reaction; TB: tuberculosis; TMS: transcranial magnetic stimulation)

CHAPTER 48: Status Epilepticus

Vishal Sondhi

The chapter is based on the definitions and guidelines for management of status epilepticus (SE) by International League Against Epilepsy (ILAE).
- *Definition:* As per the 2015 ILAE definition of SE, two time points have been defined:
  1. *T1:* T1 is the time point beyond which the seizure is unlikely to terminate on its own because of either the failure of seizure termination or the initiation of mechanisms that lead to abnormally prolonged seizures
  2. *T2:* T2 is the time point beyond which seizure persistence may result in long-term consequences such as neuronal death, injury, and alteration of neuronal networks.

  The duration of T1 and T2 for different types of SE are mentioned here:

Type of status epilepticus	T1	T2
Generalized convulsive status epilepticus	>5 minutes	≥30 minutes
Focal status epilepticus	10 minutes	>60 minutes
Absence SE	10–15 minutes	Unknown

- *Classification:* The categorization of SE is typically similar to that of individual seizures and comprises four major types:
  1. Focal SE without impairment of consciousness or awareness (simple partial SE)—continuous or repeated focal motor or sensory seizures without impaired consciousness.
  2. Focal SE with impairment of consciousness or awareness (complex partial SE)—continuous or repeated episodes of focal motor, sensory, or cognitive symptoms with impaired consciousness. This is also called nonconvulsive SE. In some patients, the clinical manifestations of seizure activity may be subtle and not apparent to the clinician.
  3. Generalized convulsive SE including tonic–clonic, tonic, and clonic—is always associated with loss of consciousness.
  4. Absence SE—generalized seizure activity, characterized clinically by altered awareness, but not necessarily unconsciousness.
- *Etiology:* SE may occur in the setting of underlying, premorbid epilepsy or as the first manifestation of epilepsy. Virtually any cause of epilepsy may have a first presentation with SE. The common causes include:
  - Febrile seizures presenting as febrile SE
  - Central nervous system (CNS) infections
  - Acute hypoxic-ischemic insult
  - Metabolic disease (e.g., hypoglycemia and inborn error of metabolism)
  - Electrolyte imbalance

- Traumatic brain injury
- Drugs, intoxication, and poisoning
- Cerebrovascular event
- *Febrile infection-related epilepsy syndrome (FIRES) and new-onset refractory status epilepticus (NORSE):*
  - Febrile infection-related epilepsy syndrome refers to a new-onset refractory SE preceded by prodromal febrile illness starting between 2 weeks and 24 hours before the onset of refractory SE, with or without fever at the onset of SE.
  - FIRES is a subtype of NORSE. NORSE is characterized by the absence of any clear acute or active structural, toxic, or metabolic cause for SE in a patient who does not have active epilepsy or any other preexisting relevant neurological disorder.
- *Management* **(Table 1)**:
  - *Immediate supportive care:*
    - Open the airway and maintain it through positioning, jaw thrust, and/or airway adjuncts as needed.
    - Suction of secretions
    - Administer 100% oxygen; use pulse oximetry
    - Establish venous access
    - *Hemodynamic support:* Initially, most children with SE have high blood pressure, but they generally do not need circulatory support. Patients with SE may have elevated heart rate and blood pressure, but these usually return to normal once the seizures subside.
  - *Initial investigations:*
    - Plasma glucose and a rapid "finger-stick" (point-of-care glucose)
    - Serum electrolytes and calcium
    - Serum antiseizure medication levels, if applicable
    - If substance use or poisoning is suspected, urine and blood toxicology
  - Correct the "correctable" metabolic derangements like hypoglycemia/hypocalcemia
  - Antiseizure treatment
    - *First therapy:* Benzodiazepines
    - *Prehospital:* Intranasal midazolam (0.2 mg/kg)
    - *In-hospital:* IV Lorazepam (0.1 mg/kg) or midazolam (0.2 mg/kg)
      - *Seizures continue after 5 minutes:* Second dose of lorazepam or midazolam
      - *Second therapy:* Antiseizure medications—if seizures persist for 10 minutes despite receiving at least two injections of lorazepam or diazepam, a secondary treatment with a long-acting antiseizure medication is necessary. Levetiracetam, phenytoin/fosphenytoin, and valproate are appropriate options in this scenario. If the SE occurred due to missing a dose of antiseizure medication, then that particular medication should be administered.
      - *Refractory SE:* In case of persistent convulsive SE, after the initial treatment measures, which include immediate benzodiazepine treatment followed by the second therapy with an antiseizure medication, further pharmacologic therapy (third therapy) is required **(Table 1)**. This therapy is usually administered through

TABLE 1: Suggested protocol for the management of status epilepticus.

Timeline	Assessment/supportive care	Antiseizure therapy
• 0–5 minutes • Stabilization phase	• Maintain patent airway; put the child in the recovery position • Check for time of seizure onset • Monitor vitals • Assess oxygenation, start oxygen by mask/nasal cannula • Attempt IV access and collect blood glucose/electrolytes/AED levels • Evaluate for sepsis/meningitis/head trauma	*IV or IO access not achieved within 3 minutes:* • IM midazolam 0.1 to 0.2 mg/kg, (maximum 10 mg) Or • Rectal diazepam (injection solution given rectally) 0.5 mg/kg (maximum 20 mg) *IV access established:* • Lorazepam 0.1 mg/kg IV (maximum 4 mg) Or • Midazolam 0.15–0.2 mg/kg IV (maximum 5 mg) Or • Diazepam 0.2 mg/kg IV (maximum 10 mg)
• 5–10 minutes • Initial therapy phase	• Reevaluate vital signs, airway, breathing, and circulation • Maintain monitoring, respiratory support, and vascular access	*Administer a second dose of benzodiazepine:* If seizures continue 5 minutes after the first dose, give the second dose • Lorazepam 0.1 mg/kg IV (maximum 4 mg) Or • Midazolam 0.15–0.2 mg/kg IV (maximum 5 mg) Or • Diazepam 0.15 mg/kg IV (maximum 10 mg)
• If seizures persist 10 minutes after administration of benzodiazepines, administer a second antiseizure medication • Established status epilepticus		
• 5–30 minutes • Second therapy phase	• Reevaluate vital signs, airway, breathing, and circulation • Maintain monitoring, respiratory support, and vascular access	*Administer second-line antiepileptic drug (AED):* • Phenytoin/fosphenytoin 20 mg PE/kg IV Or • Valproate 20–40 mg/kg IV Or • Levetiracetam 20–40 mg/kg IV Or • Phenobarbital 20 mg/kg IV (maximum 1 g)
• If seizures persist 10 minutes after administration of second antiseizure medication • Established status epilepticus		
• 5–30 minutes • Second therapy phase	• Reevaluate vital signs, airway, breathing, and circulation • Maintain monitoring, respiratory support, and vascular access	*Administer second-line AED:* • Phenytoin/fosphenytoin (if not already given) 20 mg PE/kg IV Or • Valproate (if not already given) 20–40 mg/kg IV Or • Levetiracetam (if not already given) 20–40 mg/kg IV

Contd...

Contd...

Timeline	Assessment/supportive care	Antiseizure therapy
		Or • Phenobarbital (if not already given) 20 mg/kg IV (maximum 1 g) • Pyridoxine 100 mg IV (in children <2 years of age)

- If seizures persist after administration of benzodiazepines and second antiseizure medication
- Refractory status epilepticus

Timeline	Assessment/supportive care	Antiseizure therapy
• >60 minutes • Coma induction	• Reevaluate vital signs, airway, breathing, and circulation • Maintain monitoring, respiratory support, and vascular access • May need intubation/inotropes	• IV midazolam 0.2 mg/kg bolus, then infusion @1 µg/kg/min, increasing 1 µg/kg/min, every 5–10 minutes, till seizures stop, up to a maximum of 18 µg/kg/min • Start tapering 24 hours after the seizure stops @1 µg/kg/min, every 3 hours • If seizure persists despite a midazolam infusion of 15–20 µg/kg/min, consider phenobarbitone/thiopentone coma/propofol
• >60 minutes • Coma induction	• Reevaluate vital signs, airway, breathing, and circulation • Maintain monitoring, respiratory support, and vascular access • May need intubation/inotropes	*IV phenobarbitone:* • Load 10 mg/kg • Start infusion at 1 mg/kg/h • Increase by 0.5 mg/kg/h every 6 hours and titrate with EEG *IV propofol:* • Load 1–2 mg/kg • Start infusion at 25–30 µg/kg/min • Maintain infusion between 30 and 200 µg/kg/min • Monitor for hypotension and ventilation *IV thiopentone:* • Load 3–5 mg/kg • Start infusion at 0.5 mg/kg/h • Maintain infusion between 0.5 and 3 mg/kg/h • Monitor for hypotension and ventilation

- If seizures persist after >24 hours after the onset of coma induction
- Super-refractory status epilepticus

- Ketamine 0.5–4.5 mg/kg bolus IV and start infusion up to 5 mg/kg/h
- Isoflurane or desflurane
- Topiramate 10 mg/kg on days 1 and 2 and thereafter 5 mg/kg/day per orogastric tube (if no increased stomach residuals)
- Magnesium 50 mg/kg over 20 minutes IV followed by 50 mg/kg/h infusion (keep serum levels <6 mEq/L)
- Pyridoxine 100–600 mg/day IV or via orogastric tube
- Methylprednisolone 10–30 mg/kg/day IV for 5 days, followed by prednisone 1 mg/kg day
- IVIG 0.4 g/kg/day IV for 5 days
- Plasmapheresis for five sessions
- Ketogenic diet 4:1
- Vagal nerve stimulation/deep brain stimulation/transcranial magnetic stimulation

(AED: antiepileptic drug; EEG: electroencephalography; IV: intravenous; IVIG: intravenous immunoglobulin; IM: intramuscular)

the continuous infusion of midazolam (preferred) or phenobarbitone. At this stage, the patient may require intubation and mechanical ventilation.
- Febrile seizures:
  - *Definition:* Seizure accompanied by fever (temperature 100.4°F or 38°C), without CNS infection or metabolic imbalance, that occurs in infants and children of 6–60 months of age with no history of prior afebrile seizures.
    - *Simple*—usually associated with a core temperature that increases rapidly to ≥39°C, usually generalized, tonic-clonic lasting for few seconds to 15 minutes, not recurrent within a 24-hour period and followed by brief postictal drowsiness.
    - *Complex*—seizure duration >15 minutes, more than one seizure within the same day, or when focal seizure activity or focal findings are present during the postictal period.
  - *Clinical features:* Seizure with a brief period of postictal drowsiness. Look for localizing signs/symptoms for the cause of fever. Rule out CNS involvement (bulging fontanel and signs of meningeal irritation)
  - *Investigations:* Not indicated in all patients. If clinically indicated then perform a complete blood count, urine routine examination (RE)/microscopic examination (ME), peripheral blood smear (PBS) for malarial parasite (MP), blood sugar, and electrolytes.
  - Indications of lumbar puncture (LP)—if meningeal signs are present, age of child <6 months, prior use of antibiotics, ill-appearing child, or any other suspicion in a young child. When not sure do LP in a young infant/toddler.

CHAPTER 49: Increased Intracranial Pressure

Arvind Mishra, KS Rana

- *Concepts:*
  - *Monroe-Kellie hypothesis:* The sum of the intracranial volumes of the brain (80%), blood (10%) and cerebrospinal fluid (CSF) (10%) is constant and an increase in any of the components causes a change in the volume of the others.
  - *Normal values for intracranial pressure (ICP):*
    - *Adults and older children:* <10–15 mm Hg
    - *Young children:* 3–7 mm Hg
    - *Term infants:* 1.5–6 mm Hg
  - ICP values >20 mm Hg are pathological and require treatment.
  - Sustained ICP values of >40 mm Hg indicate severe, life-threatening intracranial hypertension.
  - *Cerebral perfusion pressure = Mean arterial pressure – intracranial pressure*
- *Causes* (**Box 1**)

BOX 1: Causes of intracranial pressure.

Increased brain volume:
- *Intracranial space occupying lesions*:
  - Brain tumors
  - Brain abscess
  - Intracranial vascular malformation
  - Intracranial hematoma
- *Cerebral edema:*
  - Encephalitis (viral and inflammatory)
  - Meningitis (TB, bacterial, and viral)
  - Hypoxic ischemic encephalopathy
  - Hepatic/uremic encephalopathy
  - Traumatic brain injury
  - Stroke
- *Increased CSF volume:*
  - Hydrocephalous
  - Choroids plexus papilloma
- *Increased blood volume:*
  - Cerebral venous thrombosis
  - Vascular malformations
  - Meningitis and encephalitis

> **BOX 2:** Clinical features of intracranial pressure.
>
> - *Early indicators of raised ICP:* Subtle changes in sensorium/personality, pupillary changes, third/sixth CN palsy, constant headache increasing in intensity and aggravated by movement or straining
> - *Late indicators of raised ICP:* Deteriorating consciousness progressing to coma, projectile vomiting, bradypnea, bradycardia, hypertension, altered respiratory pattern, hemiplegia, decorticate or decerebrate posturing, loss of brain stem reflexes
> - SIADH
> - *History suggestive of increased ICP:* Occipital headache, neck pain, vomiting, irritability, visual disturbances, tonic posturing, or worsening sensorium
> - *Cushing's triad:* Hypertension/bradycardia/irregular respiration (indicates impending herniation)
> - *History suggestive of etiology:* Trauma, previous shunt surgery, fever, ataxia, overhydration, predisposing factors for SIADH
>
> (CN: cranial nerve; ICP: intracranial pressure; SIADH: syndrome of inappropriate antidiuretic hormone secretion)

- Clinical features (**Box 2**):
    - Signs of cerebral herniation:
        - Glasgow Coma Score <8
        - Abnormal pupil size and reaction (unilateral or bilateral)
        - Absent doll's eye movements
        - Abnormal tone (decerebrate/decorticate posturing and flaccidity)
        - Hypertension with bradycardia
        - Respiratory abnormalities (hyperventilation, Cheyne-Stokes breathing, apnea, and respiratory arrest)
        - Papilledema
- *Management:*
    - *Positioning*—head position in midline elevated to 15–30° to encourage jugular venous drainage. Ensure that the child is euvolemic.
    - Lumbar puncture contraindicated due to risk of herniation
    - Rapid sequence intubation if impending herniation
    - *Hyperventilate. Aim for Partial pressure of carbon dioxide ($PaCO_2$) of 30–35 mm Hg.* Use an end-tidal CO_2 monitor if available. Hyperventilation acts by constriction of cerebral blood vessels and lowering of cerebral blood flow (CBF). The effect lasts only a few hours.
    - *Maintain mean arterial pressure* to preserve cerebral perfusion.
        - Avoid hypotonic fluids.
        - Do not lower the elevated blood pressure (BP) associated with Cushing's response.
        - Do not use ketamine or succinylcholine.
    - *Mannitol (20%):*
        - *Initial dose:* 0.5–2.5 mL/kg IV fast every 4–6 hours for 48–72 hours. Avoid hypovolemia and shock.
        - Reduction in ICP occurs in 15 minutes and lasts 3–6 hours.
        - Taper dose to prevent rebound.

- *Hypertonic saline:* Continuous infusion at 0.1–1.0 mL/kg/h, to target a serum sodium level of 145–155 mEq/L
- Do not delay antibiotics if meningitis suspected

Management of raised ICP is depicted in **Flowchart 1**.

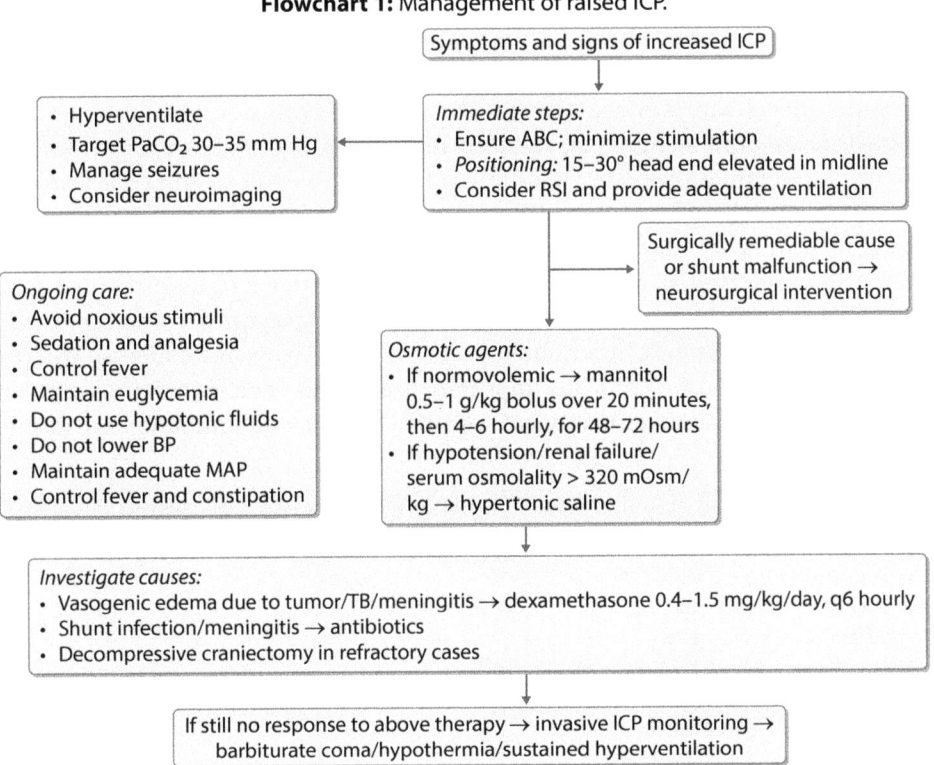

Flowchart 1: Management of raised ICP.

(ABC: airway, breathing, circulation; BP: blood pressure; ICP: intracranial pressure; MAP: mean arterial pressure; PaCO$_2$: partial pressure of carbon dioxide; RSI: rapid sequence intubation)

CHAPTER 50: Head Injury in Children

Arvind Mishra, KS Rana

- Head injury can be caused by penetrating trauma, blunt force, rotational acceleration, or acceleration-deceleration injury. They may be associated with a depressed or nondepressed skull fracture, epidural hematoma, subdural hematoma, cerebral contusion, brain edema, increased intracranial pressure (ICP), brain herniation, concussion (mild-to-moderate diffuse brain injury), and/or coma [diffuse axonal injury (DAI)].
- All patients with head injuries should be considered to have cervical spine injury unless proven otherwise. Hence, immobilize the C-spine before a careful history and physical examination. All patients presenting to an emergency department with a head injury should be assessed urgently by a trained staff who must assess and establish whether they are high risk or low risk for clinically important brain injury and/or cervical spine injury. Indications of admission, neurosurgical consult, CT scan, and intubation are discussed in **Box 1**.

BOX 1: Indications of admission, neurosurgical consult, CT scan, and intubation.

- *Indications of admission*:
  - Any indication for a CT scan
  - Suspicion of nonaccidental injury
  - Any difficulty in assessment
  - Child not accompanied by a responsible adult
  - Significant medical comorbidity
- *Indications of neurosurgical consult*:
  - GCS ≤12 after initial resuscitation
  - Deterioration postadmission
  - Definite or suspected open or penetrating injury
  - Focal neurological signs
  - Basal fracture or CSF leak
  - Seizures
- *Indications for CT scan*:
  - GCS ≤13 or decrease in GCS
  - High-speed road traffic accident
  - LOC >5 minutes or focal neurological deficit
  - Tense fontanelle
  - Open head injury or depressed skull fracture
  - Basal skull fracture
  - Laceration/contusion >5 cm diameter
  - Post-traumatic seizures
  - More than three discrete vomiting episodes
  - Amnesia lasting for >5 minutes

Contd...

Contd...

- Fall from a significant height (10 feet or five stairs)
- Abnormal drowsiness
- Suspicion of nonaccidental head injury
- Indications for intubation:
  - Loss of airway protective reflexes:
    - Loss of pharyngeal muscle activity and tone
    - Inability to clear secretions
    - Foreign body/direct trauma
    - Seizures
  - Abnormal breathing due to:
    - Chest wall/respiratory muscle dysfunction
    - Pulmonary disease: aspiration, contusion
    - Cervical spine injury
  - $PaCO_2$ >45 mm Hg or <25 mm Hg
  - Anisocoria >1 mm
  - GCS ≤8 or fall in GCS score of more than three, irrespective of initial GCS

(CT: computed tomography; GCS: Glasgow Coma Scale; $PaCO_2$: partial pressure of carbon dioxide; LOC: loss of consciousness)

TABLE 1: Pediatric Glasgow Coma Scale.

	Infants	Children	Score
Eye-opening	Spontaneous	Spontaneous	4
	In response to verbal stimuli	In response to verbal stimuli	3
	In response to pain only	In response to pain only	2
	No response	No response	1
Verbal response	Coos and babbles	Oriented, appropriate	5
	Irritable cries	Confused	4
	Cries in response to pain	Inappropriate words	3
	Moans in response to pain	Incomprehensible words or nonspecific sounds	2
	No response	No response	1
Motor response	Moves spontaneously and purposefully	Obeys commands	6
	Withdraws to touch	Localizes painful stimulus	5
	Withdraws in response to pain	Withdraws in response to pain	4
	Decorticate posturing to pain (abnormal flexion)	Responds to pain with flexion	3
	Decerebrate posturing to pain (abnormal extension)	Responds to pain with extension	2
	No response	No response	1

- Assessment of the consciousness of the patient is done by a modified Glasgow Coma Scale, which is an important tool in influencing treatment decisions and outcomes.
- Supratentorial subdural hematomas are venous in origin, are frequently bilateral, and usually occur without associated skull fracture. Supratentorial epidural hematomas are usually associated with skull fractures. Signs of basal skull fracture—hemotympanum, "panda/raccoon" eyes, cerebrospinal fluid leakage from the ear or nose, Battle's sign.

SECTION 8: Neurological Disorders

- Loss of consciousness (LOC) is not always immediate; a lucid period of several minutes may intervene between injury and the onset of neurological deterioration.
- Noncontrast computed tomography (NCCT) brain is the neuroimaging modality of choice in head injury patients, which can help the neurosurgical team to decide upon any urgent intervention.
- Avoid hyperglycemia, particularly during the early stages of brain injury. Consider the use of intravenous solutions that do not contain dextrose for early fluid and electrolyte management.

The pediatric Glasgow Coma Scale is discussed in **Table 1**.
Protocol for the management of head injury in children is described in **Flowchart 1**.

Flowchart 1: Protocol for the management of head injury in children.

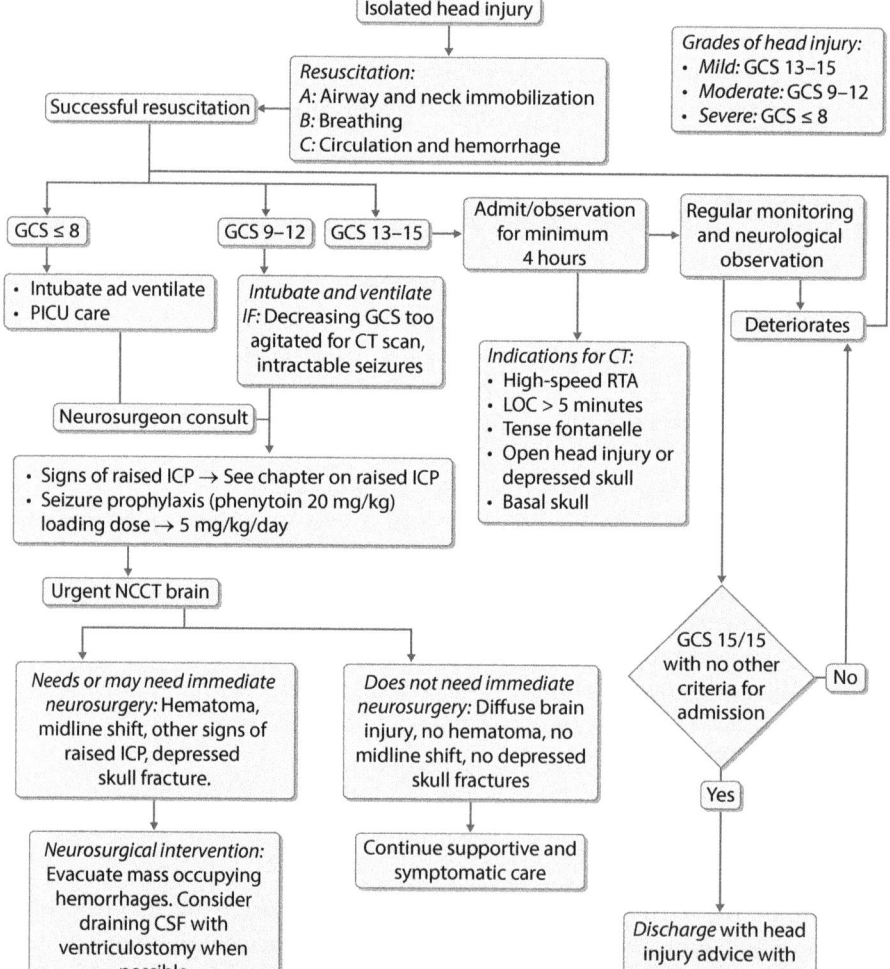

(CSF: cerebrospinal fluid; CT: computed tomography; GCS: Glasgow Coma Scale; ICP: intracranial pressure; LOC: loss of consciousness; RTA: road traffic accident; NCCT: noncontrast computerized tomography; PICU: pediatric intensive care unit)

CHAPTER 51

Acute Flaccid Paralysis

H Ravi Ramamurthy, KS Rana

- Acute flaccid paralysis (AFP) is acute onset (<4 weeks) flaccid paralysis of affected limbs. It is characterized by hypotonia of affected limbs, and areflexia/hyporeflexia.
- The common causes of AFP in children in India are poliomyelitis, Guillain–Barré syndrome (GBS), traumatic neuritis, and transverse myelitis. Other causes include botulism, diphtheritic neuritis, porphyrias, lead neuropathy, hypokalemic paralysis, hypophosphatemia, and hypermagnesemia.
- The approach to a case of AFP is described in **Flowchart 1**.
- Among the common causes, GBS is a progressive form of AFP with potential life-threatening respiratory paralysis. The timely diagnosis and treatment of GBS is essential in pediatric practice and has been described in brief below.
- GBS:
  - GBS is an autoimmune post-infectious polyneuropathy involving mainly motor but sensory, autonomic, and brainstem findings can also occur. It can affect children of any age.
  - It is usually preceded by a nonspecific viral infection by about 10–14 days. It could be a gastrointestinal (GI) infection (especially *Campylobacter jejuni*) or respiratory tract infection (especially *Mycoplasma pneumoniae*).
  - *Clinical features:* It starts as an acute or subacute onset weakness which begins usually in the lower extremities and progressively involves the trunk, the upper limbs, and finally the bulbar muscles, a pattern known as *Landry ascending paralysis*. The weakness is usually symmetric, but asymmetry is found in 9% of patients. It can be associated with pain in muscles in the initial stages. Bulbar involvement occurs in about 50% of cases and respiratory insufficiency may also result. Dysphagia and facial weakness are often impending signs of respiratory failure. Tendon reflexes are lost (areflexia), usually early in the course, but are sometimes preserved until later. GBS has three stages. There is a progression phase over several days to several weeks, a plateau phase of similar duration, and then recovery over weeks to months.
  - The autonomic nervous system may also be involved in some cases. Sinus tachycardia, postural hypotension, episodes of profound bradycardia, lability of blood pressure, diaphoresis, and occasional asystole can occur.
  - Acute inflammatory demyelinating polyradiculoneuropathy (AIDP) is the most common form of GBS. Other types are acute motor axonal neuropathy (AMAN), acute motor and sensory axonal neuropathy (AMSAN), and Miller Fisher syndrome (consists of acute external ophthalmoplegia, ataxia, and areflexia and is associated with serum anti-GQ1b antibodies).

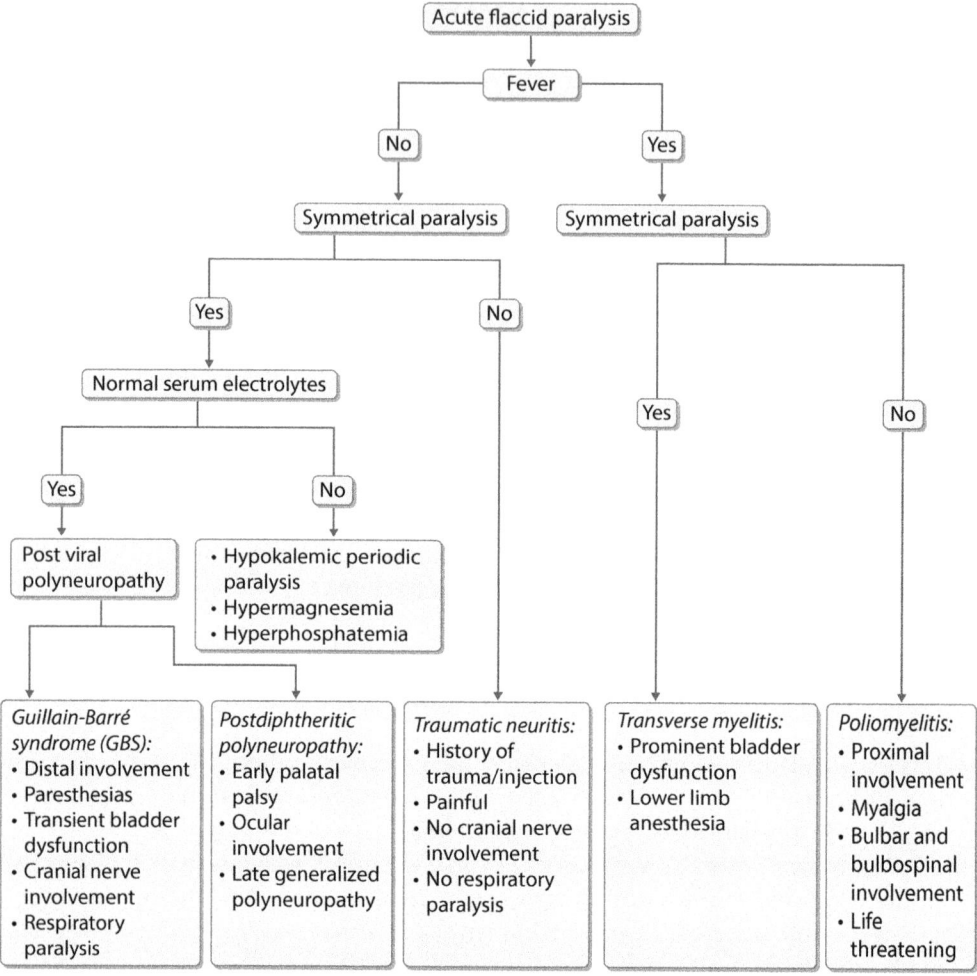

Flowchart 1: Approach to a case of acute flaccid paralysis.

- *Investigations:* Cerebrospinal fluid (CSF) shows albuminocytologic dissociation (elevated CSF protein with a normal CSF cell count) which is pathognomonic of GBS. Fewer than 10 white blood cells (WBCs)/mm^3 are found. CSF findings may be normal within the first 48 hours of symptoms, and occasionally the protein may not rise for a week. Motor nerve conduction velocities are greatly reduced, and sensory nerve conduction time is often slow. An electromyogram shows evidence of acute denervation of muscle. Serum creatine phosphokinase (CPK) level may be mildly elevated or normal.
- *Predictive models:* The Erasmus GBS Respiratory Insufficiency Scale for children (EGRIS-Kids) is a prognostic model designed to predict the risk of respiratory failure in children with GBS. The scale assigns points for age (0 for ≤5 years, 1 for 6–10 years, 2 for >10 years), GBS disability scale score at admission (1–4 for nonintubated scores in scale), and cranial nerve involvement (0 for absence, 3 for presence). The scale is

TABLE 1: Predictors at hospital admission—their categories and score.

Predictors at hospital admission	Categories	Score
Age (years)	≤5	0
	6–10	1
	11–17	2
Cranial nerve involvement	Absent	0
	Present	3
GBS disability score	1	1
	2	2
	3	3
	4	4
EGRIS-Kids		1–9

(EGRIS-Kids: Erasmus GBS Respiratory Insufficiency Score for children; GBS: Guillain–Barré syndrome)

scored from 1 to 9; results correlate with the risk of respiratory failure ranging from 4 to 50%.

Predictors at hospital admission—their categories and scores are discussed in **Table 1**.

- *Treatment:* Rapidly progressive ascending paralysis is treated with intravenous immunoglobulin (IVIG), the most common regimen used is for 5 days. Plasmapheresis, steroids, and/or immunosuppressive drugs are alternatives, if IVIG is ineffective.
- *Prognosis:* Spontaneous recovery begins within 2-3 weeks. The tendon reflexes are usually the last function to recover. Improvement usually follows a gradient inverse to the direction of involvement, with recovery of bulbar function first and lower extremity weakness resolving last.

- *Acute flaccid paralysis surveillance program*
- *AFP surveillance program:* India is on the verge of eradicating poliomyelitis. The Ministry of Health and Family Welfare, Government of India has instructed that all health facilities, clinicians, and other practitioners are required to notify all AFP cases immediately to the district immunization officer (DIO).
- *Case definition:* In the Global Polio Eradication Initiative (PEI), AFP is defined as "*Any case of AFP in a child aged <15 years, or any case of paralytic illness in a person of any age when polio is suspected*".
- *Components of AFP surveillance:*
  - The AFP surveillance network and case notification
  - Case and laboratory investigation
  - Outbreak response and active case search in the community
  - A 60-day follow-up, cross-notification, and tracking of cases
  - Data management and case classification
  - Virologic case classification scheme
  - Surveillance performance indicators
- *Stool specimen collection and transportation:* Collection of stool specimens from every AFP case is critical. Two stool specimens are collected as soon as possible after

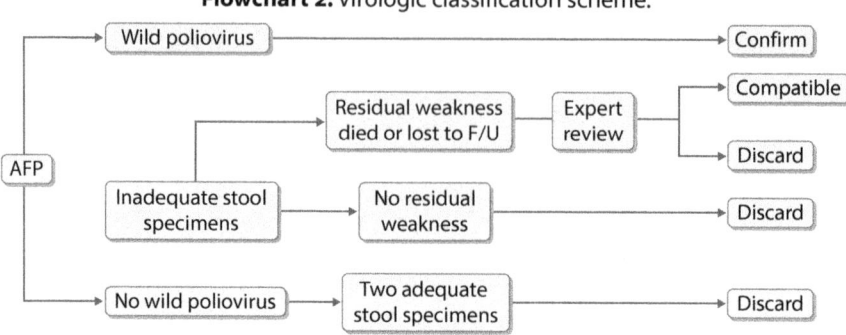

Flowchart 2: Virologic classification scheme.

(AFP: acute flaccid paralysis)

the onset of paralysis—ideally within 14 days and at least 24 hours apart. However, stool specimens should be collected from any late-reported AFP case up to 60 days from the date of paralysis onset. Each specimen should be 8 g—each about the size of one adult thumb—collected in a clean, dry, and screw-capped container. The specimens are collected, labeled, and then transported in the "reverse cold chain"—in a vaccine carrier specifically designated for this purpose to one of India's eight World Health Organization (WHO)-accredited polio laboratories.

- *Virologic classification scheme (**Flowchart 2**)*
  An overview of GBS is depicted in **Flowchart 3**.

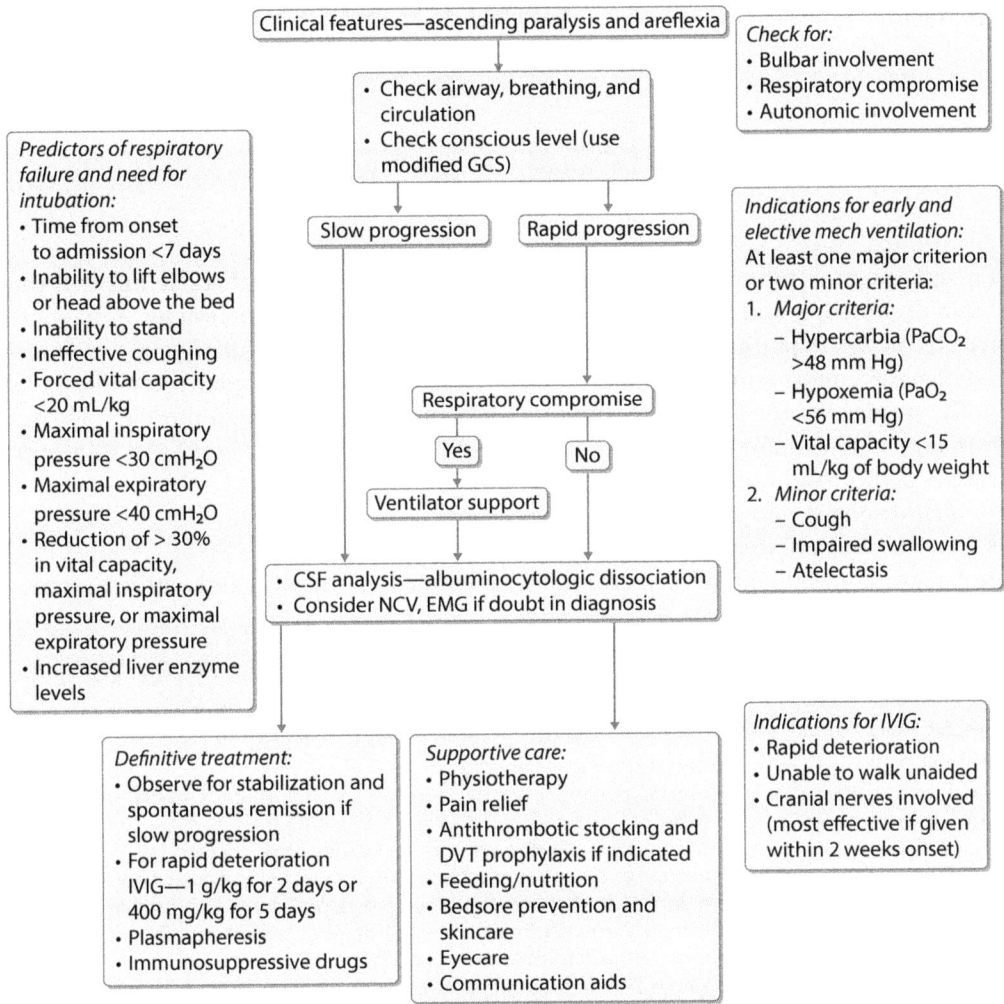

Flowchart 3: Guillain-Barré syndrome.

(CSF: cerebrospinal fluid; DVT: deep vein thrombosis; EMG: electromyography; GCS: Glasgow Coma Scale; IVIG: intravenous immunoglobulin; NCV: nerve conduction velocity)

CHAPTER 52: Febrile Encephalopathy

Vishal Sondhi

- Encephalopathy refers to dysfunction of the level or contents of consciousness due to brain dysfunction and can result from global brain insults or focal lesions. A diagnosis of febrile encephalopathy includes all patients who have a fever and altered consciousness.
- *Etiology*: The most common cause of fever-associated encephalopathy in children living in the tropics is central nervous system (CNS) infections, although there are numerous potential causes. When dealing with febrile encephalopathy, it is helpful to group the causes of this condition into:
  - Febrile encephalopathy with meningeal signs
  - Febrile encephalopathy without meningeal signs

Table 1 enumerates the parameters for febrile encephalopathy with and without meningeal irritation.

TABLE 1: Febrile encephalopathy with and without meningeal irritation.

Febrile encephalopathy with meningeal irritation[1]	Febrile encephalopathy without meningeal irritation

• Meningitis[2]
• Meningoencephalitis[2]
• Acute disseminated encephalomyelitis
	• *Infections causing encephalopathies*:
	  – *Shigella* encephalopathy, enteric encephalopathy, cerebral malaria, and dengue
	  – *Rickettsial:* Lyme disease and Rocky Mountain spotted fever
	• *Systemic infections:* Severe gram-negative sepsis and toxic shock syndrome
	• Infections with complications, such as stroke, venous thrombosis, metabolic derangements (fluid and electrolyte disturbances (dehydration, hyponatremia, hypernatremia, and hypoglycemia)
	• *Metabolic disorders (decompensated or precipitated by the intercurrent infection)*: Diabetic ketoacidosis, Reye syndrome, and inborn errors of metabolism
	• *Organ failures with intercurrent infections:* Uremia and hepatic failure
	• *Postinfectious disorders:* Acute disseminated encephalomyelitis, hemorrhagic shock, and encephalopathy syndrome
	• *Postimmunization encephalopathy:* Whole cell pertussis vaccine and Semple rabies vaccine
	• *Drugs and toxins:* Anticholinergics
	• Post prolonged convulsive status epilepticus
	• Heatstroke

[1]Infants and severely ill children with a meningeal infection or inflammation may not have meningeal signs.
[2]Etiological agent for meningitis/meningoencephalitis may vary based on season and geography and may include any but not limited to following:
- *Virus:* Japanese encephalitis virus, dengue, Nipah, *Enterovirus*, and measles
- *Bacteria:* Pneumococcal, *Haemophilus influenzae* type b, *Meningococcus*, *Salmonella*, and *Listeria*
- *Protozoa:* Malaria
- *Rickettsia:* Scrub typhus
- *Mycobacteria:* Tuberculous meningitis
- *Fungus:* Cryptococcus

- Presentation and key features for selected conditions **(Table 2)**.
- *Management*: The minimum essential workup and management of a child with acute febrile encephalopathy is highlighted in **Box 1**.

TABLE 2: Presentation and key features for selected conditions.

Condition	Key features	Key interventions
Pyomeningitis	• Acute presentation with fever and meningeal signs, CSF shows high opening pressure, often cloudy, 100–5,000 cells, predominantly polymorphic, CSF sugar <50% of blood sugar, elevated protein • Microscopy and culture of CSF and blood are important for microbe isolation	Early and high-dose antibiotics
Viral meningoencephalitis	• Epidemiological factors important for etiology • *CSF:* Clear, cells 5–1,000, lymphocytes predominate, CSF sugar normal, protein normal or mildly elevated. MRI may show diagnostic findings	Empiric treatment for HSV, until excluded by CSF, DNA, and PCR
Cerebral malaria	• Epidemiological factors important • No meningeal signs • Retinopathy • RDT have high sensitivity for diagnosis	Early use of intravenous antimalarials
ADEM	Encephalopathy and associated optic neuritis or myelitis, are clinical clues, MRI is diagnostic	High dose pulse steroids
Scrub typhus	In Asia pacific region, febrile multiorgan symptomatology, rash, eschar, transaminitis, thrombocytopenia, and/or hyponatremia	Doxycycline
Enteric encephalopathy	Two-thirds week of typhoid fever	Intravenous antibiotics and intravenous dexamethasone
Tuberculous meningitis	• Chronic febrile episode, meningeal signs, and focal neurological deficits • *CSF:* High opening pressure, 100–500 WBCs (predominantly lymphocytes), CSF sugar <50% of blood sugar, elevated protein (1–5 g) • Neuroimaging is often diagnostic depicting basal exudates, hydrocephalous, and infarcts • Perform chest X-ray for extraneural tuberculosis	Antitubercular treatment, steroids, and management of hydrocephalus

(ADEM: acute disseminated encephalomyelitis; CSF: cerebrospinal fluid; DNA: deoxyribonucleic acid; HSV: herpes simplex virus; MRI: magnetic resonance imaging; PCR: polymerase chain reaction; RDT: rapid diagnostic test; WBCs: white blood cells)

SECTION 8: Neurological Disorders

BOX 1: Essential workup and management of a child with acute febrile encephalopathy.
- *Clinical evaluation:* Thorough history and examination
- *Supportive care:*
  - Establish and maintain airway
  - Support ventilation and oxygenate as indicated
  - *Circulation:* Establish IV access, take samples
  - Fluid bolus if in circulatory failure, inotropes if required, treat electrolyte abnormalities if identified
  - Identify signs of cerebral herniation or raised ICP and manage accordingly*
  - Treat seizures and fever or hypothermia
- *Specific treatment:* Empirical treatment (Based on epidemiology, season)—
  - Ceftriaxone ± vancomycin (other antibiotics may be indicated like doxycycline for Rickettsial disease)
  - *Antimalarials (quinine/artesunate):* Smear positive, RDT positive cases, empiric treatment if resident of *Plasmodium falciparum* endemic area, short history, absent meningeal signs, anemia, hypoglycemia, and retinal hemorrhages.
  - *Acyclovir:* In sporadic meningoencephalitis with or without focal neurological findings, behavior changes, aphasia, suggestive CT (frontotemporal changes), and hemorrhagic CSF
  - *Steroids:* Meningococcemia with shock, enteric encephalopathy, ADEM

*Measures for raised ICP including nursing with head end elevated, avoiding sharp angulations of neck, sedation, controlling fever, maintaining normotension, euglycemia, and oxygenation, avoiding painful procedures and cautious use of osmotic agents like mannitol and hypertonic saline
(ADEM: acute disseminated encephalomyelitis; CSF: cerebrospinal fluid; CT: computed tomography; ICP: intracranial pressure; RDT: rapid diagnostic test)

CHAPTER 53

Autoimmune and Demyelinating Disorders

Ruchika Jha, Vishal Sondhi

- Although individually uncommon, autoimmune causes collectively comprise a significant proportion of autoimmune neurologic disorders in children, especially those with an acute or subacute presentation. The spectrum of presentation of autoimmune neurologic disorders is broad **(Flowchart 1)** based on the underlying immune dysregulation, mandating a high degree of suspicion. Moreover, their timely detection and appropriate management are of paramount importance due to the possible chronic sequelae and disease burden entailed **(Tables 1 to 3) (Box 1)**.

Flowchart 1: The spectrum of pediatric autoimmune central nervous system (CNS) disorders.

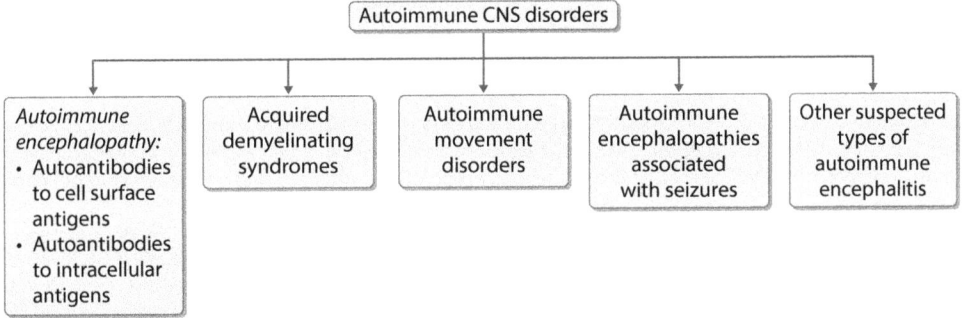

TABLE 1: When to suspect autoimmune and demyelinating disorders in children?

Disease	Clinical features
Autoimmune encephalopathy: • Anti-NMDAR encephalitis • VGKC complex • Encephalitis associated with $GABA_AR$, mGluR5, $GABA_BR$, DPPX, GlyR, and D2R antibodies • Antibodies to intracellular/intraneuronal antigens (Hu, Ma2, GAD65, and amphiphysin)	Acute or subacute onset of neuropsychiatric symptoms, abnormal behavior, decreased verbal output, sleep disorder, seizures, abnormal movements (orofacial dyskinesias, dystonia, and rigidity), autonomic dysfunction, and hypoventilation
Acquired demyelinating disorders: • Acute disseminated encephalomyelitis (ADEM) • Clinically isolated syndrome (CIS) • Optic neuritis • Transverse myelitis • Multiple sclerosis • Neuromyelitis optica spectrum disorder	Encephalopathy and polyfocal deficits (ADEM), abnormal behavior, seizures, cerebellar ataxia, decreased visual acuity, pain in ocular movements, paraparesis with sensory level, and bladder involvement

Contd...

Contd...

Disease	Clinical features
Autoimmune movement disorders: • Opsoclonus myoclonus syndrome • Sydenham chorea • Pediatric autoimmune neuropsychiatric disorders associated with streptococcal infections (PANDAS)	Opsoclonus, nonepileptic myoclonus, ataxia, sleep disturbance, cognitive dysfunction, behavioral disruption, chorea, emotional lability, obsessive-compulsive disorder, attention deficit hyperactivity disorder, and tics
Autoimmune encephalopathies associated with epilepsy and status epilepticus: • Rasmussen encephalitis • Fever-induced refractory epileptic encephalopathy syndrome (FIRES) • Acute encephalitis with refractory repetitive partial seizures (AERPS) • New-onset refractory status epilepticus (NORSE)	Refractory encephalopathy characterized by progressive refractory focal seizures, cognitive deterioration, and focal neurological deficits
Other autoimmune encephalopathies: • Bickerstaff encephalitis • Hashimoto encephalitis • Rapid-onset obesity with hypothalamic dysfunction, hypoventilation, and autonomic dysregulation (ROHHAD) • Chronic lymphocytic inflammation with pontine perivascular enhancement responsive to steroids (CLIPPERS)	Ophthalmoplegia, ataxia, and decreased level of consciousness with frequent hyperreflexia, stroke-like symptoms, tremors, myoclonus, aphasia, seizures, ataxia, sleep and behavioral problems, rapid onset obesity, hyperphagia, abnormal behavior, autonomic dysfunction and central hypoventilation, episodic diplopia or facial paresthesias with subsequent brainstem or spinal cord dysfunction

(D2R: dopamine-2 receptor; DPPX: dipeptidyl-peptidase-like protein-6; GABA$_B$R: γ-aminobutyric acid B receptor; GABA$_A$R: γ-aminobutyric acid A receptor; GAD: glutamate decarboxylase; GlyR: glycine receptor; mGluR5: metabotropic glutamate receptor 5; NMDAR: N-methyl-D-aspartate receptor; VGKC: voltage-gated potassium channel-complex)

TABLE 2: Initial investigations for suspected autoimmune encephalopathy.

Diagnostic imaging	Brain MRI with gadolinium (T1, T2, FLAIR, and DWI sequences) + MRI spine (if features suggestive of spinal cord involvement)
Blood tests	• CBC with differential, ESR, CRP, and ferritin • Serum testing for antibodies associated with AE • Vitamin B$_{12}$ and vitamin D levels • Free T3, TSH, and thyroid autoantibodies (anti-TPO, antithyroglobulin, anti-TSH receptor antibodies) • ANA and expanded nuclear antigen panel if features suggestive of systemic autoimmunity also present • Serum complements levels and immunoglobulin levels
Lumbar puncture	• Opening pressure, CSF cytology, protein, lactate, oligoclonal bands, infectious testing based on regional epidemiology • CSF testing for antibodies associated with AE • Save 5–10 mL for future testing
Respiratory tests	Nasopharyngeal swab for respiratory viruses, mycoplasma
EEG	Epileptiform discharges, changes in background activity
Others	PET/SPECT if indicated

(AE: autoimmune encephalitis; ANA: antinuclear antibody; CBC: complete blood count; CRP: C-reactive protein; CSF: cerebrospinal fluid; DWI: diffusion-weighted imaging; ESR: erythrocyte sedimentation rate; EEG: electroencephalography; FLAIR: fluid attenuated inversion recovery; MRI: magnetic resonance imaging; PET: positron emission tomography; SPECT: single-photon emission computed tomography; TSH: thyroid stimulating hormone)

TABLE 3: Initial investigations for suspected autoimmune movement disorders.

Diagnostic imaging	• Brain MRI with contrast • Whole-body imaging for tumor evaluation if positive antibody • Ovarian/testicular USG
Lumbar puncture	• CSF cell count, protein, glucose, IgG index, oligoclonal bands, neopterin, and antibodies • Also consider CSF neurotransmitters, lactate, pyruvate, amino acids
Serum autoimmune studies	• ANA and thyroid autoantibodies • Serum autoimmune antibody panel
EEG	Epileptiform discharges, changes in background activity
Genetic/metabolic evaluation	To ascertain other etiologies of movement disorders

(ANA: antinuclear antibody; CSF: cerebrospinal fluid; EEG: electroencephalography; IgG: immunoglobulin G; MRI: magnetic resonance imaging; TSH: thyroid-stimulating hormone; USG: ultrasonography)

BOX 1: Initial investigations for suspected acquired demyelination.

Investigations that should be considered for all cases with suspected acquired demyelination
- Contrast-enhanced MRI of brain + spine + optic nerves
- Serum AQP4
- Serum MOG-Ab
- CSF for:
  - Cells, glucose, and proteins
  - IgG and albumin
  - CSF IgG index
  - Oligoclonal bands

Investigations that may be considered based on case-to-case basis
- Evoked potentials:
  - Visual evoked potentials
  - Brainstem evoked response audiometry
  - Somatosensory evoked potentials
- Optical coherence tomography
- Investigations for systemic autoimmunity
  - C3 and C4
  - ANA and anti-dsDNA
  - ESR
  - CRP
- 25(OH) vitamin D
- Bacterial and viral studies

(ANA: antinuclear antibody; anti-dsDNA: anti-double stranded DNA; AQP4: aquaporin-4; CRP: C-reactive protein; CSF: cerebrospinal fluid; DNA: deoxyribonucleic acid; ESR: erythrocyte sedimentation rate; IgG: immunoglobulin G; MOG: ??; MRI; magnetic resonance imaging)

Approach to a case of suspected autoimmune disorder is given in **Flowchart 2**.

Flowchart 2: Algorithmic approach to a case of suspected autoimmune disorder.

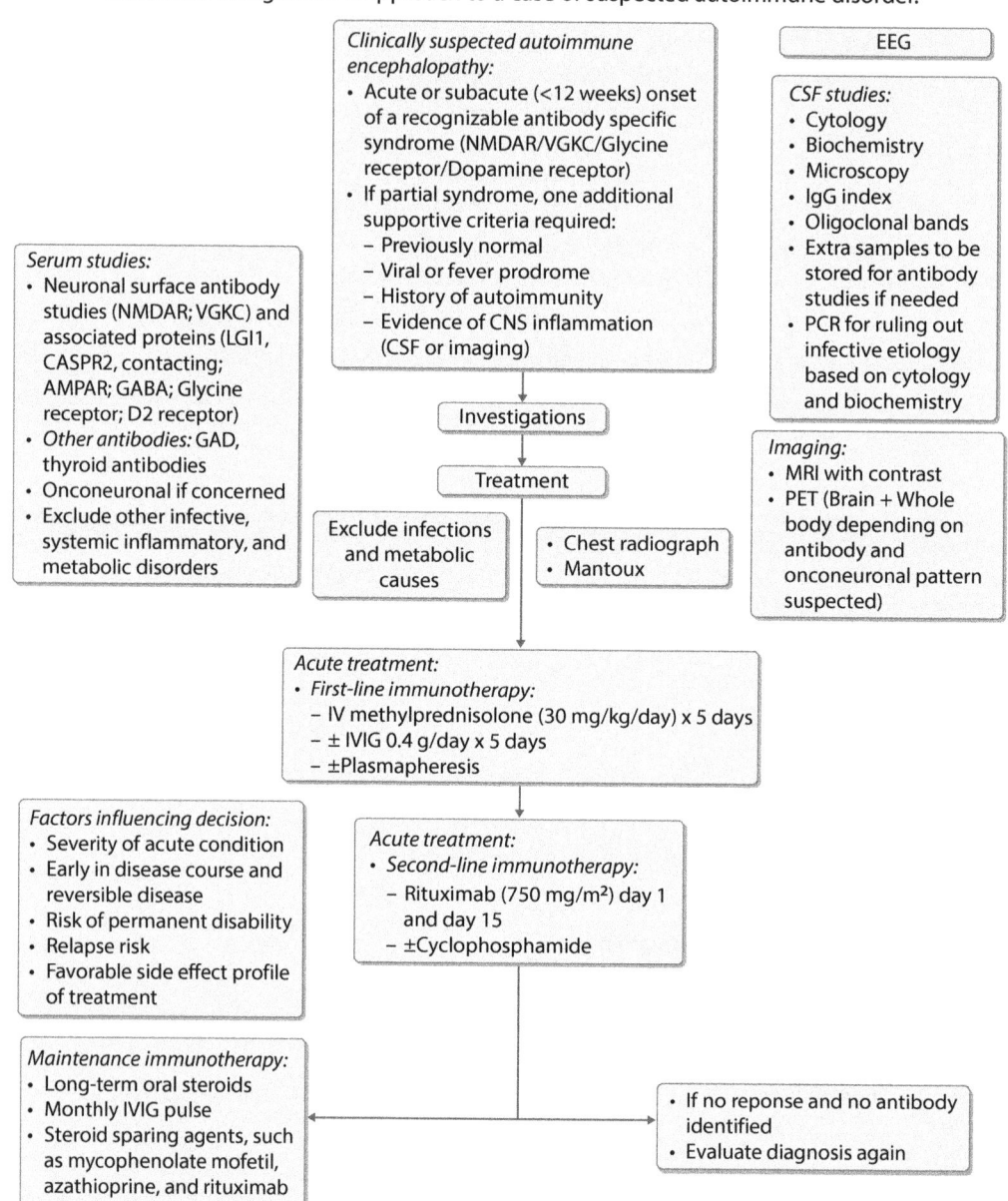

(AMPAR: α-amino-3-hydroxy-5-methyl-4-isoxazolepropionic acid receptor; CASPR2: contactin-associated protein-like 2; CNS: central nervous system; EEG: electroencephalography; GABA: gamma-aminobutyric acid; GAD: glutamate decarboxylase; IVIG: intravenous immunoglobulin; LGI1: leucine-rich, glioma-inactivated 1; MRI: magnetic resonance imaging; PCR: polymerase chain reaction; PET: positron emission tomography; NMDAR: N-methyl-D-aspartate receptor; VGKC: voltage-gated potassium channel-complex)

SECTION 9

Neonatal Disorders

- **Respiratory Distress in Neonates**
  G Shridhar
- **Neonatal Sepsis**
  G Shridhar
- **Neonatal Seizures**
  G Shridhar
- **Inborn Errors of Metabolism**
  Suprita Kalra
- **Approach to a Child with Ambiguous Genitalia**
  Sarguna K Logen

CHAPTER 54

Respiratory Distress in Neonates

G Shridhar

- Respiratory distress contributes to 30–40% of all admissions among neonates to the neonatal intensive care unit (NICU) and is more common among preterm (30%) than term (4.2%) neonates.
- The presence of any one of the following signs signifies respiratory distress:
  - *Tachypnea:* Respiratory rate >60/min
  - Lower chest (subcostal/intercostal) retractions
  - Nasal flaring
  - Grunting
  - Cyanosis
- The following are life-threatening signs of respiratory distress that require immediate intervention:
  - Gasping, choking, or stridor (signs of upper airway obstruction)
  - Apnea or poor respiratory efforts
  - Bradycardia, poor perfusion, and cyanosis

  The causes of respiratory distress in neonates are enumerated in **Box 1**.

  A good antenatal history, gestation of the neonate, onset, course of respiratory distress, and clinical evaluation along with other investigations [chest X-ray, ABG, two-dimensional echocardiogram (2D echo), etc.] as indicated help narrow down the cause of respiratory distress.
- The severity of respiratory distress in neonates can be objectively assessed by the Silverman–Andersen score (preterm neonates) OR Downes–Vidyasagar score (term neonates). A score of 0 suggests no distress; score of 1–4 mild distress; score of 5–7 moderate distress and score of >7 severe distress or impending respiratory failure **(Tables 1, 2 and Flowchart 1)**.
- The goals of treatment are:
  - To reduce the work of breathing by appropriate respiratory support.
  - To target SpO$_2$ between 90 and 95%
  - To identify and treat the underlying cause

BOX 1: Causes of respiratory distress in neonates.

Airway:
- Choanal atresia
- Pierre Robin sequence
- Tracheoesophageal fistula

Pulmonary:
- Respiratory distress syndrome (RDS)
- Transient tachypnea of newborn (TTNB)
- Meconium aspiration syndrome (MAS)
- Congenital pneumonia
- *Air-leak syndromes:* Pneumothorax
- Persistent pulmonary hypertension of newborn (PPHN)
- Congenital diaphragmatic hernia
- Lung malformations
- Pulmonary hemorrhage

Cardiac:
- Critical congenital heart disease
- Arrythmias
- Congestive cardiac failure
- Cardiomyopathy

Thoracic:
- Chest wall deformity
- Skeletal dysplasia

Neurological:
- Central nervous system (birth asphyxia, intracranial hemorrhage, meningitis)
- Sedation

Others:
- Neonatal sepsis
- Anemia/high-output failure
- Polycythemia
- Hypoglycemia
- Hypothermia/hyperthermia
- Inborn errors of metabolism

TABLE 1: Silverman–Andersen score.

Score	Upper chest*	Lower chest*	Xiphoid	Nares dilatation	Expiratory grunt
Score 0	Synchronized	No retractions	None	None	None
Score 1	Lag on inspiration	Just visible	Just visible	Minimal	Heard with stethoscope
Score 2	See-saw respiration	Marked retractions	Marked retractions	Marked	Heard with naked ear

*Upper and lower chest are above and below the mid-axillary line.

CHAPTER 54: Respiratory Distress in Neonates

TABLE 2: Downes–Vidyasagar score.

Score	Respiratory rate	Cyanosis	Air entry	Retraction	Grunt
Score 0	<60 breaths/min	Nil	Normal	None	Nil
Score 1	60–80 breaths/minute	In room air	Mild decrease	Heard with stethoscope	Mild
Score 2	80 breaths/min or apnea	In >40% oxygen	Marked decrease	Heard with naked ear	Moderate to severe

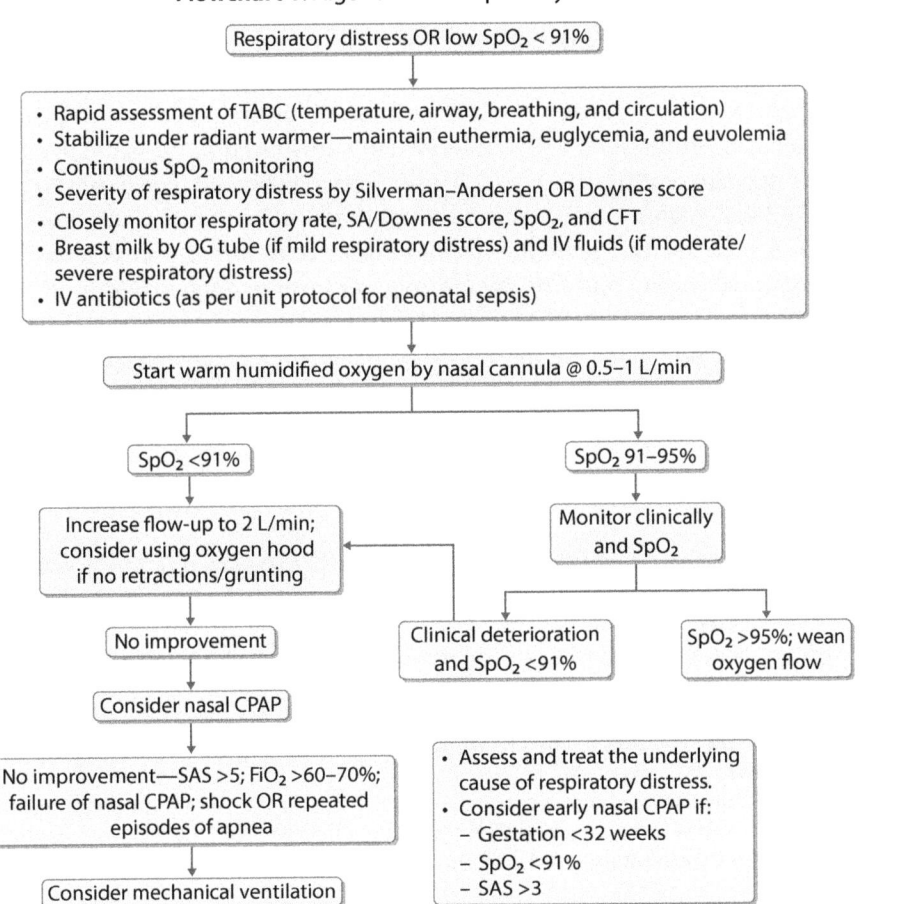

Flowchart 1: Algorithm for respiratory distress.

(CFT: capillary filling time; CPAP: continuous positive airway pressure; IV: intravenous; OG: orogastric; SA: Silverman-Anderson; SAS: Silverman-Anderson score)

CHAPTER 55

Neonatal Sepsis

G Shridhar

- Neonatal sepsis is a clinical syndrome secondary to bloodstream infection (including pneumonia, septicemia, meningitis, arthritis, osteomyelitis, and urinary tract infections) and a major causes of neonatal mortality and morbidity in low- and middle-income countries (LMICs) including India.
- *Epidemiology:* The Delhi Neonatal Infection Study group (DeNIS) in 2016 reported a 6.2% and 14.3% incidence of culture positive and total (culture positive and negative) sepsis among all NICU admissions with 25% mortality attributed to neonatal sepsis. The most common organisms causing both Early Onset Sepsis (EOS) and Late Onset Neonatal Sepsis (LONS) in Asian region (unlike the developed countries) are *Escherichia coli* (*E. coli*), *Klebsiella, Acinetobacter, Pseudomonas, Staphylococcus aureus* (*Staph aureus*), *coagulase negative Staphylococcus,* and *Candia* (among out born neonates). Group B *Streptococcus* is not a common cause of EOS in India. There is an alarming increase in the incidence of antibiotic resistance among many NICUs in Asia fueled by overuse/abuse of broad-spectrum antibiotics.
- *Terminology and classification:*
  - *Probable sepsis:*
    - Clinical and laboratory features consistent with bacterial infection without a positive culture
  - *Clinical sepsis:*
    - High clinical suspicion with suggestive history, but negative sepsis screen, blood/cerebrospinal fluid (CSF) culture
  - *Culture positive sepsis:*
    - Systemic clinical features with pure growth of bacteria from one or more normally sterile sites
  - *Suspect sepsis/ruling out sepsis:*
    - Sepsis is suspected based on risk factors/clinical features, but the clinical course is not consistent (rapid recovery within a few hours) and sepsis screen is negative
  - *Early onset sepsis (EOS):*
    - Clinical features at <72 hours after birth—in severe cases may be symptomatic at birth
    - Traditionally believed to be caused by ascending infection from maternal genital tract
    - Manifests with respiratory distress, pneumonia and/or shock
  - *Risk factors:*
    - Prolonged rupture of membranes (PROM) >24 hours
    - Prolonged labor (I stage + II stage >24 hours)
    - Intrauterine inflammation, infection or both (Triple I)/maternal chorioamnionitis
    - Foul smelling liquor
    - Single unclean PV examination during labor
    - Spontaneous preterm labor in absence of PROM
    - Severe perinatal asphyxia (Apgar score <4 at 1 minute)

- *Late onset sepsis (LONS):*
  - Clinical features after 72 hours of birth
  - Community-acquired infection or healthcare-associated infection (HAI)
  - Manifests with septicemia, pneumonia and/or meningitis
  - Predisposing factors
    - *Community-acquired infection:* Poor hygiene, poor cord care, pre-lacteal feeds, and bottle feeding
    - *Healthcare-associated infection:* Prematurity/low birth weight, admission to NICU, invasive lines/use of parenteral fluids/stock solutions/parenteral nutrition, mechanical ventilation

- Clinical features
  - *Nonspecific features:* The earliest signs are often subtle and nonspecific. A high index of suspicion is required for early diagnosis.
    - Hypothermia or fever
    - Lethargy, poor feeding
    - Respiratory distress, apnea
    - Brady cardia/tachycardia
    - Poor perfusion, prolonged capillary refill time (CRT)
    - Hypotonia
    - Hypoglycemia/hyperglycemia
    - Metabolic acidosis
  - *Systemic features:* Organ specific
    - *Central nervous system:* Bulging anterior fontanelle, vacant stare, high pitched cry, irritability, stupor/coma, and seizures
    - *Cardiovascular:* Cyanosis, hypotension, and shock
    - *Gastrointestinal:* Increased gastric residuals, vomiting, and abdominal distension
    - *Hepatic:* Direct hyperbilirubinemia
    - *Renal:* Acute renal failure
    - *Hematological:* Bleeding, petechia, and purpura
    - *Skin:* Pustules, abscess, sclerema, mottling, umbilical redness, and discharge
- Choice of antibiotics:
  - The choice of antibiotics must ideally be based on local culture and antibiotic sensitivity data and profile of organisms for last 6–12 months. The most appropriate and rational combination of antibiotics must be selected:
    - *First line:* Must cover approximately 75–80% of organisms
    - *Second line:* Must cover approximately 90–95% of organisms
    - *Third line:* Must cover approximately 95–100% of organisms
  - The initial combination of antibiotics should cover both gram-negative and gram-positive organisms.
  - Avoid cephalosporins as first-line antibiotics.
  - Each NICU should have a written antibiotic policy and practice antibiotic stewardship (reasons for starting antibiotics, modify antibiotics based on culture reports and clinical course, have clear plan for de-escalation/stopping, do not use third line drugs without consultation)

- **Duration of antibiotics:**
  - *Culture negative sepsis (clinical course consistent with sepsis):* 5–7 days
  - *Blood culture positive but no meningitis:* 14 days
  - *Meningitis [with or without positive blood/cerebrospinal fluid (CSF) culture]:* 21 days

The algorithm for early onset sepsis is given in **Flowchart 1**.
The algorithm for late onset sepsis is given in **Flowchart 2**.

Flowchart 1: Algorithm for early onset sepsis.

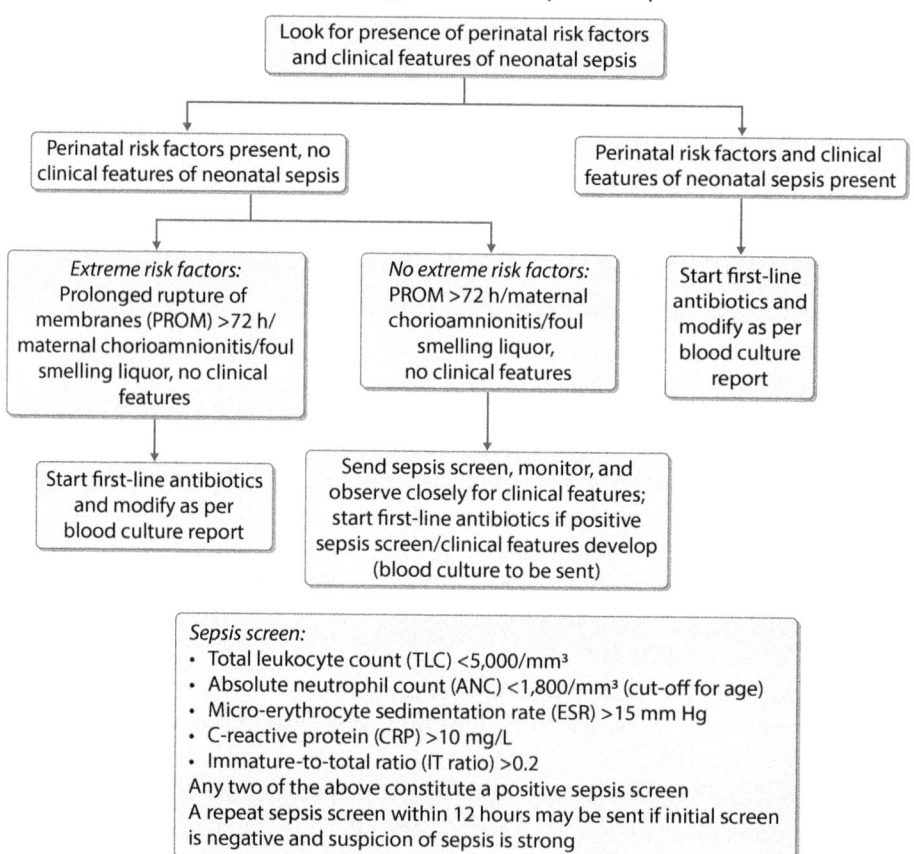

Sepsis screen:
- Total leukocyte count (TLC) <5,000/mm³
- Absolute neutrophil count (ANC) <1,800/mm³ (cut-off for age)
- Micro-erythrocyte sedimentation rate (ESR) >15 mm Hg
- C-reactive protein (CRP) >10 mg/L
- Immature-to-total ratio (IT ratio) >0.2

Any two of the above constitute a positive sepsis screen
A repeat sepsis screen within 12 hours may be sent if initial screen is negative and suspicion of sepsis is strong

Flowchart 2: Algorithm for late onset sepsis.

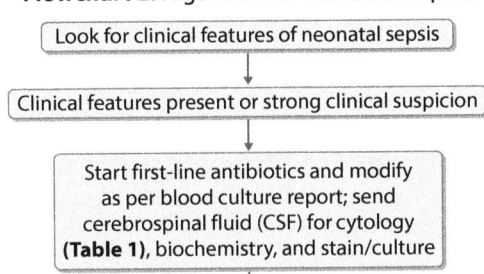

TABLE 1: Normal cerebrospinal fluid (CSF) parameters in term and preterm neonates (median with range).

CSF parameter	Term neonates	Preterm neonates
Cells/mm^3	8 (0–32)	5 (0–44)
Polymorphonuclear (PMN) (%)	60%	8% (0–66)
CSF protein (mg/dL)	90 (20–170)	148 (54–370)
CSF glucose (mg/dL)	52 (34–119)	67 (33–217)

CHAPTER 56

Neonatal Seizures

G Shridhar

- Neonatal seizures are the most striking clinical manifestation of neurological dysfunction in neonates with a significant risk of mortality and long-term morbidity. The mortality ranges from 7 to 20%, while around 30% neonates develop cerebral palsy, 15 to 35% develop epilepsy and 50% have developmental delay.
- *Epidemiology:* The incidence increases with decreasing gestational age and birth weight. The reported incidence among preterm and term neonates is 20.8 and 8.4 per 1,000 live births, respectively, while the incidence is 36.1 per 1,000 live births among very low birth weight (VLBW) neonates.
- *Definition:* A sudden alteration in motor, behavioral or autonomic activity, with or without alteration in consciousness. Neonatal seizures can be of the following types:
  - *Electrographic seizures:* Paroxysmal electrical activity that evolves over time.
  - *Electroclinical seizures:* Electrographic seizures with associated clinical signs.
    Video-electroencephalography (EEG) recordings have shown that up to 80% of electrographic seizures in neonates lack a clinical correlation and are EEG-only seizures.
- *Classification:* Traditionally, there are four clinically recognizable types of neonatal seizures:
  1. *Subtle seizures:* Often missed, these are usually mild motor, behavioral or autonomic paroxysms and the most common (50%) type:
     - *Ocular:* Tonic horizontal eye deviation (term), sustained eye opening with ocular fixation (preterm) or cycled fluttering
     - *Oro-facial-lingual movements:* Chewing, tongue thrusting, lip smacking, pouting of lips etc.
     - *Limb movements:* Cycling, rowing, paddling, swimming etc.
     - *Autonomic:* Tachycardia or bradycardia
     - Apnea may be a rare manifestation of seizures in term neonates. This is usually associated with a normal heart rate or tachycardia initially, followed later by bradycardia due to prolonged hypoxemia.
  2. *Clonic seizures:* Rhythmic movements of muscle groups with a rapid phase followed by a slow return, occurring at a frequency of 1–3 jerks/s and commonly associated with EEG changes. They may be focal clonic, multifocal clonic, or rarely generalized clonic seizures.
  3. *Tonic seizures:* Sustained flexion or extension of axial or appendicular muscle groups. They may be focal or generalized and resemble decerebrate (tonic extension of all limbs) or decorticate (flexion of upper limbs and extension of lower limbs) posturing. In about 85% cases, they are not associated with EEG changes and represent brainstem release phenomena secondary to severe brain injury.

4. *Myoclonic seizures:* Single or multiple, lightning-fast jerks of the upper or lower limbs with a predilection of flexor muscle groups. EEG correlates commonly include burst suppression, focal sharp waves, or hypsarrhythmia.

Focal clonic seizures have the best long-term prognosis, while myoclonic seizures carry the worst prognosis in terms of recurrence and neurodevelopmental outcome.

The International League Against Epilepsy (ILAE) in 2021 has classified neonatal seizures as electrical or electroclinical seizures. Clinical events without an EEG correlate have been defined as non-seizure episodes. However, many neonatal intensive care units (NICUs) in the country do not use continuous EEG recording and the clinical classification is still widely used.

- *Causes:*
  - Hypoxic ischemic encephalopathy (HIE) secondary to perinatal asphyxia (38%)
    - Most seizures manifest by 12–24 hours, the rest by 48 hours
    - Subtle seizures are the most common type.
    - Additional causes such as hypoglycemia, hypocalcemia, or intracranial hemorrhage may coexist
  - Metabolic (12–15%)
    - Hypoglycemia
    - Hypocalcemia (early and late onset)
    - Hypomagnesemia
    - Hyponatremia or hypernatremia
    - Inborn errors of metabolism
  - Intracranial hemorrhage (11%) and stroke (18%)
    - Intraventricular hemorrhage (preterm) and subarachnoid, intraparenchymal, or subdural hemorrhage (term)
    - Usually manifest between 2 and 7 days
    - Ischemic stroke and cerebral sinus venous thrombosis (CSVT) are often missed
  - Infections (5%)
    - Bacterial meningitis
    - TORCH (toxoplasmosis, rubella cytomegalovirus, herpes simplex, and HIV) infections
    - Cerebral dysgenesis (4%)
  - Miscellaneous (9%)
    - Polycythemia
    - Maternal narcotic withdrawal
    - *Drug toxicity:* Accidental injection of local anesthetic into scalp

Seizures due to subarachnoid hemorrhage and hypocalcemia have a good prognosis, while seizures due to hypoglycemia, meningitis and cerebral malformations have a high risk of poor neurodevelopmental outcome.

- *Investigations:*

Essential investigations (in all neonates)	*Additional investigations*
- Blood glucose - Serum calcium - Serum sodium - Cerebrospinal fluid (CSF) examination - Cranial ultrasound (USG) - EEG and/or amplitude-integrated EEG	- PCV (plethoric/at-risk for polycythemia) - Serum bilirubin (if icteric) - Serum magnesium - Arterial blood gas (ABG) (lethargy, vomiting, family history) - CT scan or MRI brain (as indicated) - TORCH (toxoplasmosis, rubella cytomegalovirus, herpes simplex, and HIV) screen - Workup for inborn errors of metabolism (IEM)

- The decision to stop antiepileptic drugs is individualized based on the underlying cause of neonatal seizures, neurological examination at discharge, and EEG findings (if available). The algorithm for neonatal seizures is given in **Flowchart 1**.

Flowchart 1: Algorithm for neonatal seizures.

```
                    Neonate with seizures
                            │
                            ▼
    • Ensure temperature, airway, breathing, and circulation (TABC)
    • IV access and samples for blood glucose, calcium, magnesium,
      sodium, potassium, PCV, ABG, and sepsis screen
    • Check blood glucose by bedside glucometer
                            │
            ┌───────────────┴───────────────┐
            ▼                               ▼
    Blood glucose <45 mg/dL      IV 10% dextrose bolus @ 2 mL/kg,
            │                    followed by GIR @ 6 mg/kg/min
            ▼
    IV 10% calcium gluconate @ 2 mL/kg,    IM injection 50% MgSO4 @ 0.25
    diluted 1:1 with 5% or 10% dextrose OR  mL/kg if seizures persist
    DW over 10–15 minutes under cardiac  → despite correction of
    monitoring                              hypocalcemia
            │
            ▼
    IV injection phenobarbitone 20 mg/kg infusion over 20 minutes
            │
            ▼
    Repeat IV injection phenobarbitone 10 mg/kg/dose
    aliquots until cumulative dose of 40 mg/kg is reached
            │
            ▼
    IV injection phenytoin 20 mg/kg slowly over 20 minutes under cardiac
    monitoring OR IV injection levetiracetam 20 mg/kg slowly over 20 minutes
            │
            ▼
    Repeat IV injection phenytoin 10 mg/kg OR repeat IV injection levetiracetam
    20 mg/kg/dose until a maximum dose of 60 mg/kg
            │
            ▼
    Consider IV injection lorazepam 0.05 mg/kg over 2–5 minutes
    OR IV injection midazolam 0.1 mg/kg bolus followed by
    infusion @ 1 µg/kg/minute up to 18 µg/kg/min
            │
            ▼
    Consider other anti-epileptic drug OR IV injection pyridoxine
            │
            ▼
    Wean AED slowly to maintenance phenobarbitone
```

(ABG: arterial blood gas; AED: antiepileptic drug; DW: distilled water; GIR: glucose infusion rate; IM: intramuscular; IV: intravenous; PCV: packed cell volume)

CHAPTER 57

Inborn Errors of Metabolism

Suprita Kalra

- Inborn errors of metabolisms (IEMs) involve defects in function of specific enzymes in a metabolic pathway, leading to either accumulation or deletion of metabolites.
- Early diagnosis is essential for treatment and prognostication. Treatment modalities are largely supportive except for few disorders. Low threshold for suspicion is required for early diagnosis to prevent complications.

Clinical features	1st-line investigations	2nd-line investigations
Asymptomatic except during intercurrent illness	Complete blood count	Tandem mass spectrometry for plasma amino acids and acyl carnitine—for organic acidemias, urea cycle disorders, aminoacidopathies, and fatty acid oxidation (FAO) defects
Consanguinity of parents	Blood gas analysis and electrolytes	Gas chromatography mass spectrometry of urine for organic acidemias
History of unexplained neonatal deaths in family	Blood glucose	High performance liquid chromatography for analysis of amino acids in blood/urine—for organic acidemia and aminoacidopathies
Seizures of unclear etiology and progressive encephalopathy	Plasma ammonia	Elevated arterial lactate
Severe metabolic acidosis	Arterial lactate	Urine orotic acid—urea cycle defects
Persistent vomiting	Liver function tests	Enzyme assay
Peculiar odor of urine, cerumen	Urine for ketones and reducing substances	*Neuroimaging:* Magnetic resonance imaging (MRI) for diagnosis of IEMs associated with specific central nervous system abnormalities
Acute fatty liver or hemolysis, elevated liver enzymes, and low platelets (HELLP) syndrome	Serum uric acid	Plasma very long chain fatty acids—increased in peroxisomal disorders

  - Cerebrospinal fluid (CSF) glycine levels
  - Mutation analysis

- Asymptomatic newborn with a previous sibling death with suspected IEM:
  - Baseline metabolic screen at birth followed by oral dextrose feeds
  - Repeat screening at 2nd day of life, if normal start breastfeeds with strict vigil on blood sugar, blood ammonia, blood gas, and urine ketone 6 hourly
  - Repeat screening after 48 hours of life along with samples for tandem mass spectrometry (TMS) and urine gas chromatography mass spectrometry (GCMS)

- Medium chain triglycerides in the form of medium chain triglyceride (MCT) oil may be started if tolerated by the baby.
- Monitor infant carefully for the first few months of life as late presentation of IEM is possible.

- Newborn with a suspected inborn error of metabolism **(Flowchart 1)**
- Emergency management **(Flowchart 2)**

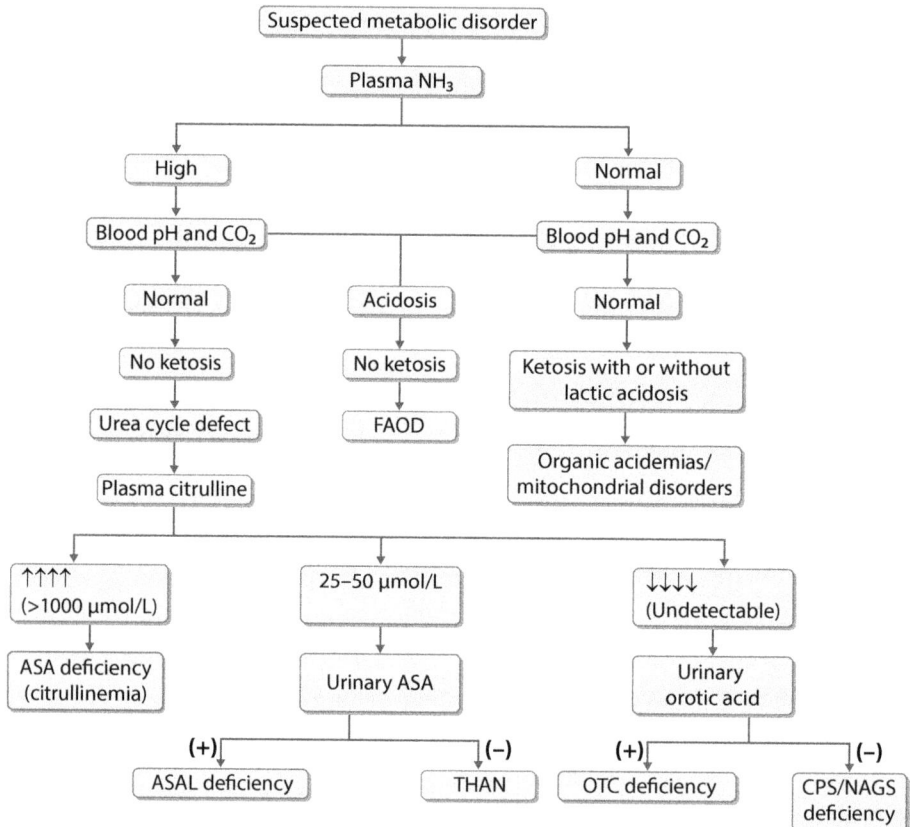

Flowchart 1: Suspected metabolic disorder.

(FAOD: fatty acid oxidation defects; PKU: phenylketonuria; NKH: nonketotic hyperglycinemia; ASA: argininosuccinic acid; OTC: ornithine transcarbamoylase; CPS: carbamoyl phosphate synthetase I; NAGS: N-acetylglutamate synthetase; THAN: transient hyperammonemia of newborn; ASAL: argininosuccinic acid lyase)

CHAPTER 57: Inborn Errors of Metabolism

Flowchart 2: Emergency management.

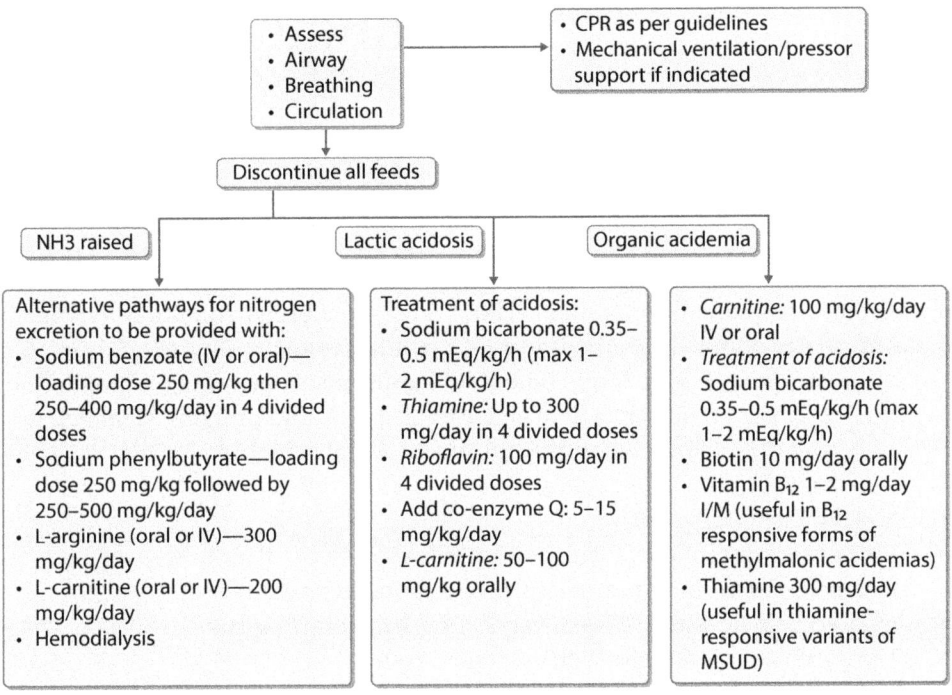

(CPR: cardiopulmonary resuscitation; IV: intravenous)

CHAPTER 58

Approach to a Child with Ambiguous Genitalia

Sarguna K Logen

- *Disorders of sexual development:*
  - Disorder of sexual development (DSD) represents broad condition in which there is atypical development of chromosomal, gonadal, or anatomical sex. Around 6–7 weeks of age, urogenital ridge forms bipotential gonads and then the differentiation occurs which is based on presence or absence of *SRY* gene and proteins, signaling molecules, endocrine stimuli. Incidence ranges from 1:1,500 live births.
- *When to suspect:*
  - Bilateral cryptorchidism
  - Unilateral cryptorchidism with hypospadias
  - Bilateral testes with perineoscrotal/penoscrotal hypospadias
  - Apparent female with clitoromegaly (>1 cm)/inguinal hernia
  - Overtly abnormal genitals such as cloacal exstrophy
  - Asymmetry of labioscrotal folds
  - Micropenis
- Etiological classification of disorder of sexual development
  - *46,XX disorder of sexual development*

Excess androgen production: • 21 alpha hydroxylase deficiency • 11 beta hydroxylase deficiency • 3 beta hydroxysteroid dehydrogenase type 2 deficiency	*Defect in androgen metabolism:* – Placental-fetal aromatase deficiency • *Maternal steroid exposure:* – Maternal androgen production – Progestational agents
• Ovotesticular DSD • 46,XX (70%) • 46,XY (10%) • 46,XX/46,XY	*Sex chromosome DSD:* • 45,XO sex chromosomal • 47,XXY sex chromosome aneuploidy • 46,XX testicular DSD • 46,XY complete gonadal dysgenesis

The events involved in sex determination and differentiation are shown in **Flowchart 1**.

Flowchart 1: Events involved in sex determination and differentiation.

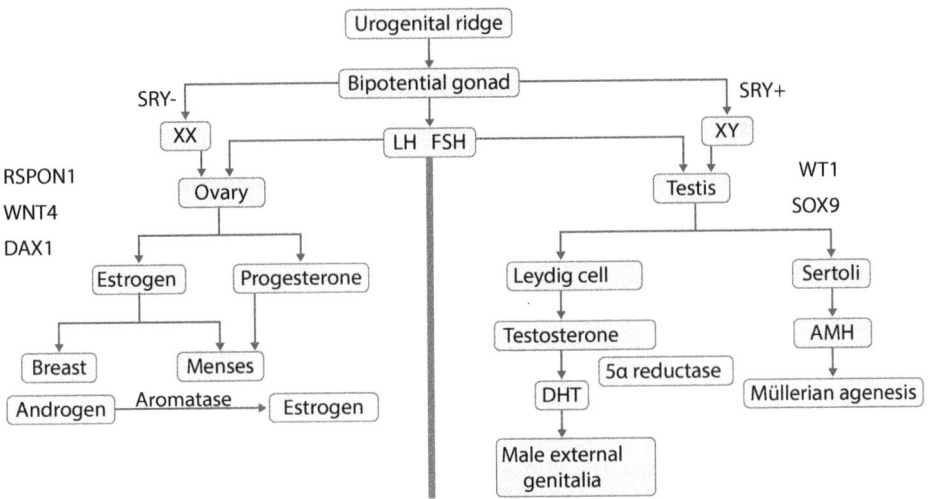

(AMH: anti-Müllerian hormone; DHT: dihydrotestosterone; FSH: follicle-stimulating hormone; LH: luteinizing hormone)

- **46,XY disorder of sexual development**
    - *Defects in testosterone production:*
        - Leydig cell hypoplasia or agenesis (human chorionic gonadotropin (hCG)/LH receptor mutation)
        - Testicular 17 beta hydroxysteroid dehydrogenase type 3 deficiency
        - Defects in testicular and adrenal steroidogenesis [steroidogenic acute regulatory protein (StAR)] protein deficiency, 3 beta hydroxysteroid dehydrogenase deficiency, 17 alpha/17,20 lyase deficiency
    - *Defects in testosterone metabolism:*
        - 5 alpha reductase type 2 deficiency
    - *Defects in testosterone action:*
        - Complete androgen insensitivity syndrome
        - Partial androgen insensitivity syndrome
    - *Defect in testicular development:*
        - Denys–Drash syndrome
        - Wilms tumor, aniridia, genitourinary malformations and a range of mental disabilities (WAGR)
        - XY pure gonadal dysgenesis
        - Mutation in *SRY* gene
    - Persistent mullerian duct syndrome

Clinical importance of history in disorder of sexual development
- **Consanguinity,** order of birth, sibling history/*antenatal history:* Maternal drugs/increased facial hair/acne in pregnancy.
- **Birth history:** Progressive weight loss, failure to thrive, salt wasting features (CAH). Childhood—inguinal hernia in a girl child with bilateral undescended testes, abnormal position of urethral meatus, and small penis (46,XY DSD).
- **Adolescence:** Failure to develop puberty or attain menarche, virilization at puberty or infertility (46,XY DSD).
- **Family history:** Unexplained neonatal death, ambiguous genitalia, infertility, primary amenorrhea, short stature.

Genital examination
- *Clitoromegaly:* Clitoral index >35 mm^2, clitoral length >9 mm/labioscrotal fold and scrotal rugosity/site of palpable gonads/anogenital ratio—ratio of the distance between the anus and posterior fourchette divided by the distance between the anus and clitoris, >0.5 suggestive of virilization/posterior labial fusion.

Defect in steroid synthesis: Congenital adrenal hyperplasia includes a group of disorders with deranged adrenal corticosteroid biosynthesis due to deficiency one or multiple enzymes [21α-hydroxylase (most common cause of ambiguous genitalia, it is an emergency)/11 beta-hydroxylase/3 beta hydroxysteroid dehydrogenase/17 alpha hydroxylase and cholesterol desmolase]. Most common DSD in neonatal period is 46XX CAH with virilization with features of severe adrenal insufficiency and shock (with or without salt wasting crisis).

Clinical features:
- Congenital adrenal hyperplasia (CAH) presents as an acute life-threatening illness in neonates. Lethargy, poor feeding, vomiting, abdominal pain, features of shock. History of preceding viral/minor illness.

1st-line investigations	2nd-line testing
• Plasma glucose, electrolytes, 17 OH-P, ACTH, CORTISOL • Dehydroepiandrosterone (DHEA), testosterone, androstenedione, DHT, plasma renin secretion • Karyotyping/FISH/USG pelvis—Gonads Mullerian structures • Hormonal work up LH, FSH, AMH, estrogen • Human chorionic gonadotropin (hCG) stimulation tests	• MRI pelvis • T/DHT ratio/cystourethrography • Gonadal biopsy-detects steroidogenic defects such as congenital adrenal hyperplasia (CAH)

Treatment:
- Maintain airway, breathing, and circulation.
- Restoration of hydration by IV fluids using a wide bore needle. Infusion of isotonic saline at 20 mL/kg over 10 minutes, if signs of shock are present (maximum up to 60 mL/kg), fluid replacement to be decided by clinical signs of shock. In newborns, 1.5–2 times fluid maintenance therapy can be given (half normal saline in 5% dextrose solution).
- Correction of hypoglycemia (5 mL/kg of 10% dextrose in case of low blood sugar)
- Glucocorticoid replacement is the cornerstone, IV hydrocortisone at 50–100 mg/m^2 bolus followed by 50–100 mg/m^2/day in divided doses (6 hourly). 25 mg bolus followed by 5–6 mg every 6 hourly. Fludrocortisone is used for infants with classical CAH.
- Correction of electrolytes/intake output monitoring/restriction of salt.
  The algorithm of 21α-hydroxylase deficiency is given in **Flowchart 2**.
  The algorithm of 11β-hydroxylase deficiency is given in **Flowchart 3**.

Goals of management in all disorders of sexual development—multidisciplinary team involvement
- Urgent detection of underlying endocrinopathy and management/gender assignment/psychological assessment/psychosocial support to parents.

CHAPTER 58: Approach to a Child with Ambiguous Genitalia

Medical management in disorders of sexual development

Drug used	Indication
• Testosterone (IM/oral/transdermal) • Topical dihydrotestosterone (DHT) cream • Estrogen replacement	• Testosterone biosynthetic defects • 5-alpha reductase deficiency • Complete androgen insensitivity syndrome (AIS) (after gonadectomy)

Surgical management

- Clitoral reduction surgery should only be considered in cases of severe virilization (Prader III, IV, and V) in 46,XX by 1 year. Orchidopexy should be performed 6–12 months. Reconstructive surgery—options left for future by avoiding irreversible surgeries until child can give consent.

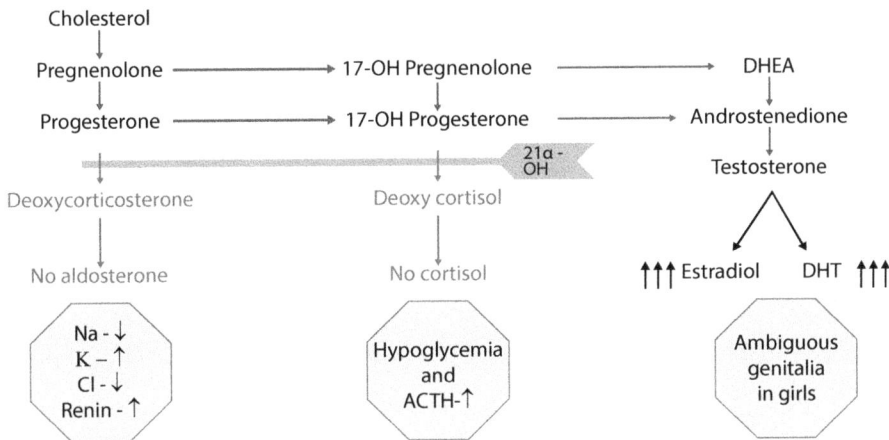

Flowchart 2: 21α–hydroxylase deficiency.

(ACTH: adrenocorticotropic hormone; DHEA: dehydroepiandrosterone; DHT: dihydrotestosterone)

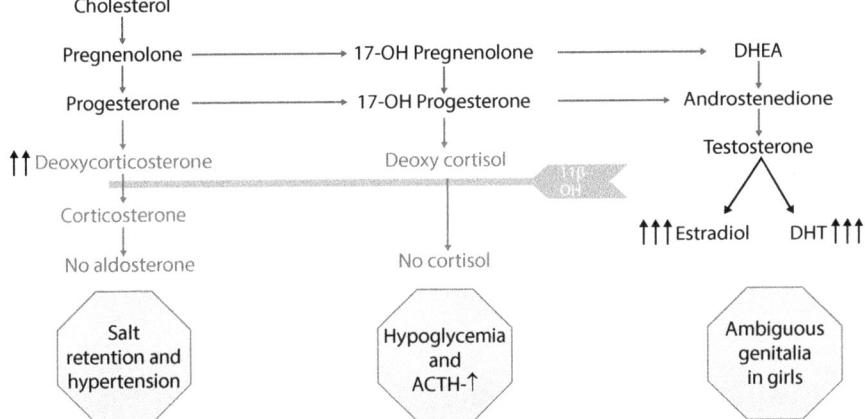

Flowchart 3: 11β–hydroxylase deficiency.

(ACTH: adrenocorticotropic hormone; DHEA: dehydroepiandrosterone; DHT: dihydrotestosterone)

SECTION 10

Infections

- **Severe Dengue**
  Anjali Gautam
- **Complicated Malaria**
  Sucheta K Menon
- **Rickettsial Disease**
  Giridharan

CHAPTER 59: Severe Dengue

Anjali Gautam

- Dengue fever is one of the common causes of fever in children. It is caused by dengue virus which belongs to the Flaviviridae family and has four serotypes.
- Based on the clinical symptoms and signs, dengue fever is further classified as dengue with or without warning signs. The warning signs of dengue are:
  - Pain abdomen or tenderness on palpation
  - Fluid accumulation in third space (pleural effusion, ascites)
  - Persistent vomiting
  - Bleeding from mucosal sites
  - Lethargy, restlessness
  - Increase in liver size of >2 cm
  - Laboratory increase in hematocrit (HCT) along with rapid decline in platelet count
- Severe dengue is a term used to denote shock due to plasma leak or severe bleeding or severe organ involvement.
- Principle of management is mainly based on initial classification at the time of presentation, based on which the patient is classified into different groups as given in **Flowchart 1**:
  - Management of dengue with shock is given in **Flowcharts 2 and 3**

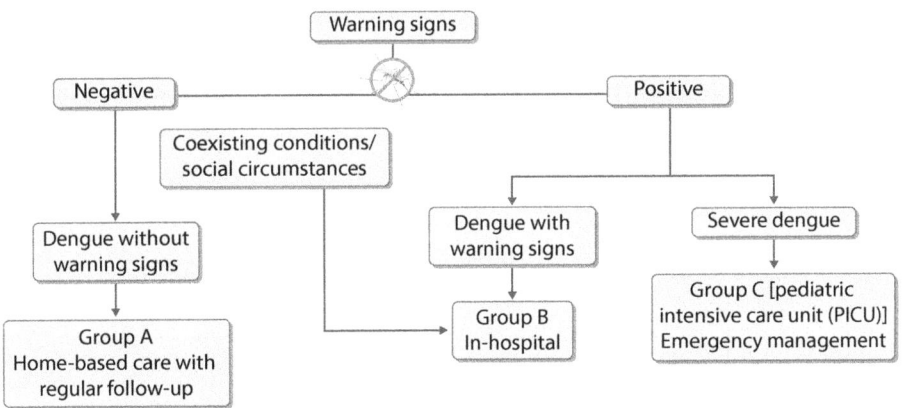

Flowchart 1: Classification of dengue based on warning signs.

Flowchart 2: Management of compensated shock.

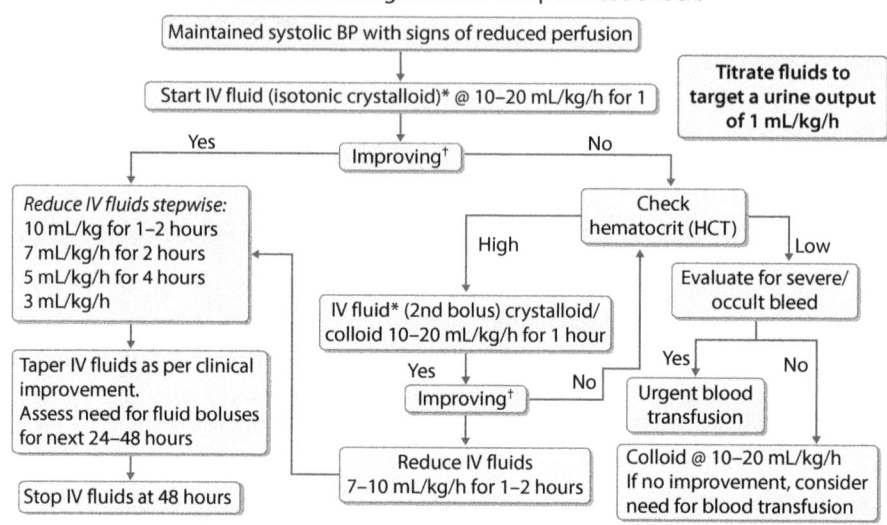

*In cases where child has already received crystalloid, colloid is preferable.
†Reassess the patients vital signs, temperature of peripheries, capillary refill time, pulse pressure, and sensorium.
(BP: blood pressure; IV: intravenous)

Flowchart 3: Management of hypotensive shock.

*In cases where child has already received crystalloid, colloid is preferable.
†Reassess the patients vital signs, temperature of peripheries, capillary refill time, pulse pressure, and sensorium.
(ABG: arterial blood gas; IV: intravenous; RBS: random blood sugar; VBS: venous blood gas)
Source: Adapted from World Health Organization. (2009). Dengue guidelines for diagnosis, treatment, prevention, and control.

CHAPTER 60: Complicated Malaria

Sucheta K Menon

- Complicated malaria is most commonly caused by infection with *Plasmodium falciparum*, risk of which is increased if treatment of an uncomplicated attack of malaria is delayed. Sometimes, however, especially in children, severe *P. falciparum* malaria may develop so rapidly that early treatment of uncomplicated malaria is not feasible.
- *Risk factors:*
  - Young children
  - Visitors (of any age) from nonendemic areas
  - Second and third trimesters of pregnancy
  - Immunocompromised states like HIV/AIDS (human immunodeficiency virus/acquired immunodeficiency syndrome)
  - Postsplenectomy status
  - *Low endemicity:* Parasitemia >2.5%/>20% in any endemicity
- *Clinical features:* Complicated malaria is defined by clinical or laboratory evidence of vital organ dysfunction (one or more of the criteria in the presence of asexual parasitemia)

  - Impaired consciousness
  - Prostration
  - *Seizures:* More than two episodes in 24 hours
  - Respiratory distress/pulmonary edema
  - Shock
  - Acute kidney injury (AKI)
  - Jaundice + signs of other organ dysfunction
  - Abnormal bleeding

- *Laboratory features:*

  - Hypoglycemia (<40 g/dL)
  - Metabolic acidosis
  - Severe normocytic anemia [hemoglobin (Hb) <5 g/dL, packed cell volume (PCV) <15% in children]
  - Hemoglobinuria
  - Hyperlactatemia (lactate >5 mmol/L)
  - Renal impairment
  - Pulmonary edema (radiological)

- *Diagnosis:*
  - *Diagnosis of malaria:*
    - *Microscopy:* Gold standard
    - Rapid diagnostic tests

- *Cerebral malaria:*
    - *Earliest symptom:* Fever, failure to feed, vomiting, lethargy
    - Altered sensorium (coma), seizures, retinal changes
    - Transient abnormalities of eye movement
    - Bruxism
    - *Motor abnormalities:* Decerebrate and decorticate rigidity

The treatment of malaria is given in **Flowchart 1**.

Flowchart 1: Treatment of severe malaria.

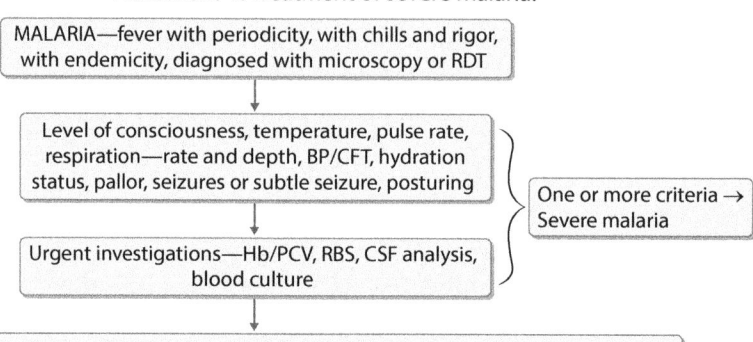

Drug	Dosage
Artesunate	2.4 mg/kg IV stat → @ 12 hours, @ 24 hours, then once a day, once able to swallow, the complete course of 7 days with: • Artesunate + sulfadoxine–pyrimethamine in all states other than northeast • Artemether + lumefantrine in northeastern state
Artemether	3.2 mg/kg → 1.6 mg/kg daily once the patient is able to swallow, complete the course: • Artesunate + sulfadoxine–pyrimethamine in all states other than northeast • Artemether + lumefantrine in northeastern state
Quinine salt	LD—20 mg salt/kg by infusion over 4 hours MD—10 mg salt/kg q 8 hours × 7 days Tetracycline or doxycycline or clindamycin added as soon as patient able to swallow for 7 days

(BP: blood sugar; CFT: capillary filling time; CSF: cerebrospinal fluid; Hb: hemoglobin; LD: loading dose; IV: intravenous; MD: maintenance dose; NG: nasogastric; PCV: packed cell volume; RBS: random blood sugar; RDT: rapid diagnostic test)

CHAPTER 61: Rickettsial Disease

Giridharan

- Rickettsial disease is a zoonotic disease caused by a gram-negative bacteria belonging to order Rickettsiales and family Rickettsiaceae. It is an obligate intracellular parasite.
- It is one of the of emerging and reemerging diseases. Humans are the accidental hosts. They are classified as follows:

Typhus group	Scrub typhus (endemic in India)	Spotted fever group	Others
• Epidemic typhus • Murine typhus	• *Agent: Rickettsia tsutsugamushi* • *Vector:* Mite • *Mammalian reservoir:* Rodent	• Indian tick typhus • Rocky mountain spotted fever	• Rickettsial pox • Q fever • Trench fever • Ehrlichiosis • Anaplasmosis

- The disease has a wide spectrum of presentation posing a challenge in diagnosis. Usual clues to diagnosis are as follows:

  One or more of the following:
  - Fever without focus for >5 days
  - Toxic-looking child with unclear etiology
  - Fever associated with any of the following—rash or eschar or edema or headache with myalgia or organomegaly or lymph node enlargement
  - Fever with multisystem involvement like acute kidney injury or hepatitis or pneumonia/pulmonary infiltrates/gastrointestinal (GI) involvement
  - Features resembling other tropical diseases

- Workup

Hematological and biochemical parameters	• Thrombocytopenia/leukopenia (neutropenia) • Elevated transaminases/hyponatremia/hypoalbuminemia
Serology (in the second week of illness)	• *Gold standard:* Immunofluorescence antibody • Fourfold rise in two serum samples, 2–4 weeks apart • *Weil–Felix:* Titers >1:80 on a single occasion is significant (low sensitivity and high specificity) • *IgM ELISA:* Highly sensitive and specific
Polymerase chain reaction	• In first week of diagnosis • Done on whole blood, eschar or skin biopsy, and eschar scrapings
Chest X-ray	Bilateral lung infiltrates
RGA scoring system may be utilized; score >14 significant	
(IgM ELISA: immunoglobulin M enzyme-linked immunosorbent assay; RGA: Rathi–Goodman–Aghai)	

- Differential diagnosis

Viral etiology	*Enterovirus*, measles, dengue, chikungunya, and infectious mononucleosis
Bacterial diseases	Enteric fever, meningococcemia, leptospirosis, scarlet fever, syphilis, and infective endocarditis
Protozoal diseases	Malaria
Noninfective causes	Kawasaki disease and thrombotic thrombocytopenic purpura

- *Management*:
  - Start empirical treatment with high index of suspicion, not to wait till laboratory confirmation
  - More emphasis on clinical parameters rather than laboratory-based results
  - *Drug of choice:* Doxycycline
    - *Route:* Oral or intravenous
    - *Dose:* 40 kg to 100 mg twice daily
    - *Duration:* Total of 7 days or 3 days of afebrile period or 10 days in complicated cases
  - Other drugs:
    - Oral clarithromycin or azithromycin
    - Chloramphenicol
    - Azithromycin—dose at 10 mg/kg/day for 5 days
  - If no improvement in 48 hours after starting antibiotics, consider alternate diagnosis or doxycycline resistant strains.
  - Continue management of complications

  Approach to rickettsial disease is given in **Flowchart 1**.

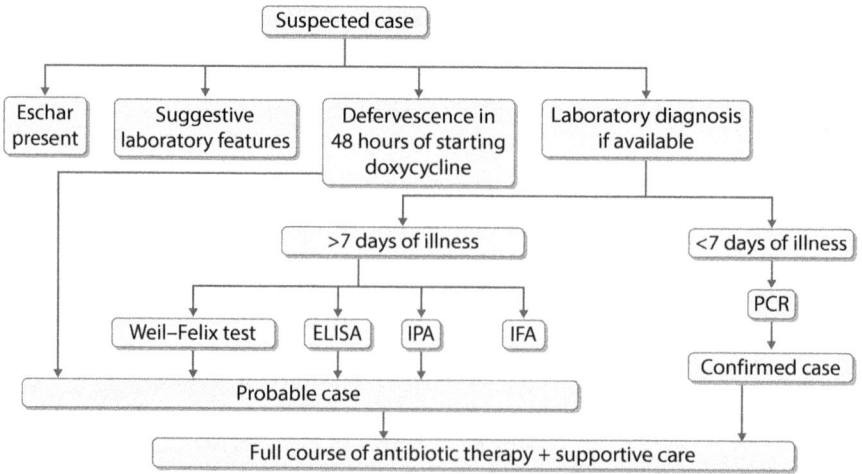

Flowchart 1: Approach to rickettsial disease.

(ELISA: enzyme-linked immunosorbent assay; IFA: immunofluorescence assay; IPA: immunoperoxidase assay; PCR: polymerase chain reaction)

SECTION 11

Toxicology and Environmental Hazards

- ◈ **Clinical Approach to a Suspected Case of Poisoning**
  Sachendra Badal, Shuvendu Roy
- ◈ **Hydrocarbon Poisoning**
  Sachendra Badal, Shuvendu Roy
- ◈ **Acetaminophen Toxicity**
  Sachendra Badal, Shuvendu Roy
- ◈ **Organophosphorus Poisoning**
  Sachendra Badal, Shuvendu Roy
- ◈ **Iron Poisoning**
  Sachendra Badal, Shuvendu Roy
- ◈ **Snake Bite Treatment Protocol**
  Sachendra Badal, Shuvendu Roy
- ◈ **Approach to Scorpion Bite**
  Sachendra Badal, Shuvendu Roy
- ◈ **Drowning**
  Suprita Kalra, Ranjit Ghuliani
- ◈ **Burns**
  Ranjit Ghuliani, Suprita Kalra
- ◈ **Electrical Injuries**
  Sarvesh Kohli

Clinical Approach to a Suspected Case of Poisoning

CHAPTER 62

Sachendra Badal, Shuvendu Roy

- Most of the pediatric poisoning is accidental. Suspect this in the following situations:
  - Encephalopathy, acidosis, shock, multiple organ dysfunction syndrome (MODS)
  - Circumstantial evidences
  - History of ingestion of poisonous substance
- *Clinical clues to suggest poisoning:* These are given in **Table 1**.
- *Different toxidromes are helpful to identify the toxin*: These are given in **Table 2**.

TABLE 1: Clinical clues to suggest poisoning.	
Odor	
Garlic	Organophosphates
Camphor	Mothballs
Bitter almond	Cyanides
Acetone	Salicylate
Skin	
Cyanosis	Nitrates, nitrites
Sweating	Organophosphates, scorpion bite
Dry	Anticholinergic
Bullae	Barbiturates
Jaundice	Acetaminophen
Purpura	Aspirin, snake bite, warfarin
Temperature	
Hypothermia	Sedatives, hypnotics, alcohol
Hyperthermia	Anticholinergic, salicylates, theophyllines
Pulse	
Bradycardia	Digitalis, beta blocker, sedatives, hypnotics, scorpion bite
Tachycardia	Anticholinergic, sympathomimetics (decongestants), theophyllines
Respiration	
Depressed	Sedatives, hypnotics, barbiturates, alcohol
Tachypnea	Salicylates, scorpion bite
Kussmaul	Methanol, salicylates
Wheezing	Organophosphates
Pneumonia	Hydrocarbons
Blood pressure	
Hypertension	Sympathomimetics (decongestants), organophosphates
Hypotension	Sedatives, hypnotics, alcohol, beta blocker

Contd...

Contd...

Ocular signs

Miosis	Sedatives, hypnotics, organophosphates, opioids
Mydriasis	Alcohol, atropine
Nystagmus	Phenytoin, barbiturates
Lacrimation	Organophosphates, irritant gases, scorpion bite
Poor vision	Methanol
Ptosis	Snake bite

Oral signs

Salivation	Organophosphates, salicylates
Dry mouth	Anticholinergics, antihistaminics

Intestinal signs

Cramps	Organophosphates
Diarrhea	Iron, arsenic
Constipation	Narcotics, lead
Hematemesis	Iron, salicylates, corrosives, theophyllines

Central nervous system (CNS) signs

Ataxia	Alcohol, antidepressants, anticholinergics, phenytoin
Coma	Sedatives, hypnotics, barbiturates, organophosphates, salicylates
Altered behavior	Anticholinergics, alcohol
Fasciculation	Organophosphates, theophyllines
Increased tone	Anticholinergics, phenothiazines, tricyclic antidepressants (TCAs), haloperidol
Seizure	Carbamazepine, aminophylline, organophosphates, salicylates

TABLE 2: Toxidromes for identification of toxin.

	Adrenergic	Anticholinergic	Anticholinesterase (cholinergic)	Opioids	Sedatives hypnotics
Heart rate	Increased	Increased	Decreased	Decreased	• Arrhythmia • QT prolongation
Temperature	Increased	Increased	No change	No change	No change
Pupil	Dilated	Dilated	Constricted	Constricted	Dilated
Mucosa	Wet	Dry	Wet	No change	No change
Skin	Diaphoresis	Dry	Diaphoresis	Normal or low	No change
Respiratory	Tachypnea	• Tachypnea • Secretion ++	• Tachypnea • Wheeze	Hypoventilation	Hypoventilation
Neurologic	Agitated, tremors, seizures, hallucinations	Agitated, hallucinations	Coma, fasciculation	Sedations	Convulsion, coma, hyperreflexia
Examples	• Cough/decongestants • Amphetamine, cocaine	Antihistaminics, tricyclic antidepressant	Organophosphates, carbamates	Morphine derivatives	Benzodiazepines

CHAPTER 62: Clinical Approach to a Suspected Case of Poisoning

- *General management of a suspected case of poisoning:*
  - Supportive care is the mainstay of management in any poisoning.
  - Initial stabilization and basic life support (PRIORITY).
  - After stabilization of airway, breathing, circulation (ABC), main goals for the management of a patient with suspected poisoning are:
    - Preventing absorption
    - Enhance excretion
    - Specific antidote
  - Circumstantial history and physical examination
  - Initial sampling for drug/toxins:
    - Gastric aspirate
    - Blood
    - Urine
- Clues on investigations and possible poisoning are given in **Table 3**.
- *Prevention of further absorption of poison*:
  - Dilution:
    - *Skin decontamination:* Remove cloth and wash with copious water and soap (corrosive poison, organophosphates)
    - *Ocular decontamination:* Irrigate with plenty of free-flow water for 20 minutes
    - *Respiratory decontamination:* Move the patient to fresh air and provide oxygen
  - *Gastrointestinal decontamination:* Majority of poison is ingested. So this is the most important decontamination.
    - *Emesis:* It is not recommended for the very young children.
    - *Gastric lavage:* It has very limited role and should only be used in older children in selected circumstances (iron, lithium, TCAs, calcium channel blocker) with proper care of airway; 10–15 mL/kg of saline or water can be used.

TABLE 3: Investigations and clues.

Investigation	Possible poisoning
Hypoglycemia	Alcohol, OHA, salicylates, INH
Hyperglycemia	Iron, theophyllines, calcium channel blocker, salicylates
Hypocalcemia	Ethelene glycol
Hypokalemia	Beta agonist, diuretics
Hyperkalemia	Beta blocker, digoxin
Metabolic acidosis	Methanol, iron, INH, alcohol, salicylate
Radiopaque substances in X-ray	Chloral hydrate, $CaCO_3$, heavy metals, irons, phenothiazines, play-doh, enteric-coated tablet, dental amalgam
Pneumonia, pulmonary edema in chest X-ray	Hydrocarbon, irritant gas, CO, cyanides
ECG abnormality	Anticholinergics, antihistaminics, theophylline, beta blocker, digoxin, calcium channel blocker

(CO: carbon monoxide; ECG: electrocardiogram; INH: isoniazid; OHA: oral hypoglycemic agent)

- *Whole-bowel irrigation:* It is done by instilling polyethylene glycol electrolyte solution, @ 30 mL/kg. It removes sustained released agents, iron, and foreign body. It is used with care for the risk of dehydration and dyselectrolytemia.
- *Binding agents:* Ingested liquids are absorbed within 30–45 minutes and the solids are absorbed within 1–2 hours. Gastrointestinal decontamination, mentioned above, is therefore not very useful in most circumstances.
    - Activated charcoal is used @ 1 g/kg and it adsorbs most toxins (except iron, heavy metals, alcohol, lithium). It is usually administered in a slurry form through nasogastic (NG) tube with proper care of airway.
    - Other agents (kaolin–pectin, fuller's earth) are less effective.
- *Enhanced elimination of the already absorbed poison*:
    - *Diuresis:* Renal clearance of the toxins is achieved by increasing urine volume and altering the urinary pH. Increasing the pH of urine by IV bicarbonate augments the elimination of weak acids (salicylates, phenobarbitone).
    - *Dialysis:* Hemodialysis is more effective than peritoneal dialysis. Substances removed by dialysis are alcohol, methanol, ethylene glycol, salicylates, and theophylline.
    - *Hemoperfusion:* Blood is pumped through activated charcoal. It is preferred method for removal of substances such as phenytoin, carbamazepines, theophyllines, and phenobarbital.
- Inactivating the action of already bound toxin/poison by specific antidotes **(Table 4)**
- *Prevention of reexposure*:
    - Health education regarding poisoning is to be stressed during well-baby clinic visit.

TABLE 4: Poison and their antidotes.

Poison	Antidotes
Acetaminophen	N-acetylcysteine
Anticholinergic	Physostigmine
Benzodiazepines	Flumazenil
Digoxin	Digoxin immune antibody
Opioids	Naloxone
Organophosphates	Atropine, pralidoxime
Salicylates	Sodium bicarbonate
Iron	Deferoxamine
Sulfonylurea	Octreotide, glucagon
Beta blocker, calcium channel blocker	Atropine, glucagon
Warfarin	Vitamin K
Phenothiazines	Diphenhydramine
Methanol, ethylene glycol	Fomepizole, ethanol
Carbon monoxide	Oxygen
Cyanide	Amyl nitrite

- Medications, insecticides, pesticides, alcohol, kerosene oil, cleaning agents, detergents, cosmetics, and perfumes are to be kept beyond the reach of the children.
- Toxic nonconsumable liquids should never be stored in the conventional soft drink bottles.
- Adolescence with suicidal poisoning or drug addiction needs to be counseled properly before discharge.

Utilize AIIMS Poison Information Helpline
Poison Information Centre: 1800116117 (toll free) and 011-26593677, 26589391, (functions round the clock)

CHAPTER 63: Hydrocarbon Poisoning

Sachendra Badal, Shuvendu Roy

- *Introduction:*
  - Petroleum distillate hydrocarbons are present in many household products. The most important adverse effect of hydrocarbons is aspiration pneumonitis.
  - Substances with low viscosity and high volatility (kerosene, gasoline, mineral spirits, lighter fluid/naphtha, lamp oil, and kerosene) rapidly spread and cover a large area of lungs when aspirated. The most common accidental poisoning is due to kerosene.
- *Clinical features:*
  - Cough is the first clinical finding followed by dyspnea. Cough usually begins within 2-5 minutes of the aspiration.
  - Following aspiration patient may deteriorate in the next 24–72 hours with resolution of symptoms in 3–6 days.
  - Mechanism of pulmonary injury is by inflammation, capillary leaking, alveolar edema, and hemorrhage. It reduces the activity and production of surfactant leading to respiratory failure. Respiratory failure is the most common cause of death.
  - Fever occurs (within 24 hours is because of direct tissue toxicity and not infection) and may persist for as long as 10 days after aspiration. Accompanying leukocytosis is usually due to chemical pneumonitis.
  - *Central nervous system (CNS) manifestations:* Initial transient mild CNS depression is common after hydrocarbon ingestion. Subsequent CNS manifestations including lethargy, irritability, confusion, seizures, and coma are due to hypoxia.
  - *Other manifestations:* Hepatic involvement (chlorinated hydrocarbon), renal tubular damages, myocardial toxicity, bone marrow depression
- *Management:*
  - Ensure airway, breathing, circulation (ABC)
  - Chest X-ray should be done after 6 hours of ingestion in asymptomatic patient and immediately in symptomatic patient.
  - Emesis/gastric lavage is contraindicated.
  - If gastric lavage is to be performed (in case of large-volume ingestion exceeding 1 mL/kg and ingestion of highly toxic hydrocarbons or with co-mixed poisons), the patient should be intubated with a cuffed tube to protect the airway from further aspiration.
  - All gastrointestinal (GI) decontamination procedures are contraindicated in hydrocarbon poisoning (high risk of aspiration and ineffective).
  - Management of respiratory failure is mainly supportive. All symptomatic patients should receive humidified oxygen.

- Noninvasive ventilation (NIV) [high-flow nasal cannula (HFNC), bilevel positive airway pressure (BiPAP)] may be required if child develops features of respiratory distress.
- Corticosteroids and prophylactic antibiotics have no role.

Management of a patient presenting with exposure to hydrocarbon is given in **Flowchart 1**.

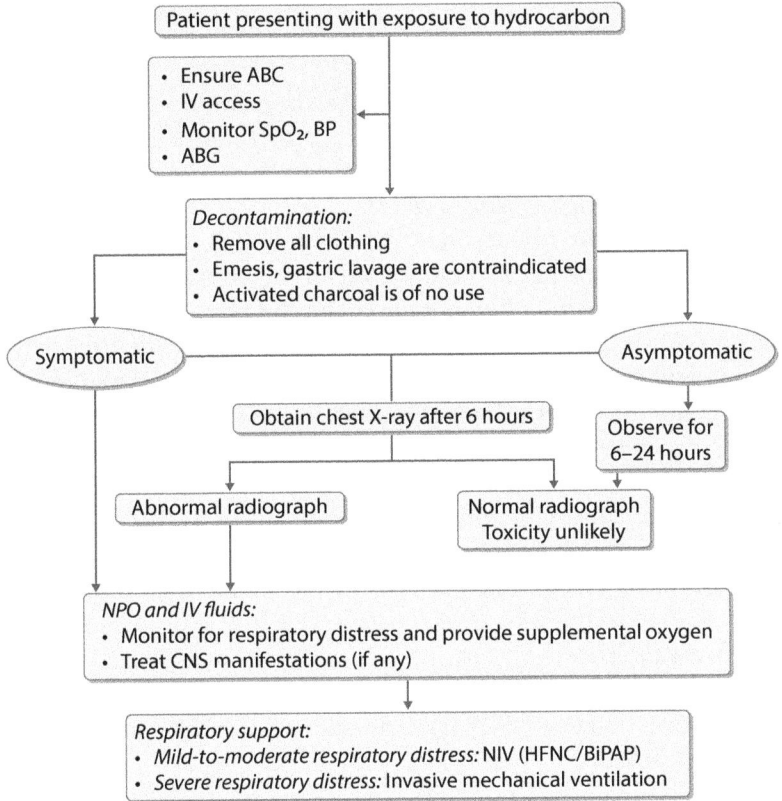

Flowchart 1: Management of a patient presenting with exposure to hydrocarbon.

(ABC: airway, breathing, circulation; ABG: arterial blood gas; BP: blood pressure; CNS: central nervous system; HFNC: high-flow nasal cannula; IV: intravenous; NPO: nil by mouth; SpO$_2$: peripheral oxygen saturation)

CHAPTER 64: Acetaminophen Toxicity

Sachendra Badal, Shuvendu Roy

- *Introduction:*
  - Acetaminophen is a safe antipyretic/analgesic drug available over the counter.
  - Toxic dose is generally considered to be:
    - *Acute ingestion:* >200 mg/kg
    - *Repeated supratherapeutic ingestion:*
      - 200 mg/kg or more over a single 24-hour period, or
      - 150 mg/kg or more per 24-hour period for the preceding 48 hours, or
      - 100 mg/kg or more per 24-hour period for the preceding 72 hours or longer
  - Acetaminophen is predominantly metabolized by *conjugation* with sulfate and glucuronide and 5–10% of the drug is *oxidized* by CYP450-dependent pathways to a toxic metabolite, N-acetyl-p-benzoquinone imine (NAPQI). NAPQI is immediately bound by intracellular glutathione and eliminated in the urine as mercapturic adducts. With increased paracetamol doses, greater production of NAPQI may deplete glutathione stores. When glutathione depletion reaches a critical level, NAPQI binds to other proteins, causing damage to the hepatocyte.
- *Clinical features:* Acetaminophen intoxication typically includes four stages as shown in **Table 1**.
- *Laboratory investigations:*
  - Complete blood count, platelet
  - Glucose, liver function test (LFT), renal function test (RFT), electrolytes
  - Coagulation parameter
  - Urinalysis
  - Drug level at or after 4 hours

TABLE 1: Stages of acetaminophen intoxication.

Stage I (<24 hours)	Stage II (24–72 hours)	Stage III (72–96 hours)	Stage IV (4 days to 2 weeks)
• Asymptomatic • Anorexia • Nausea • Vomiting • Diaphoresis • Pallor	• Resolution of stage I symptoms • Right upper quadrant pain • *LFT:* Elevated liver enzymes • Oliguria	*Worsening with:* • Coagulopathy • Jaundice • Encephalopathy • Renal failure • Myocardial pathology, death	Complete resolution of hepatic dysfunction

- The same investigations need repeating daily for a minimum of 48 hours postingestion. Normal results at 48 hours exclude hepatic damage.
- *Management:*
  - Ensure airway, breathing, and circulation (ABC).
  - *Confirm following information:*
    - The maximum possible dose and calculation of the dose per kg
    - The time of ingestion
    - Possible other drugs ingested
    - Risk factors that may lead to increased hepatotoxicity (fasting, taking other hepatotoxic drugs)
- A minimum of two plasma acetaminophen concentrations should be obtained. The first at least 4 hours after the exposure and a second sample 4-6 hours after the first sample. This is plotted in Rumack–Matthew Nomogram **(Fig. 1)**.
- If it is above the treatment line, decontamination followed by further management is to be started.
- There is no role for gastric lavage in ingestion of paracetamol syrup. Most of the drug is absorbed within 15 minutes of intake. Activated charcoal can be administered within 1 hour of ingestion of tablets.

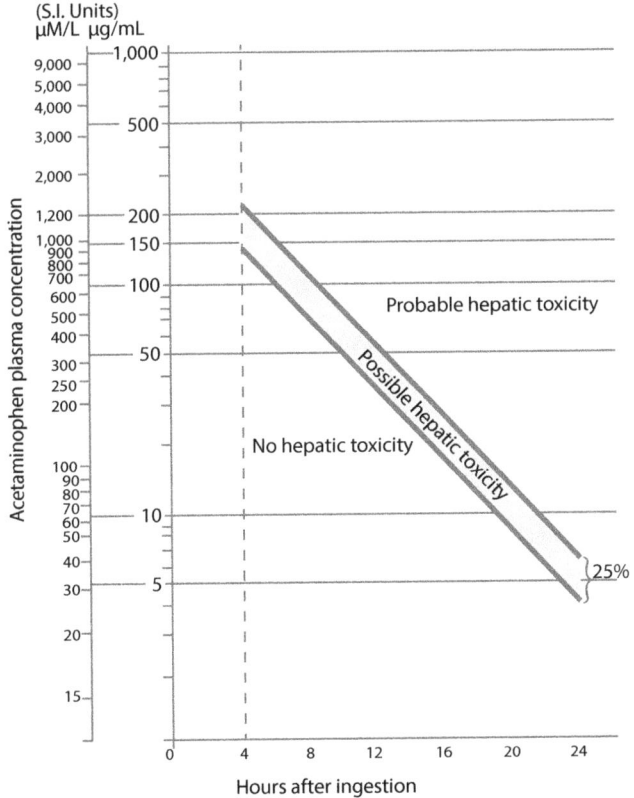

Fig. 1: Rumack–Matthew nomogram.

- Correction of hypoglycemia by glucose infusion
- *Antidote—N-acetylcysteine (NAC):* NAC serves as a precursor for hepatic glutathione synthesis, replenishes glutathione stores, and prevents the reaction of NAPQI with hepatocytes.
    - *Oral:* 140 mg/kg loading dose, followed by an additional 17 doses of 70 mg/kg every 4 hours (for a total of 1330 mg/kg over 72 hours)
    - *Intravenous (IV):* initial IV loading dose of 150 mg/kg is infused over 15–60 minutes, followed by an initial maintenance dose of 50 mg/kg infused over 4 hours, followed by 100 mg/kg infused over 16 hours.
- Treatment with NAC is indicated for those children with levels above the threshold shown on the Rumack–Matthew Nomogram. It is extremely effective if started within 8 hours of ingestion.
- At the end of therapy, repeat the LFT and the prothrombin time/international normalized ratio (INR). If any laboratory studies are abnormal, continue the infusion. In the setting of liver dysfunction, continue until liver function improves.
- *Do not wait for acetaminophen levels to commence treatment if definite history of toxic ingestion.*

Algorithm for acetaminophen poisoning is shown in **Flowchart 1**.

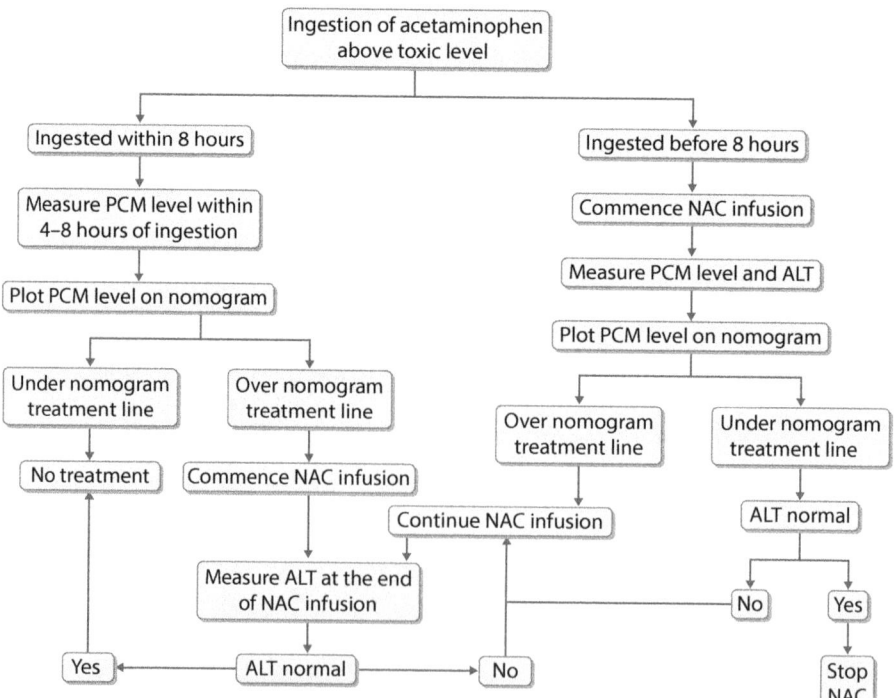

Flowchart 1: Algorithm for acetaminophen poisoning.

(ALT: alanine transaminase; NAC: N-acetylcysteine; PCM: paracetamol)

CHAPTER 65

Organophorus Poisoning

Sachendra Badal, Shuvendu Roy

- *Organophosphorus (OP) compounds are classified as:*
  - Highly toxic compounds (e.g., tetraethyl pyrophosphates, parathion); these are mainly used as agricultural insecticides.
  - Intermediately toxic compounds (e.g., coumaphos, chlorpyrifos, trichlorfon); these are used as animal insecticides.
  - Low toxicity compounds (e.g., diazinon, malathion, dichlorvos); these are used for household application and as field sprays.
  - *Carbamates:* Propoxur (Baygon)
- *Mode of action:*
  - Organophosphates cause irreversible inhibition of the enzyme acetylcholinesterase (AChE), present in red blood cell (RBC) (true AChE) and serum (pseudocholinesterase).
  - Inhibition of AChE allows acetylcholine (ACh) to remain active in the synapse—resulting in sustained depolarization of the postsynaptic neuron.
  - Accumulation of ACh causes overstimulation of both muscarinic and nicotinic receptors, and subsequently disrupts the transmission of nerve impulses in both the peripheral and central nervous system (CNS).
- *Clinical features:* The toxic features are usually obvious within 30 minutes to 3 hours. Early cases present predominantly with parasympathetic overactivity, and a characteristic garlic smell. The end result may be a multiorgan dysfunction. Most fatalities occur within 24 hours and those who recover usually do so within 10 days.
  Organophosphorus poisoning causes four distinct clinical syndromes (toxidromes):
  - Acute OP poisoning
  - Intermediate syndrome
  - OP-induced delayed neuropathy
  - Chronic OP-induced neuropsychiatric disorder
- The most common symptoms of cholinergic excess (mnemonic) are: *DUMB BELS*, which stands for *d*iarrhea/*d*efecation, *u*rination, *m*iosis, *b*ronchorrhea, *b*radycardia, *e*xcitation (muscle)/*e*mesis, *l*acrimation and *s*alivation, and gastrointestinal cramps. Common symptoms and signs are given in **Table 1**
- *Laboratory investigations*:
  - *Blood:* Complete blood count (CBC), peripheral blood smear (PBS), glucose, electrolytes, blood urea nitrogen (BUN), creatinine, liver function test (LFT), and arterial blood gas (ABG)
  - *Urine:* Glucose, protein, drug level
  - *Imaging:* Chest X-ray (CXR) if indicated

TABLE 1: Common symptoms and signs.		
Muscarinic	**Nicotinic**	**Central nervous system effects**
Cardiovascular: • Bradycardia, hypotension *Respiratory:* • Rhinorrhea, bronchorrhea • Bronchospasm, cough, wheeze *Gastrointestinal:* • Nausea/vomiting • Increased salivation • Abdominal cramps, diarrhea *Genitourinary:* • Urinary incontinence *Eyes:* • Miosis • Blurred vision • Lacrimation *Skin:* • Diaphoresis	*Cardiovascular:* • Tachycardia, hypertension *Musculoskeletal:* • Fasciculations • Paralysis • Muscle weakness	• Anxiety, restlessness • Confusion, dizziness • Toxic psychosis • Ataxia, seizures • Fatigue, unconsciousness • Respiratory depression • Circulatory collapse

- *Others:* Baseline electrocardiogram (ECG) (prolongation of QTc, torsades de pointes)
- *Specific enzyme levels:* RBC acetylcholinesterase and plasma pseudocholinesterase. Clinical features of OP poisoning appear when RBC cholinesterase activity is <75% of normal and in clinical overt poisoning, it is generally <10%.
- *Management:*
    - Ensure airway, breathing, and circulation
    - Skin decontamination—wash with copious soap and water
    - Gastric lavage—if victims reach within 1 hour; airway protection to be taken with a cuffed endotracheal tube
    - Activated charcoal @ 0.5-1 g/kg every 4 hours
    - Injection atropine reverses the muscarinic effects; dose @ 0.05 mg/kg/dose repeated every 5-10 minutes until atropinization is complete [increased heart rate (>100 beats/min), moderately dilated pupils, reduction in bowel sounds, dry mouth, and decrease in bronchial secretions. It has no effect on CNS symptoms as it does not cross the blood-brain barrier.
    - Start atropine infusion @ 10-20% of total atropine required every hour
    - Injection pralidoxime hydrolytically cleaves the OP from the enzyme AChE restoring the enzyme function. It is highly effective in reversing the nicotinic actions. It acts synergistically with atropine. It should be only used in patients after complete atropinization, as it has intrinsic muscarinic activity and can worsen the condition. The dose is 25-50 mg/kg IV infusion in 30 minutes, followed by 10-20 mg/kg/h till reversal of CNS symptoms or achievement of spontaneous respiration. It has no role in carbamate poisoning.
    Management of patient presenting with suspected organophosphate/carbamate ingestion is given in **Flowchart 1**.

CHAPTER 65: Organophosphorus Poisoning

Flowchart 1: Management of patient presenting with suspected organophosphate/carbamate ingestion.

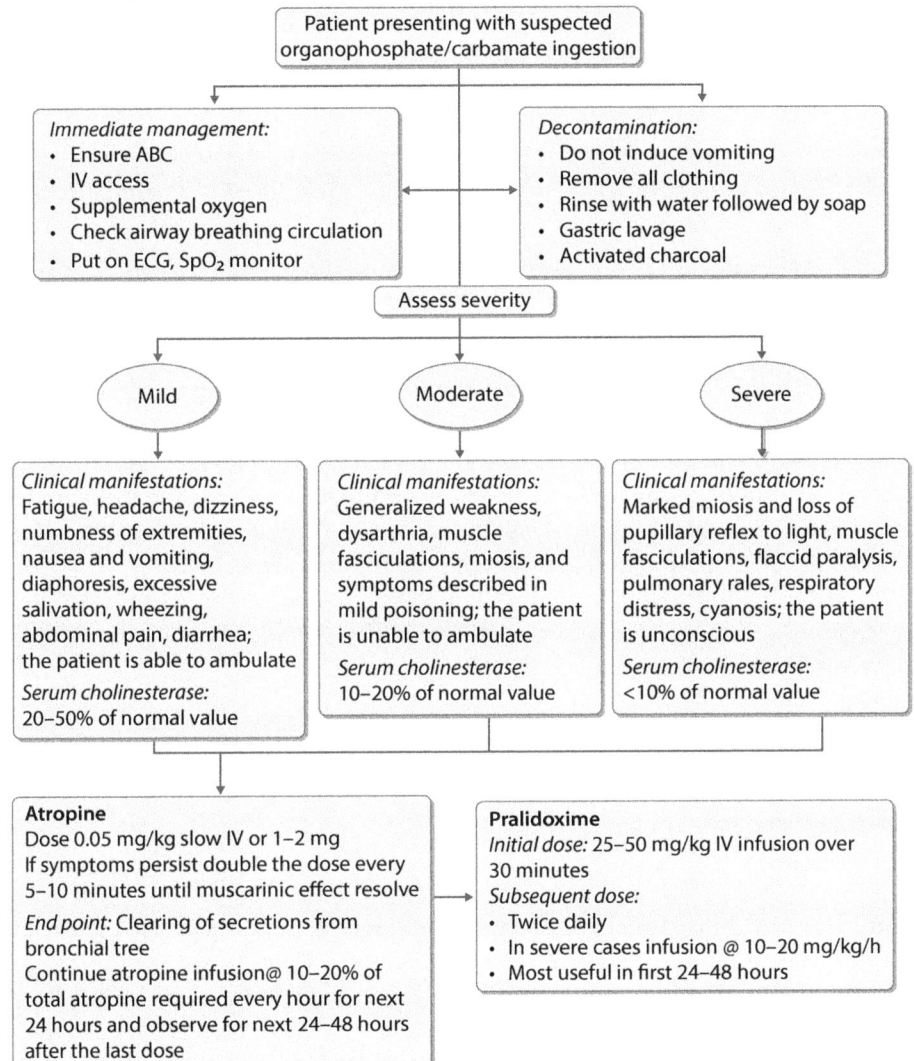

(ABC: airway, breathing, circulation, ECG: electrocardiogram; IV: intravenous; SpO$_2$: peripheral oxygen saturation)

CHAPTER 66: Iron Poisoning

Sachendra Badal, Shuvendu Roy

- **Introduction:**
    - Iron is one of the most common causes of poisoning in children due to its easy availability and bright-colored appearance with sugarcoating resembling candy. Ingestion of elemental iron >20 mg/kg have risk of mild toxicity involving mostly gastrointestinal (GI) symptoms. Systemic toxicity occurs when it is >60 mg/kg.
    - Iron is irritant and corrosive to the GI mucosa, leading to nausea, vomiting, diarrhea, ulceration, and bleeding. In large doses, iron directly damages the mitochondria and interferes with aerobic cellular respiration, thereby producing metabolic acidosis.
    - Availability of elemental iron in different preparations are as follows:

Form of iron	Elemental iron (%)
Ferric hydroxide (colloidal)	50
Ferrous fumarate	33
Ferric pyrophosphate	30
Ferrous sulfate	20
Ferric ammonium citrate	15
Ferrous gluconate	12

- **Clinical features:** Clinical features appear in five stages depending on the ingested iron.

Stage I	Stage II	Stage III	Stage IV	Stage V
• <6 hours • Gastrointestinal (GI) toxicity	• 6–24 hours • Relative stability	• 12–48 hours • Circulatory collapse	• 48–96 hours • Hepatic phase	• 2–4 weeks • Gastric scarring
• Nausea • Vomiting • Abdominal pain • Diarrhea • Hematemesis	• Resolution of GI symptoms • Persisting tachycardia	• Shock • Hypoglycemia • Metabolic acidosis	• Jaundice • Liver failure	GI obstruction due to strictures

- **Laboratory investigations:**
    - Complete blood count (CBC), glucose, liver function tests (LFTs), PT/aPTT (prothrombin time/activated partial thromboplastin time), blood urea nitrogen (BUN), creatinine, electrolytes, arterial blood gas (ABG)
    - Chest and abdomen radiographs (iron being radiopaque)

- Serum iron level to be done after 4 hours

Iron level (µg/dL)	Significance
50–120	Normal
120–350	Mild-to-moderate toxic features
350–1,000	Severe toxic features
>1,000	Fatal toxicity

- *Management*:
    - History of ingestion <30 mg/kg of elemental iron usually does not require hospitalization
    - Ensure airway, breathing, and circulation (ABC)
    - Activated charcoal has no role. Gastric lavage is done as soon as possible. Whole-bowel irrigation is indicated if shadows of undissolved tablets are seen on abdominal X-ray.
    - Gastric lavage is not recommended in young infants. Whole-bowel irrigation using polyethylene glycol may be tried.
    - *Management of GI toxicity:* H_2 blocker, proton-pump inhibitors, antacids
    - *Management of shock/cardiovascular instability:* Judicious fluid therapy, transfusion (if required); inotropes if hypotension uncorrected after adequate fluid replacement
    - *Management for metabolic acidosis:* Injection sodium bicarbonate
    - *Hepatic toxicity:* Injection vitamin K, blood component therapy (if indicated)
    - Serum iron level are done 4 hours after ingestion
    - Removal of iron by chelation therapy using deferoxamine infusion.
        - Indications of chelation:
            - Serum iron >500 µg/dL regardless of symptom
            - *Symptoms of stage III and above:* Regardless of serum iron concentration
    - In case of renal failure, hemodialysis may be helpful to remove the chelated iron.

Approach for iron poisoning is mentioned in **Flowchart 1**.

SECTION 11: Toxicology and Environmental Hazards

Flowchart 1: Approach for iron poisoning.

```
                   ┌─────────────────────────────────────┐
                   │ Patient presenting with iron toxicity│
                   └─────────────────────────────────────┘
                                    │
        ┌──────────────────────────┐
        │ • Ensure ABC             │
        │ • IV access              │
        │ • Blood sampling including│
        │   serum iron (after 4 hours)│
        └──────────────────────────┘
                                    │
             • Whole-bowel irrigation, gastric lavage
             • No emesis to be induced
```

- Symptomatic and/or serum iron >500 µg/dL
  - Treat shock
  - Treat metabolic acidosis
  - Treat GI bleed
  - Treat coagulopathy
  - Treat hypo/hyperglycemia
  - Chelation with deferoxamine

- Asymptomatic
  - Observe for 24 hours
  - Asymptomatic investigations normal
  - No treatment required

Deferoxamine infusion:
- Start IV infusion in 5% D at a slow rate and gradually reach @ 15 mg/kg/h (maximum 6 g/24 h)
- Monitor urine for pink-to-red orange discoloration
- Continue infusion till serum iron level returns normal, metabolic acidosis is corrected, urine becomes normal color and child is asymptomatic

(ABC: airway, breathing, circulation; 5% D: 5% dextrose; GI: gastrointestinal; IV: intravenous)

CHAPTER 67: Snake Bite Treatment Protocol

Sachendra Badal, Shuvendu Roy

- Venomous snakes are only 10% of all the snakes. Two important groups of venomous snakes are:
    1. *Elapidae:* Cobras, kraits, and sea snakes (short permanently erect fangs, spectacle marking on the hood—cobra)
    2. *Viperidae:* Typical viper and pit viper (long fangs normally folded up against upper jaw and pit organ between eye and nostril)

  The difference between venomous and nonvenomous snakes is discussed in **Table 1 and Figure 1**.

  Comparative clinical features and treatment for snake bite are mentioned in **Table 2**.
- First aid

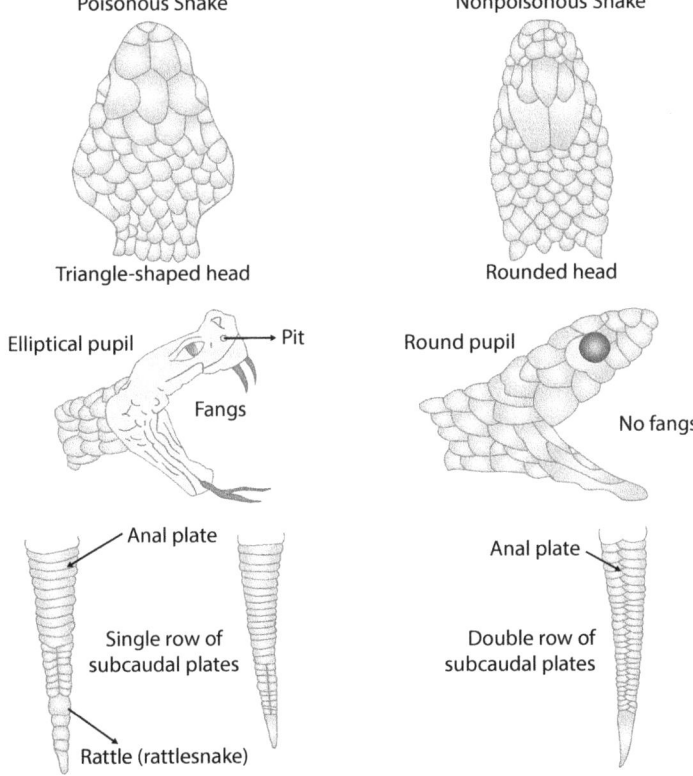

Fig. 1: Poisonous and nonpoisonous snakes.

TABLE 1: Difference between venomous and nonvenomous snakes.

	Venomous	**Nonvenomous**
Head	Triangular	Rounded
Pupil	Elliptical	Round
Fangs	Present	Absent
Subcaudal plates	Single row	Double row

TABLE 2: Comparative clinical features and treatment.

Clinical features and treatments	Cobra	Krait	Russell's viper	Saw scaled viper	Other vipers
Local pain/tissue damage	Yes	No	Yes	Yes	Yes
Ptosis/neurotoxicity	Yes	Yes	Yes; in South India	No	No
Coagulation	No	No	Yes	Yes	Yes
Renal problems	No	No	Yes	No	Yes
Neostigmine and atropine	Yes	Can be tried	Can be tried	No	No
Mechanical vent	Often	Often	No	No	No
Component support	No	No	Yes	Yes	Yes
Dialysis	No	No	May be	May be	May be

- "Do it Right"
  (*R*eassure, *I*mmobilize with bandage and splint as done for fractured bone, *G*et to the *H*ospital immediately, and *T*ell the doctor of systemic symptoms)
- *Immediate assessment:*
  - Care of airway, breathing, and circulation, if required.
  - Admission and observation for 24 hours.
  - *History*—type of snake, time of bite, any local medication or tourniquet application.
  - *Local examination*—fang marks and local swelling
  - Injection tetanus toxoid
  - *Analgesic:* Paracetamol and tramadol
  - Handling tourniquet—distal pulse to be checked before release. Sudden removal may cause a massive release of venom from the site into the circulation. It can be released after starting antisnake venom (ASV) administration.
  - Monitoring—pulse, blood pressure (BP), respiration, and oxygen saturation.
  - Intravenous (IV)—line placement and blood sampling
- *Urgent investigation:*
  - 20-minute whole blood clotting test (20 WBCT)—2 mL of fresh venous blood is taken in a sterile glass tube and kept for 20 minutes. No clotting after 20 minutes, Viperidae bite is likely.
  - Routine hemogram, peripheral smear
  - Prothrombin time (PT), activated partial thromboplastin time (aPTT), fibrinogen degradation product (FDP), and D-dimer
  - Urine for red blood cell (RBC), hemoglobinuria, and myoglobinuria
  - Serum creatine phosphokinase (CPK), urea, creatinine, and potassium
- *Detailed evaluation for clinical features suggesting envenomation:*
  - *Viper bites*—local pain and enlarging swelling, tender lymphadenopathy, bleeding from IV sites, gingival bleeding, epistaxis, petechiae, purpura, hematuria, and oliguria

- *Elapid bites*—local pain and swelling, paresthesia, descending paralysis starting from ptosis, diplopia, dysphagia leading to paresis of respiratory muscles manifested as desaturation and paradoxical respiration.
- *Krait bite* may be painless.
■ ASV—ASV in India is polyvalent (effective against Russell's viper, common cobra, common krait, and saw-scaled viper).
  - *Indications of ASV:*
    ◆ *Local sign:*
      – Local swelling of more than half of the bitten limb (e.g., beyond the knee or ankle)
      – The rapid extension of local swelling
      – Severe local blistering/bruising/necrosis
    ◆ *Systemic signs:*
      – *Evidence of coagulopathy:* Prolonged 20-minute whole blood clotting test (20 WBCT), visible spontaneous bleeding
      – *Evidence of neurotoxicity:* Ptosis, external ophthalmoplegia, resp distress, muscle paralysis
      – *Cardiovascular system (CVS) abnormality:* Shock, hypotension, arrhythmia, and abnormal electrocardiogram (ECG).
      – Persistent and severe vomiting and abdominal pain.
  - *ASV administration:*
    ◆ There is no need for administering an ASV test dose (a reaction can occur even after a negative test dose)
    ◆ Initial dose—dilute 10 vials of ASV in 10 mL/kg of isotonic fluid and give it slowly over 1–2 hours
    ◆ 10 mL of ASV neutralizes 6 mg of venom. Children receive the same ASV dose as adults.
    ◆ *If the child has known sensitivity, in addition to the above premedicate with:*
      – Injection adrenaline 0.01 mg/kg (1:10,000) SC
      – Injection of hydrocortisone 5 mg/kg IV
  - *Patient should be closely monitored for 2–3 hours:*
    ◆ Urticaria, itching, tachycardia, hypotension, and desaturation
    ◆ Single breath count test
    ◆ Amount of iris covered by the descending eyelid
    ◆ Distance between upper and lower incisor
    ◆ Length of time upward gaze can be maintained
    ◆ 20-WBCT
  - *Recovery phase:*
    ◆ Spontaneous bleeding stops within 15–30 minutes
    ◆ Blood coagulability is usually normalized within 6 hours
    ◆ Cobra-induced neurotoxicity starts resolving within 30–60 minutes
    ◆ Krait-induced neurotoxicity improves much later
  - *Repeat doses:*
    ◆ *Antihemostatic:* 10 vials given over 1 hour IV infusion, if 20-WBCT is abnormal after 6 hours of the initial dose. 25–30 vials is the maximum dose to be administered in total.
    ◆ *Neurotoxic:* 10 vials repeated after 1–2 hours if symptoms have worsened. No further dosing (total 20 vials) of ASV is recommended.

- **Supportive therapy:**
  - Tetanus prophylaxis
  - Injection of neostigmine (0.04 mg/kg) and injection of atropine (0.02 mg/kg) for elapid bites.
  - Respiratory paralysis is managed with assisted ventilation.
  - Fresh-frozen plasma (FFP), cryoprecipitate, and platelet concentrate for hemostatic disturbances.
  - Broad-spectrum antibiotics to be started in severe local envenomation.
  - *Renal failure:* Dialysis may be required. Hemodialysis preferred
  - Avoid intramuscular injections
  - Appropriate pain management
  - Avoid sedation as it will mask neurotoxic manifestations.

Treatment of patients presenting with suspected snake bite is discussed in **Flowchart 1**.

Flowchart 1: Treatment of patient presenting with a suspected snake bite.

```
Patient presenting with suspected snake bite
```

- Ensure ABC
- IV access × two lines, 20-WBCT
- Evaluate for shock, acute respiratory failure, and acute renal failure
- Put on ECG, SpO₂ monitor, and O₂ if required

- Reassure, rest, lie still, and immobilize limb
- Remove tight clothing
- Mark proximal level of swelling and measure circumference of limb, observe bite marks
- Avoid tourniquet

Snake brought to hospital → Yes → Snake identified → Yes → Snake nonpoisonous beyond doubt → Yes → Reassure discharge and give TT
No → Envenomation signs present
No → Hospitalize 24 hours observation → Envenomation signs present

- Polyvalent ASV 10 vials IV over 1 hour
- Be ready with anaphylactic tray with adrenaline loaded
- Monitor for ASV reaction
- Monitor for envenomation signs
- CBC, coagulation studies in 6 hours

Check response and assess circulation, i.e., need of component support and colloid support

Signs of persistent systemic envenomation → Yes → Repeat dose of antivenom (elapid after 2 hours and viperid after 6 hours)
No → 24-hour observation

(ASV: antisnake venom; CBC: complete blood count; ECG: electrocardiography; SpO₂: saturation of peripheral oxygen; TT: tetanus toxoid; 20-WBCT: 20 minutes whole blood clotting test)

CHAPTER 68: Approach to Scorpion Bite

Sachendra Badal, Shuvendu Roy

- *Introduction:* There are around 1,400 species of scorpions but only 46–50 of these are potentially lethal to humans. Most scorpion envenomations have similar cardiovascular manifestations with an autonomic storm. Mesobuthus tamulus (Indian red scorpion) is the most common scorpion bite in India.
- *Pathophysiology (Flowchart 1):*
  - Scorpion venom causes an autonomic storm. There is intense and persistent depolarization of autonomic nerves with massive release of neurotransmitters from the adrenal medulla and parasympathetic and sympathetic nerve endings, leading to toxic cardiovascular manifestations.
  - Initially parasympathetic system is stimulated (excessive sweating, vomiting, salivation) which usually lasts for 1–2 hours and is followed by sympathetic overactivity (α > β, tachycardia, hypertension, and cold peripheries)

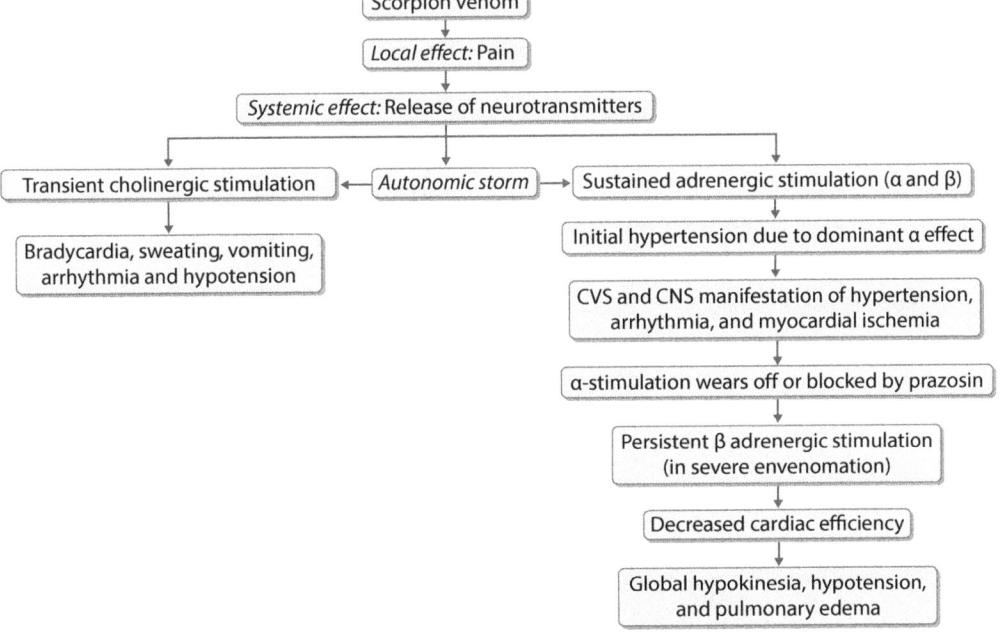

Flowchart 1: Pathophysiology and clinical features.

(CNS: central nervous system; CVS: cardiovascular system)

- *Clinical features:*
  - Clinical grade of scorpion sting envenomation (**Box 1**).
  - Central nervous system (CNS) effects (hypertensive encephalopathy, hemorrhagic stroke, altered consciousness, and convulsions) are however invariably fatal.
  - Alpha-receptor stimulation causes hyperkalemia and hyperglycemia (by inhibiting insulin secretion).
- *Investigations:* Since most of the toxic manifestation involves the cardiovascular system; electrocardiography (ECG), chest X-ray, and cardiac enzymes are required to rule out arrhythmia, pulmonary edema, myocardial enzyme, and heart failure.
- *Management* (**Flowchart 2**):
  - *Supportive therapy:*
    - Fluid-restoration of volume status is required. Use of afterload-reducing agents/diuretics can cause hypotension

---

BOX 1: Clinical grade of scorpion sting envenomation.

- *Mild:* Severe, excruciating local pain at the sting site (due to serotonin of the venom) radiating along with corresponding dermatomes, mild local oedema with sweating at the sting site, without systemic involvement.
- *Moderate:* Signs and symptoms of *autonomic storm* characterized by parasympathetic stimulation (vomiting, profuse sweating from all over body, salivation, bradycardia, premature ventricular contraction, hypotension, and priapism in men) and sympathetic stimulation (hypertension, tachycardia, cold extremities, and transient systolic murmur).
- *Severe:* Tachycardia, hypotension with pulmonary edema, and *shock*.

Flowchart 2: Treatment of scorpion sting.

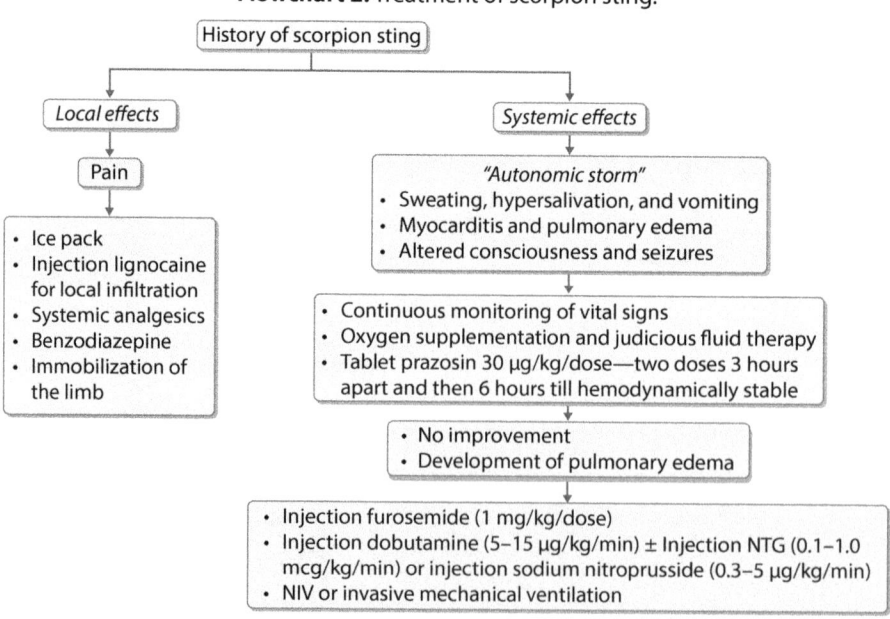

(NIV: noninvasive ventilation; NTG: nitroglycerine)

- Oxygen
- *Analgesia:* Cold ice application, local infiltration with lignocaine (1%), and systemic analgesics are indicated to relieve the excruciating pain at the sting site. Benzodiazepines can also be used.
- *Prazosin:* Since alpha receptor stimulation plays a major role in the evolution of the clinical spectrum, prazosin, a competitive postsynaptic alpha1, adreno-receptor antagonist is the first line of management.
  - This is given as an immediate measure in all with evidence of autonomic storm. It should not be given as prophylaxis in children when pain is the only symptom.
  - *Dose:* 30 µg/kg/dose. The drug should be repeated in the same dose at the end of 3 hours according to clinical response and later every 6 hours till extremities are warm, dry, and peripheral veins are visible.
  - *Monitoring:* Pulse, blood pressure, and respiration must be monitored every 30 minutes for 3 hours, every hour for the next 6 hours, and later every 4 hours till improvement.
- *Inotropic support:* Despite prazosin administration, some children develop marked tachycardia, hypertension, and pulmonary edema. Furosemide infusion can be given in this condition followed by vasodilators, such as sodium nitroprusside (0.3–8 µg/kg/min) and nitroglycerine (5–8 µg/kg/min). Prazosin is to be given one hour before termination of sodium nitroprusside drip. Dobutamine/milrinone infusion are required in case of cardiogenic shock.
- *Other drugs:* Oxygen therapy along with frusemide can be added for treating pulmonary edema. Morphine, a standard therapy in pulmonary edema, should be avoided in scorpion stings since narcotics worsen dysrhythmias.
- *Antivenom therapy:* Scorpion antivenin can be administered intravenously, 30 mL (3 vials) if the victim reports within half an hour of the sting with an autonomic storm. However, its use is debatable.

CHAPTER 69

Drowning

Suprita Kalra, Ranjit Ghuliani

- *Definition:* The World Congress of Drowning has defined drowning as respiratory impairment from immersion/submersion in a liquid.
- *Pathophysiology:*
  - After initial breath holding, when the victim's airway lies below the liquid's surface, a reflex laryngospasm is triggered by the presence of liquid in the oropharynx or larynx which leads to hypoxia, hypercarbia and acidosis, and aspiration of water into the lungs.
  - Approximately 10–20% of individuals maintain tight laryngospasm until cardiac arrest occurs and inspiratory efforts have ceased. These victims do not aspirate any appreciable fluid.
  - Damage to an alveolar-capillary membrane by aspirated water leads to loss of surfactant, decreased lung compliance, significant V/Q mismatch, and profound hypoxemia.
  - In young children suddenly immersed in cold water (<20°C), the mammalian diving reflex may occur and produce apnea, bradycardia, and vasoconstriction of non-essential vascular beds with shunting of blood to the coronary and cerebral circulation.
  - The most important contributory factors to morbidity and mortality from drowning are hypoxemia, acidosis, and the multiorgan effects of these processes.
- *Rescue and management:* Its primary aim is rapid restoration of oxygenation and spontaneous circulation. If the victim is unresponsive start cardiopulmonary resuscitation (CPR) as per pediatric advanced life support (PALS). Hypothermia can mimic cardiac arrest. So, continue advanced life support until the patient has been warmed. Transfer patient to the pediatric intensive care unit (PICU) for definitive care.
- *Indications to withhold/cease CPR:* Victim submerged for >60 minutes and showed no ROSC on CPR of >25–30 minutes
- *Prognosis:* Outcome largely depends upon the duration of submersion and the success of resuscitative measures. Patients who are conscious at arrival to the hospital after successful resuscitation tend to have a favorable prognosis for survival. On the other hand, generalized edema, and cardiac and respiratory arrest are markers of poor outcomes.
- *Management (Flowchart 1):*

Flowchart 1: Management for drowning.

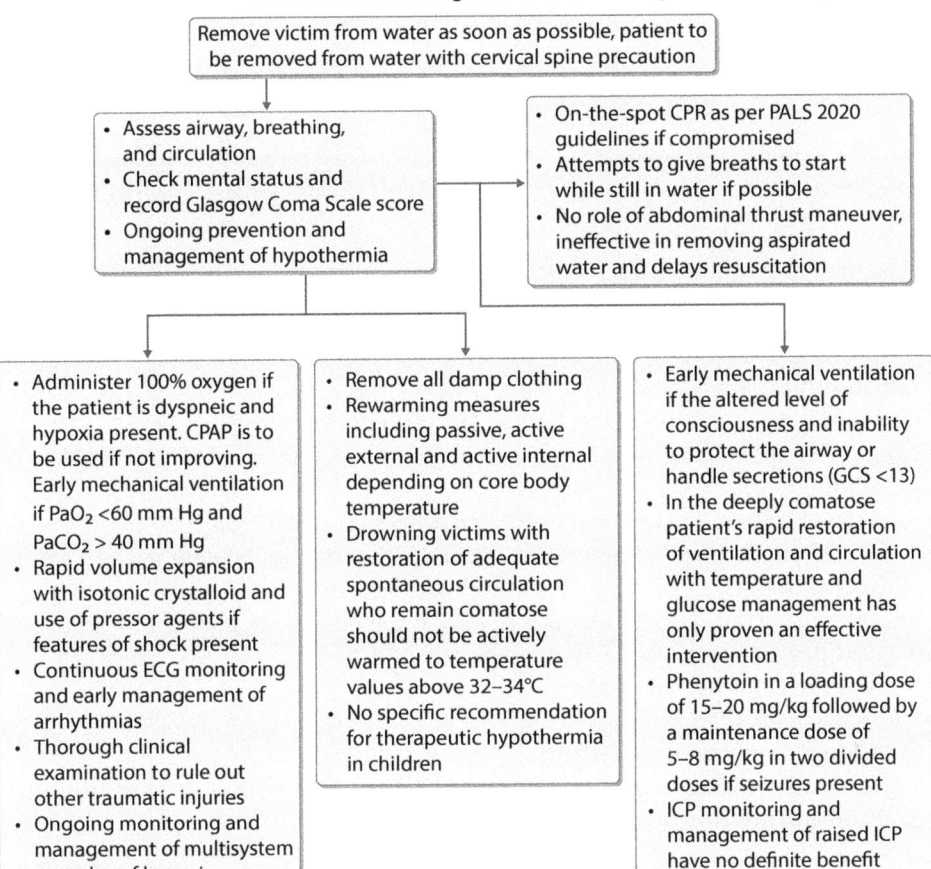

(CPAP: continuous positive airway pressure; CPR: cardiopulmonary resuscitation; ECG: electrocardiography; ICP: intracranial pressure; PaCO$_2$: partial pressure of carbon dioxide; PALS: pediatric advanced life support)

CHAPTER 70

Burns

Ranjit Ghuliani, Suprita Kalra

- *Serious burn requiring hospitalization:*
  - >10% burns in a child
  - Any burn in infants
  - Any full-thickness burn
  - Burns of special regions—face, hands, feet, and perineum
  - Circumferential burns
  - Inhalation injury
  - Associated trauma or significant preburn illness, e.g., diabetes
- *Evaluation of burn wounds:* Depending upon the depth of involvement, burn wounds can be categorized into:
  - First-degree burns—erythematous, no blistering but severe pain
  - Second-degree burns can be divided into:
    - Superficial partial thickness
    - Deep partial thickness
  - They are painful and have blistering
  - Third-degree burns—involve all skin layers. Not sensitive to pain. Require early excision and grafting

"Rule of nine" often overestimates burn size in children. Age-specific body surface area charts may be used in children to estimate total body surface area (TBSA).

- *Early management and resuscitation of burn injuries:* Establish adequate oxygenation, ventilation, and normal circulation. Burns should be initially washed with tepid water. Ensure adequate pain control, initiate fluid resuscitation, give injection tetanus prophylaxis, and avoid hypothermia
- *Fluid: Fluid resuscitation:* TBSA >20% burn requires fluid resuscitation with balance crystalloid [Ringer's lactate (RL) or plasmalyte]
  - *Fluid requirement:* Parkland formula—2–4 mL/kg/% TBSA + maintenance fluid. Half of the calculated fluid requirement is given over 8 hours from the time of burn and the remaining half in the next 16 hours.
- *Topical antimicrobial therapy:* Prophylactic systemic antibiotics have no role in thermal injury, topical antimicrobial therapy is effective.
- *Nutrition:* Burn injury produces hypermetabolic response with protein and fat catabolism. Management of hypermetabolic response include:
  - Reduce heat loss
  - Excision and closure of burn wound
  - Early enteral feeding
  - Recognition and treatment of infection

- *Analgesia:*
  - Children with burns have background pain and procedural pain.
  - Opiate analgesia along with anxiolytic agents in conjunction with nonpharmacological measures for pain relief is required.
  - For background pain preemptive control morphine sulfate in a dose of 0.3–0.6 mg/kg orally every 4–6 hours or 0.05–0.1 mg/kg IV until wound cover is achieved is used.
  - Lorazepam in a dose of 0.05–0.1 mg/kg is given 6–8 hourly for anxiety.
  - Oral morphine 0.3–0.6 mg/kg 1–2 hours before along with IV morphine 0.05–0.1 mg/kg given immediately before giving optimum pain control before procedures like dressings.
  - Midazolam in doses of 0.01–0.02 mg/kg in nonventilated and 0.05–0.1 mg/kg in ventilated patients is used for sedation.
  - During weaning opiate dose is to be reduced by 25% every 1–3 days with the addition of acetaminophen if a patient experiences pain.
  Management of burns is shown in **Flowchart 1**.
  - Estimation of burns in children **(Fig. 1)**.

Flowchart 1: Burns intervention.

- CPR as per AHA 2020 guidelines if compromised

Assess:
- Airway
- Breathing
- Circulation

- Admit if BSA >10%
- IV fluid if BSA >15%
- IV fluid as per Parkland formula, i.e., first 24 hours 2–4 mL/kg/%TBSA–Ringer's lactate (RL), 1/2 of this in first 8 hours postburn, rest in next 16 hours PLUS maintenance fluids. Titrate to maintain pulse and BP and urine output >1 mL/kg/h
- Fluid required in next 24 hours 1/2 of first day's RL in 5% dextrose
- Fresh frozen plasma if prothrombin time >1.5 times control or >1.2 times control before any invasive procedure

Assess exposure: Percentage area of burns as per Lund and Browder's method

Assess the depth of burns

Immediate management

Admit if any full thickness burn

- Extinguish flames
- Cover the burned area with a clean, dry sheet, and cold compress on small burns
- Tetanus prophylaxis
- Debride all bullae
- Cleanse burn with 0.25% chlorhexidine solution or 0.1% cetrimide solution
- Topical application of silver sulfadiazine/mafenide acetate to prevent bacterial colonization
- Early debridement and grafting in second and third-degree burns.
- Systemic antibiotic prophylaxis has no role in the prevention of bacterial infections
- In established burns wound sepsis systemic antibiotics to cover predominant organisms isolated in the unit and modified later as per culture results

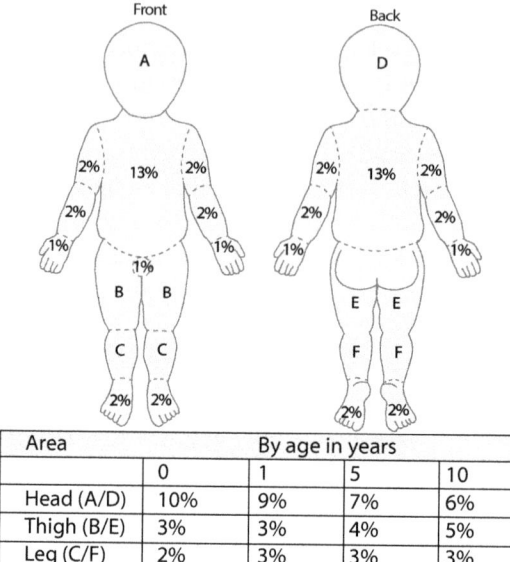

Fig. 1: Estimation of burns in children.

CHAPTER 71

Electrical Injuries

Sarvesh Kohli

- *Introduction:* Electrical injuries in children may be uncommon but can be fatal. Severity depends on various factors such as the source of electricity, site, and duration of contact, and pathway of current in the body.
- *Epidemiology:* Deaths due to electrocution injuries account for almost 3.2% of total accidental deaths in India across all ages.
- *Types of electrical injuries* **(Table 1)**:
  - Minor electrical burns (extension cord)
    - Nonconductive injuries usually do not extend beyond the site of contact.
  - High-tension wire (voltage >1,000 V)
    - Admit patient regardless of the extent of the injury for observation
    - Mortality 3–15%
  - Lightening (direct strike or adjacent/in-contact object)
    - Linear burns (first or second degree)
    - Feathering/arborescent pattern
- *Factors influencing the severity of electrical injury include:*
  - Whether the current is alternating current (AC) or direct current (DC):
    - Alternating current may cause tetanic contraction of skeletal muscle and prevent release from the source of electricity and respiratory arrest. It may also cause ventricular fibrillation (VF) (R-on-T phenomenon).
    - Asystole is more common after DC shock.
  - Voltage
  - Magnitude of energy delivered
    - High current (15–20 mA) causes muscle spasm

TABLE 1: Comparison of types of electrical injuries.

Characteristic	Low voltage	High voltage	Lightning
Voltage	<1,000 V	>1,000 V	>30 × 10⁸ V
Current	<240A	<1,000A	2,00,000A
Respiratory arrest (cause)	Tetany of respiratory muscles	Indirect trauma, tetanic contractions of respiratory muscles, burns causing eschar	Direct central nervous system (CNS) injury, tetanic contractions of respiratory muscles
Cardiac arrest (cause)	Ventricular fibrillation	Ventricular fibrillation	Asystole
Burns	Usually, superficial	Common, deep	Rare, superficial
Rhabdomyolysis	Possible	Common	Uncommon
Blunt injury (cause)	Uncommon	Injury from being thrown away from the source	Blast effect (shockwave)
Mortality risk	Low risk	Moderate risk	Very high

- *Resistance to current flow:*
  - Moisture decreases resistance
  - Nerves and blood vessels are good conductors
  - Muscle, skin, tendon, fat, and bone have more resistance
- *Pathway of current:*
  - Transthoracic (hand to hand or opposite leg)—higher risk of mortality
  - Vertical (hand to foot) or straddle (foot to foot)—lesser risk
- Area and duration of contact
- *Mechanisms of electrical injury:*
  - Direct effect of electrical current on tissues (dysrhythmia and respiratory arrest)
  - *Electrical to thermal energy:* Electrothermal burn at the point of contact. Current follows the path of least resistance.
  - Electroporation
  - Secondary mechanical trauma
- *Lightening injuries:* Direct strike, contact strike (current from another object in contact), side flash or splash, ground strike (contact points, e.g., feet are separate creating potential difference)
- Burns are most commonly present at the site of electrical contact or places in contact with the ground. They are generally not predictive of the pathway of current and may significantly underestimate the extent of internal injury.

Flowchart 1 describes clinical considerations for electrical injuries.

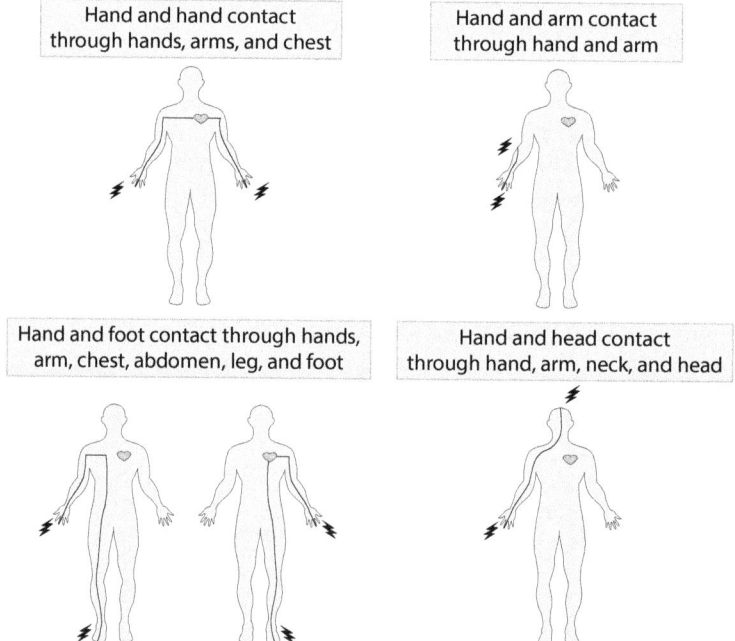

Fig. 1: Paths followed by electrical current through the body based on entry and exit sites. (transthoracic, vertical, straddle).
Source: https://www.robsonforensic.com/articles/electrocution-expert-witness https://www.robsonforensic.com/images/uploads/articles/Electrical-Shock-Electrocution-Expert-Witness4.jpg

Flowchart 1: Clinical considerations of electrical injuries.

Electrical injuries: Clinical considerations

Genral considerations:
- Primary assessment as per PALS
- Manage airway, breathing, circulation
- Immobilize spine
- *History:* Voltage, type of current
- CBC, electrolytes, BUN, creatinine, glucose

Cardiac:
- Dysrhythmias, ST-T wave changes
- Cardiac monitor, ECG, chest radiograph
- CK-MB
- Arrhythmia specific treatment

Renal:
- Acute kidney injury, myoglobinuria
- Urinalysis, BUN, creat, urine myoglobin
- Aggressive fluid management
- Maintain urine output >1 mL/kg/h
- Central venous/pulmonary arterial pressure monitoring – if available

Cutaneous/oral:
- Oral commissure burns, tongue, dental injuries
- Look for entry/exit wounds, cardiac involvement
- Observe eschar till it sloughs
- Reconstructive surgery opinion

Musculoskeletal:
- Compartment syndrome, long bone fracture, spine injury
- Monitor, fasciotomy if required
- Immobilization if fracture
- Orthopedic/surgery consult

Pulmonary:
- Respiratory arrest, aspiration syndrome
- Protect and maintain airway
- CXR, ABG
- Respiratory support/mechanical ventilation - if indicated

Neurologic:
- Paralysis/paraplegia, intracranial, hematoma, SIADH, cerebral edema, autonomic disturbance
- Treat seizures (Restrict fluids if needed)
- Spine radiographs, MRI
- *Delayed:* Seizures, headache, peripheral neuropathy

Abdominal:
- Viscous perforation, solid organ damage, ileus
- Place NG tube
- ALT, AST, amylase, BUN creatinine,
- CT scan if needed
- Pediatric surgery consult

Ocular:
- Visual changes, optic neuritis, extraocular muscle paresis
- Ophthalmology consultation

(ABG: arterial blood gas; ALT: aminotransferase; AST: aspartate aminotransferase; BUN: blood urea nitrogen; CBC: complete blood count; CK-MB: creatine kinase-myoglobin binding; CT: computed tomography; CXR: chest X-ray; ECG: electrocardiography; MRI: magnetic resonance imaging; PALS: Pediatric Advanced Life Support; SIADH: syndrome of inappropriate anti-diuretic hormone)

Source:
1. Adapted from NHSGGC guidelines (Electrical Injury guideline RHCG), Pediatric Emergency Medicine Practice (Pediatric Electrical Injuries in the Emergency Department: An Evidence-Based Review) and Uptodate.
2. Electrical injuries guideline RHCG (no date) www.clinicalguidelines.scot.nhs.uk. Available at: https://www.clinicalguidelines.scot.nhs.uk/nhsggc-guidelines/nhsggc-guidelines/burns/electrical-injuries-guideline-rhcg/
3. Pediatric Electrical Injuries in the Emergency Department: An Evidence-Based Review (Trauma CME) | EB Medicine (no date) www.ebmedicine.net. Available at: https://www.ebmedicine.net/topics/trauma/pediatric-electrical-injuries

SECTION 12

Procedures

- **Use of Bedside Ultrasonography in PICU**
  Arvind Kumar
- **Endotracheal Intubation**
  Sanjeev Khera
- **Rapid-sequence Intubation**
  Sanjeev Khera
- **Central Venous Line (Femoral Vein)**
  Sanjeev Khera
- **Intraosseous Cannulation**
  Sanjeev Khera
- **Peripherally Inserted Central Catheter Insertion**
  Sanjeev Khera, Gaurav Ray
- **Radial Artery Cannulation**
  Sanjeev Khera
- **Umbilical Vein Catheterization**
  Sanjeev Khera, Gaurav Ray
- **Intercostal Drainage Tube Insertion**
  Mithlesh Kumar Tiwari
- **Thoracocentesis: Needle Aspiration of Pneumothorax**
  Sanjeev Khera
- **Abdominal Paracentesis**
  Sanjeev Khera

CHAPTER **72**

Use of Bedside Ultrasonography in PICU

Arvind Kumar

- *Introduction:* In last few decades, use of ultrasonography (USG) in critical patient management has been increased. It provides more safe, cost-effective, focused, and rapid dynamic images, which are very useful for treating physician to take efficient and early treatment decision. Two types of uses are: (1) Diagnostic USG and (2) therapeutic USG in intensive care unit (ICU).
- *Diagnostic USG:*
  - *Cardiovascular status:* Cardiac finding that could be provided by it, includes myocardium contractility, regional wall motion abnormality, volume and size of chambers, valvular stenosis, or regurgitations. It identifies life-threatening conditions like pericardial tamponade or aortic dissection too. For estimation of intravascular volume status and predicting fluid responsiveness inferior vena cava (IVC) diameter, IVC collapsibility index, cardiac output, and variability of blood flow or velocity can be measured by using two-dimensional, motion or Doppler mode of imaging in USG, instead of using traditionally central venous pressure (CVP) monitoring, which is invasive and has more risks of complications **(Fig. 1)**.

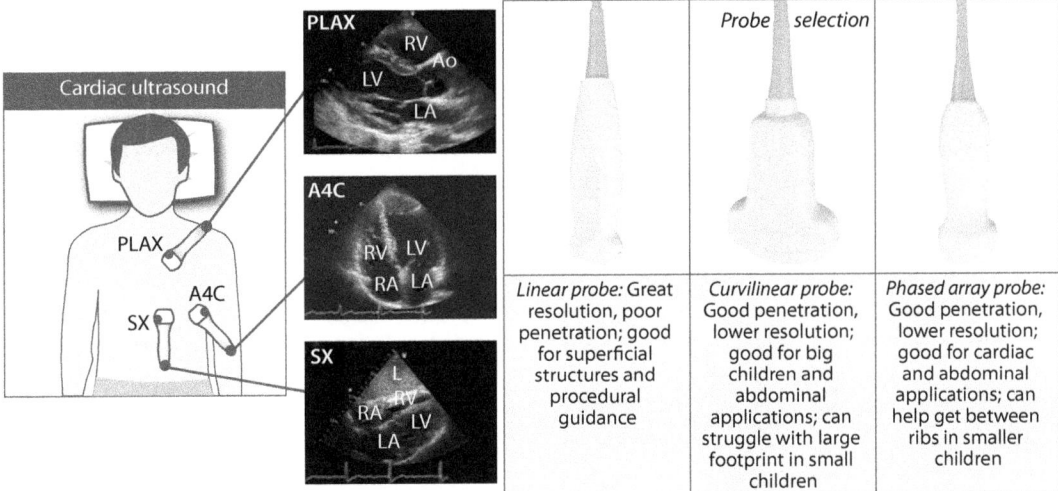

Fig. 1: Three cardiac views for volume and cardiac function. (A4C: apical four-chamber view; Ao: aorta; LA: left atrium; LV: left ventricle; PLAX: parasternal long-axis view; RA: right atrium; RV: right ventricle; SX: parasternal short-axis view)

- *Thoracic cavity:* Lung and pleural pathology can be diagnosed with the use of USG. High frequency (7–12 MHz) linear probe is used for pleural and superficial lung pathology and lower frequency probe is needed for deeper structure. Sliding of visceral pleura over parietal pleura, known as sliding sign, is normal finding. Absence of sliding sign indicates pneumothorax and lung point is the transition point where normal sliding pattern changed to pneumothorax pattern (absent sliding) **(Figs. 2 and 3)**. Vertical hyperechoic lines in lung USG are "B" lines and these are mostly consistent with interstitial pneumonia and pulmonary edema. USG findings

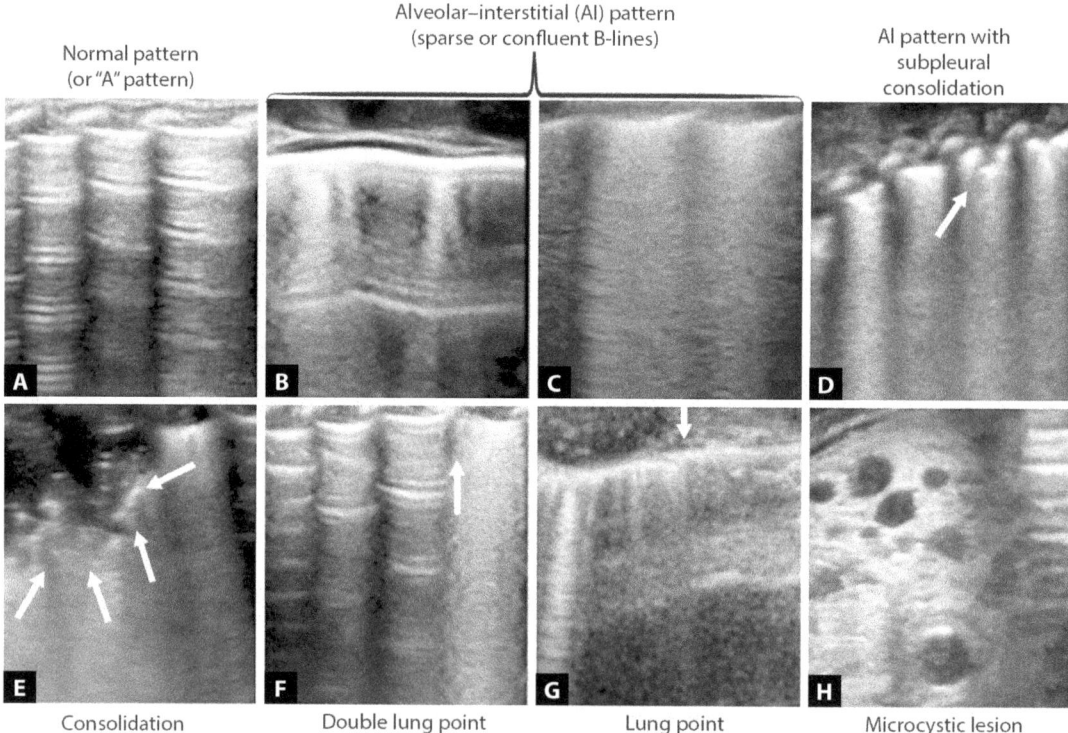

Figs. 2A to H: Lung ultrasound findings.

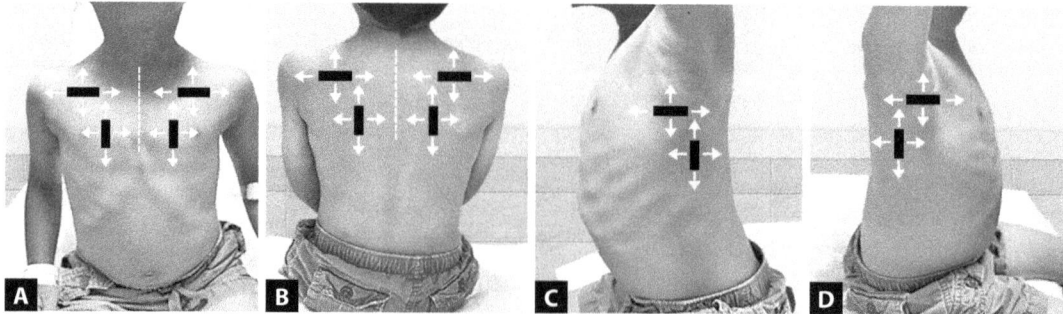

Figs. 3A to D: Twelve examination regions.

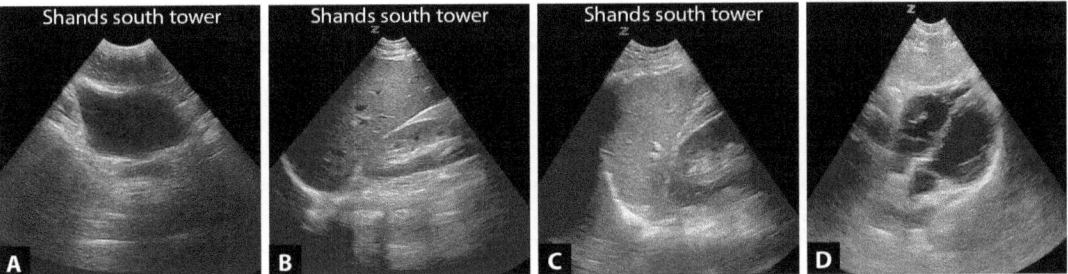

Figs. 4A to D: (A) Bladder view; (B) Hepatorenal view; (C) Splenorenal view; and (D) Subxiphoid view.

for superficial pneumonia are subpleural consolidation, lobar consolidation, dynamic air bronchogram, and multiple small hyperechoic lines at interface of air and water. Lower frequency probe (3–5 MHz) is used for diaphragmatic sonography. It will help for assessment of readiness for extubation in case prolonged ventilated patient includes diaphragm movement, serial monitoring of thickness, amplitude, and velocity of contraction.
- *Abdomen:* Focused assessment with sonography in trauma (FAST) has been used to diagnose and treat intra-abdominal pathology in case of critical patient with traumatic injury. It is used to detect dependent fluid in peritoneal cavity with the help of four view (left upper quadrant, right upper quadrant, and suprapubic regions, as well as a subxiphoid view of the pericardium). If thoracic view is added to above to detect pneumothorax as well, it is known as extended FAST (e-FAST) **(Figs. 4A to D)**.
- *USG-guided procedure/therapeutic USG:*
  - *Vascular access:* Use of USG for central venous cannulation has become standard of care. High-frequency linear probe with short-axis view is used for direct visualization of vein.
  - *Intra-abdominal fluid paracentesis:* Sonography provides direct visualization of intra-abdominal structures while paracentesis to avoid injury and decrease complications.
  - *Thoracentesis:* Indicated in case of pleural effusion causing respiratory distress and empyema. USG guidance will help in small effusion, complicated effusion, and obese and ventilated children.
  - *Nutritional assessment:* In case of prolonged pediatric intensive care unit (PICU) stay or critically sick children, USG helps in serial monitoring of muscle mass for nutritional assessment. Lower limb muscle gets affected in initial 5 days, subsequently upper limbs muscle too undergo atrophy.
  - *Neurological assessment:* Use of USG in pediatric neurology includes transcranial USG for hydrocephalous, hemorrhage, brain death, and intracranial pressure assessment. Measurement of optic nerve sheath diameter (ONSD) is noninvasive method to assess intracranial pressure.

CHAPTER 73: Endotracheal Intubation

Sanjeev Khera

- An emergency endotracheal (ET) intubation may be required in prehospital or emergency room/critical care area setting for securing the airway or as a part of ongoing resuscitation. In other cases, it may be an elective procedure anticipating the requirement of a controlled secure airway.
- *Indications:*
  - To secure an unstable airway (airway infections, syndromic child, facial dysmorphism, micrognathia, macroglossia)
  - Neurological dysfunction [depressed or deteriorating sensorium, comatose, Glasgow Coma Scale (GCS) <8 or rapid fall in GCS—14 to 10)
  - Respiratory failure (impaired gas exchange, hypoxia, hypercarbia)
  - Surgical procedures or diagnostic procedures requiring general anesthesia
  - Patient transport
- *Precautions/relative contraindication:* No absolute contraindication
  - Anticipated difficult airway
  - Laryngeal fracture (known or suspected) or facial trauma, penetrating laryngeal trauma
- *Materials:*
  - Intravenous (IV) access, monitoring equipment
  - *Suction apparatus:* Wall suction/portable device
  - Oropharyngeal, nasopharyngeal airways
  - Nonrebreather mask
  - Oxygen source
  - Self-inflating bag and mask (ambu) or JC circuit
  - *Appropriate size ET tube (cuffed or uncuffed):*
    - Size calculation: $(n/4) + 3.5$ cm internal diameter for cuffed tube, $(n/4) + 4$ cm for uncuffed tube (n = age in years)
    - For neonates: <1 kg (2.5 mm), 1-2 kg (3.0 mm), >2 kg (3.5 mm)
  - Laryngoscope blade and handle (Miller 0-1 up to 1 year, Miller or Mac (2) 2-8 years, (2-3) 8-12 years)
  - Pediatric stylet
  - Spare batteries and bulbs
  - ET tube fix adhesive tape
  - *Medicines for rapid sequence intubation:*
    - Atropine (0.02 mg/kg IV)
    - Fentanyl
    - Ketamine or midazolam
    - Vecuronium or rocuronium

Mnemonic: SOAP ME [suction, oxygen, airway equipment, pharmacopeia/position, monitor, end tidal CO_2 ($EtCO_2$) equipment]

- *Preprocedure steps:*
  - *Personnel:* Ideally at least three persons should be present for performing and assistance during the procedure.
  - *Preoxygenation with 100% oxygen:*
    - *Spontaneously breathing:* Nonrebreather mask
    - *Not breathing:* Bag and mask
  - *Position:* Sniffing position (a towel roll may be placed under the shoulder) to align the oral, pharyngeal, and tracheal axes
  - Deflate the cuff of ET tube before use
  - Sedation and neuromuscular block
  - Ensure availability of alternate airway like laryngeal mask airway (LMA) in case of failed procedure
- *Procedure:*
  - The clinician/intubator stands at patient's head end with the assistant usually on the right side of patient.
  - Open the mouth using the thumb and index and middle finger (scissor technique) or pushing the chin caudally.
  - *Laryngoscopy:*
    - With the laryngoscope held in left hand, insert blade from the right side of mouth and pass it along the base of tongue pushing the tongue to the left to reach the midline of the hypopharynx.
    - Once in the oropharynx, lift the mandible while putting force along the direction of the axis of the handle. Note, not to use the teeth, maxilla, or palate as the fulcrum for lifting the mandible.
    - After retracting adequately, identify the epiglottis, which is usually the first structure to be visualized. If the glottic structures or epiglottis are not visualized, the blade of laryngoscope may be either too deep or superficial (adjust accordingly).
    - Use external laryngeal manipulation (cricoid pressure) if the glottic structure is difficult to visualize or expected to be placed anteriorly.
    - Suction secretions if required.
    - As the epiglottis is visualized, it is lifted by placing it under the laryngoscope blade or by placing the blade in the vallecula and lifting the mandible.
    - Identify the glottic opening by visualizing the inverted "V"-shaped vocal cords.
    - Keeping the glottic opening under vision, pass the ET tube from the right side of mouth through the vocal cords.
    - Advance the ET tube to premeasured depth to ensure the tube tip lies between the carina and glottic inlet.
    - Secure the ET tube with the index finger of right hand against the palate and remove the laryngoscope blade.
    - Connect the ET tube with a bag and mask and check for chest rise with positive pressure breaths. Look for misting in the tube and auscultate chest bilaterally (axilla) to confirm equal air entry.

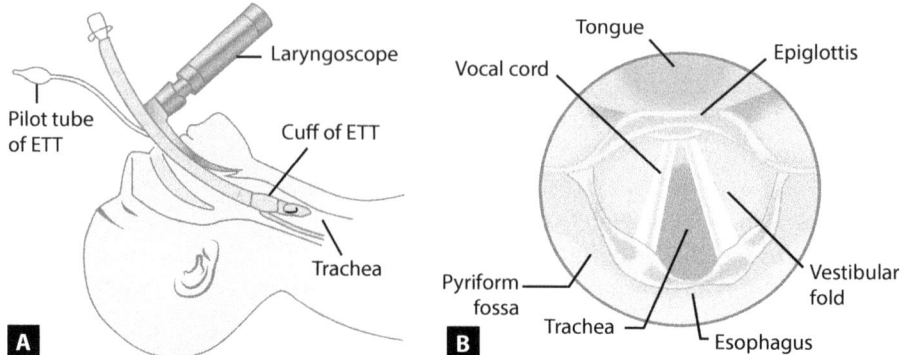

Figs. 1A and B: (A) Endotracheal intubation and (B) Laryngeal anatomy as seen during endotracheal intubation. (ETT: endotracheal tube)

- A colorimetric $EtCO_2$ monitor may also be used for guiding correct placement.
- On confirming, fix the ET tube with adhesive tape and connect to the ventilator.
- *Documentation:*
  - Procedure note describes indications, equipment, and technique.
  - Number of attempts
  - Confirmation of placement
  - Complications if any and management

CHAPTER 74: Rapid-sequence Intubation

Sanjeev Khera

- *Indications:* Patients who are at high risk of pulmonary aspiration of gastric content during tracheal intubation
    - Full stomach
    - Intestinal obstruction/ileus
    - Tense abdominal distension
- *Contraindications:*
    - *Relative:*
        - Anticipated "difficult airway"
        - Upper airway obstruction
        - Raised intracranial pressure
        - Lack of expertise or inexperience in the technique
    - *Material and equipment:*
        - Laryngoscope appropriate size
        - Endotracheal (ET) tube appropriate size
        - Stylet
        - Syringe 10 mL (to inflate ET tube balloon)
        - Suction catheter
        - Carbon dioxide detector
        - Oral and nasal airways
        - Ambu bag and mask attached to oxygen source
        - Assistant for cricoid pressure
- *Steps of rapid-sequence intubation (RSI):*
    - Evaluation
    - Preparation
    - Preoxygenation for 3–5 minutes (avoid positive pressure ventilation)
    - *Premedication:*
        - Lidocaine [1.5 mg/kg intravenous (IV)]
        - Opioid analgesic (fentanyl 3 µg/kg IV)
        - Atropine (0.02 mg/kg IV)
        - A "defasciculating" dose of a nondepolarizing agent (e.g., 0.01 mg/kg vecuronium)
    - *Induction (any one agent to be used):*
        - Etomidate (Amidate) (0.3 mg/kg IV)
        - Ketamine (Ketalar) (1–2 mg/kg IV)
        - Propofol (Diprivan) (2 mg/kg IV)
        - Midazolam (Versed) (0.3 mg/kg IV)

- *Paralysis:*
    - Depolarizing neuromuscular blocker [e.g., succinylcholine at 2 mg/kg IV or 4 mg/kg intramuscular (IM)]
    - Nondepolarizing neuromuscular blocker (e.g., rocuronium at 1–1.2 mg/kg IV)
- *Complications:* Cardiovascular collapse following RSI
- *Modified RSI:* In very sick children who cannot tolerate short period of desaturation and hypoxemia, RSI can be modified by providing positive pressure ventilation.

The protocol for rapid-sequence intubation is given in **Flowchart 1**.

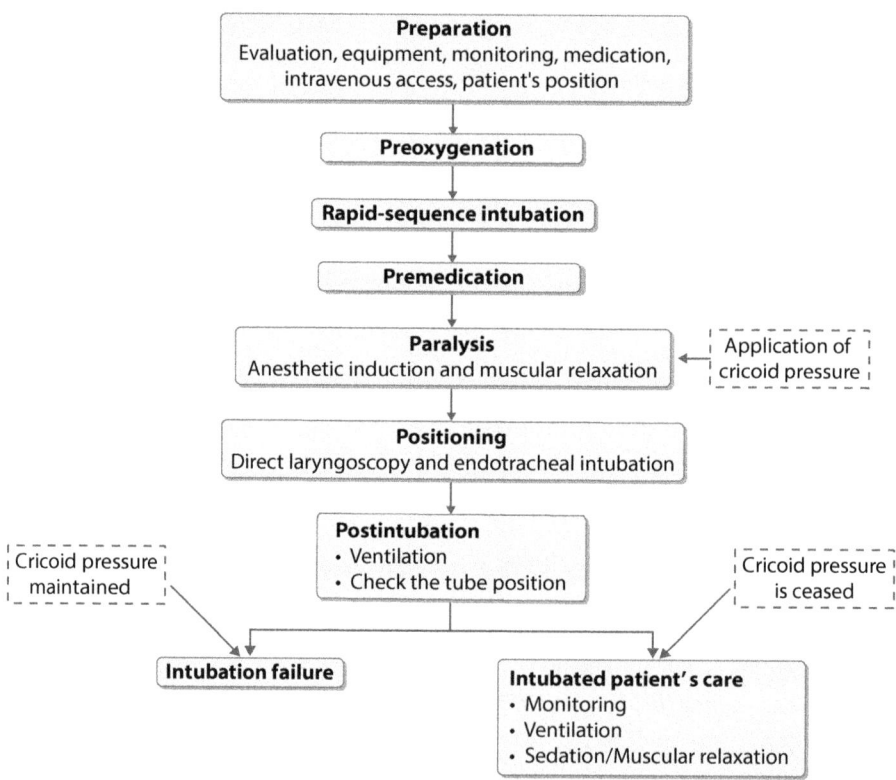

Flowchart 1: Protocol for rapid-sequence intubation.

CHAPTER 75

Central Venous Line (Femoral Vein)

Sanjeev Khera

- A central venous access is the process of placing a catheter into a centrally located vein like femoral, internal jugular, or subclavian.
- *Indications:*
  - Difficult access to peripheral veins
  - Venous access required for longer duration
  - Resuscitation (rapid large fluid boluses)
  - *Critically ill patient:* Repeated investigations required, monitoring of mechanical ventilation [arterial blood gas (ABG)], need for multiple inotropic supports or hypertonic solutions.
  - Central venous pressure monitoring
  - *Renal replacement therapy:* Hemodialysis or continuous renal replacement therapy (CRRT)
  - Cardiac pacing (transvenous)
- *Relative contraindications:*
  - No absolute contraindication
  - Abdominal trauma (penetrating) or disruption of inferior vena cava
  - Coagulopathy or thrombus (venous)
  - Vascular compromise of the limb
  - Local infections, burns
  - Structural malformations, deformities
- *Equipment:*
  - Universal precautions: Sterile gown, gloves, mask, cap
  - *Asepsis:* Skin disinfectant (povidone iodine/chlorhexidine gluconate), sterile drape, sterile gauze pieces (2 × 2 inch or 4 × 4 inch)
  - *Procedural sedation:* Midazolam (1 mg/mL dilution), ketamine (10 mg/mL dilution)
  - *Central venous catheter kit (appropriate size):* Central venous catheter (double or triple lumen), guidewire, introducer needle, dilator, blade, hubs for access port
  - Rolled towel or saline bottle for positioning of lower limb
  - Syringes (2 mL, 5 mL, 10 mL)
  - Local anesthetic [lignocaine or lidocaine without adrenaline or topical eutectic mixture—EMLA (eutectic mixture of local anesthetics)]
  - Ultrasound (USG) for guidance if available (sterile probe cover and gel)
  - Suture (nonabsorbable, 3-0 or 4-0, silk or nylon)
  - Needle holder

- Three-way connector
- Sterile clear dressing (Tegaderm)
- *Procedure:*
  - *Position:* Child is placed supine with the lower limb flexed and abducted at the hip joint to make the vessel more prominent and easily accessible. A rolled towel can also be placed beneath the ipsilateral hip thus making the inguinal region flatter and ensure ease of access during needle insertion.
  - The child may be given procedural sedation to minimize pain and avoid movement (if already comatose—only pain relief required).
  - Check the central venous catheter kit for any inadequacies or faulty equipment. Flush all ports of the catheter with normal saline and keep all lumens in locked position after checking.
  - Palpate the femoral artery by the nondominant hand. The femoral vein is placed medially to the femoral artery, just below the inguinal ligament. USG may be used to identify the vein during the procedure and perform a guided insertion if available.
  - Local anesthesia with 1% lignocaine without adrenaline or topical EMLA may be used before the procedure at the site.
  - Clean the insertion site thoroughly with povidone iodine and alcohol-based disinfectant followed by securing the site with a sterile surgical drape to ensure asepsis.
  - *Catheterization—landmark technique:*
    - Modified Seldinger technique is used for insertion of the central catheter.
    - Arterial pulsations are localized around the midpoint between anterior superior iliac spine and pubic symphysis along the inguinal ligament by the index and middle finger of nondominant hand.
    - Move 1–2 cm inferior and 1–2 cm medial to the localization of arterial pulsations to access the course of femoral vein.
    - With the fingers palpating the femoral artery, insert the introducer needle attached with a saline filled syringe medial to the index finger at approximately 30–45° angle to the skin, toward the umbilicus or cephalad, keeping gentle negative suction while advancing.
    - As the needle enters the venous lumen, a flash of blood may be noted inside the syringe. Hold the needle hub still at this point and carefully remove the syringe. Observe for free backflow (not pulsatile) of blood in the needle.
    - Insert and advance guidewire through the needle hub and notice for free movement of the wire during insertion. Any resistance may indicate displacement of needle or incorrect position. Avoid forcing guidewire against resistance. Insert guidewire leaving only 2–3 cm behind the needle hub.
    - Hold the guidewire in place and gently remove the needle. Apply sterile gauze at insertion site for hemostasis.
    - A small stab incision with tip of blade at the site of insertion can be made before introducing the dilator.
    - Introduce dilator over the guidewire in a rotating manner to create a track for passage of the catheter.

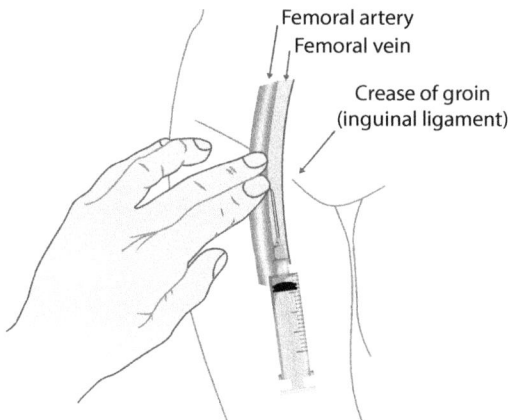

Fig. 1: Femoral vein catheterization.

- Remove the dilator and thread the venous catheter over the guidewire completely, advancing till the hub is in contact with the skin. Identify the access port through which the guidewire is exiting.
- Check for backflow of blood from the empty ports using a saline filled syringe for confirming correct placement of the catheter.
- Once confirmed, remove the guidewire, and check the remaining port for patency.
- Secure the catheter in place with nonabsorbable sutures and a sterile transparent dressing (to identify any bleeding at insertion site and intervene).
- Secure the hubs with sterile disinfectant-soaked gauze pieces and ensure sterility by "scrub the hub" technique before and after handling of the catheter.

- *Complications:*
  - Hematoma, hemorrhage
  - Arterial puncture
  - Thrombosis (deep vein thrombus) or embolus
  - Transient occlusion of catheter
  - Central line-associated blood stream infections
  - Insertion site infections
  - Dysrhythmia
  - Arteriovenous fistula formation

CHAPTER 76: Intraosseous Cannulation

Sanjeev Khera

- Intraosseous (IO) cannulation is a well-recognized alternative procedure for emergency administration of fluids and drugs in conditions where peripheral access is difficult or impossible. It provides access to the central venous canal inside the marrow cavity of the long bones receiving blood from Haversian's and Volkmann's canals which subsequently drains into venous circulation by intramedullary and emissary veins.
- *Indications:*
  - Circulatory access in cardiac arrest
  - Difficult intravenous (IV) access (>90 seconds or three failed attempts to establish IV access)
- Contraindications **(Table 1)**
- *Equipment:*
  - Procedure tray (povidone iodine, sterile drapes, 1% lignocaine without adrenaline, syringes 5 mL, 10 mL)
  - IO needle (manual trocar 16 G, spring-loaded devices, drill-based devices)
  - Fluids and resuscitation drugs
- *Sites for insertion:*
  - *Proximal tibia:* Infants and children, 1–2 cm below anterior tibial tuberosity and 1 cm medially on tibial plateau
  - *Distal tibia:* 2–3 cm proximal to medial malleolus over flat central aspect, 90° to skin
  - *Humeral head:* For older children, 1 cm above the greater tubercle and 2–3 cm lateral to biceps tendon, inserted at 45° angle aiming toward the opposite scapula
  - *Distal femur:* Only children under 6 years, in a fully extended knee, insert 2 cm above patella, and 1–2 cm medial to the anterior midline
- *Procedure:*
  - Assess the patient and record vital parameters
  - Explain procedure to the parent/caretaker
  - Observe universal precautions and ensure adequate assistance

TABLE 1: Absolute and relative contraindications of intraosseous (IO) cannulation.

Absolute	Relative
Trauma (proximal to insertion)	Previous orthopedic surgery (at site)
Bone disease (osteogenesis imperfecta, osteomyelitis, osteoporosis)	IO cannulation at same site in past 48 hours
Insertion site infections (skin/surrounding tissue)	Clotting disorders

CHAPTER 76: Intraosseous Cannulation

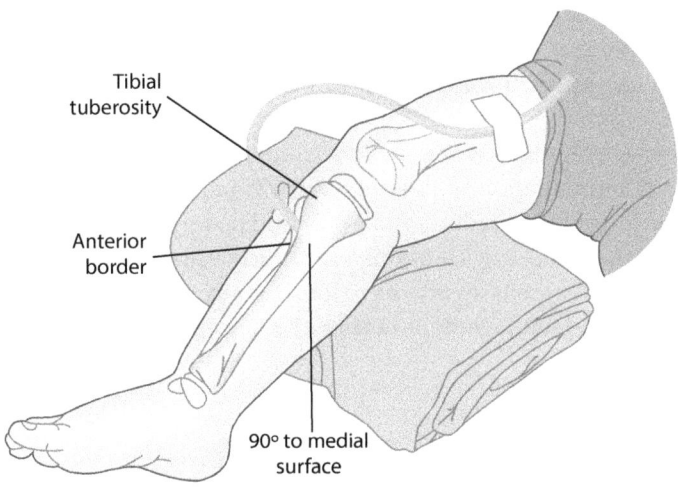

Fig. 1: Intraosseous cannulation site.

TABLE 2: Complications, prevention, and management of intraosseous (IO) cannulation.

Complication	Prevention	Management
Dislodgement	• Stabilize needle with adequate tape and dressing • Frequently reassess position and depth of needle	• Adjust depth of insertion • Flush the cannula
Infection/osteomyelitis	• Ensure asepsis during procedure • Avoid keeping IO access beyond 24 hours	Treat with antibiotics
Extravasation	Ensure fixation of canula properly and assess for extravasation before starting fluids	Discontinue IO access
Pain	Local anesthesia during procedure	Pain relief medication
Others: Skin necrosis, growth plate injury		

- Identify insertion site, mark important landmarks, and position and stabilize the limb adequately
    - *Proximal tibia:* Place firm support behind knee like a rolled towel with knee slightly flexed and palpate the anteromedial surface below the tibial tuberosity. Confirm site of insertion and insert needle at 90° to the skin surface **(Fig. 1)**.
- Check required equipment before initiating procedure [IO needle, fluids, drugs, and intravenous (IV) sets].
- Insert the needle perpendicular to the skin surface in a corkscrew motion till a give-away in the resistance is noted usually observed as a "pop".
- Remove trocar and check for spontaneous backflow of blood or confirm by gentle aspiration.
- Stabilize needle with dressing material.

- Aspirate blood for sampling followed by flushing the needle with 5–10 mL saline to ensure patency.
- Palpate calves on both the legs to check for any extravasation of fluids from the IO site.
- Administer bolus/fluids and drugs as required.
- Ensure documentation of the procedure in patients case records (indication, person/team performing procedure, vitals pre- and postprocedure, steps of procedure, number of attempts, fluids/drugs administered, and samples taken).
- Perform frequent reassessments to look for any complications postprocedure.
- Complications and management **(Table 2)**

CHAPTER 77: Peripherally Inserted Central Catheter Insertion

Sanjeev Khera, Gaurav Ray

A peripherally inserted central catheter (PICC) is a catheter that is placed in peripheral vein, inserted to reach the central venous system.

- *Indications:*
  - Total parenteral nutrition (TPN) (due to prematurity, congenital GI malformation, and bowel obstruction)
  - Presumed long duration of intravenous drugs
  - High osmolarity fluids through IV access

The veins used for access are:
- Basilic or cephalic vein in cubital fossa
- Saphenous vein
- *Scalp veins:* Temporal or posterior auricular
- External jugular vein
- Axillary vein

Basilic and cephalic veins in right cubical fossa are preferred as the route to the central veins is short and direct.

- *Equipment:*
  - Radio-opaque central venous catheter of appropriate size
  - Break-away or peel-away needle introducer
  - Non-toothed forceps
  - Gauze piece
  - Drapes
  - Povidone–iodine or chlorhexidine solution for skin preparation (based on institutional policy)
  - Normal saline or sterile water
  - Dressing adhesives, preferably transparent
  - Heparinized normal saline (0.5–1 U/mL heparin)
  - 5 mL and 10 mL syringes
  - Three-way cannula, or "t-connector"
  - Measuring tape
  - Sterile gown, gloves along with mask, and head cover
- *Preparation:*
  - Explaining the procedure to the caregiver and receiving informed consent.
  - Comfort measures such as nonnutritive sucking, facilitated tucking, and swaddling.

- Identification of a suitable vein for peripherally inserted central catheter (PICC) insertion.
- Positioning of the patient.
- Measurement of the distance from insertion point to the site supposed location of catheter tip. For basilic and cephalic veins, from insertion site, proximally to shoulder joint, to 3rd right intercostal space at the lateral border of sternum.
- Apply head cover and mask.
- Prepare a sterile tray for equipment.
- Wear a sterile gown and gloves after performing strict hand hygiene.
- Flush the catheter using a 5–10 mL syringe, with heparinized saline and leave the syringe attached.
- Holding extremity with gauze, clean the insertion site with the prep solution, covering larger area by coming out in concentric circles. Wait for the field to dry and repeat this process. Place the extremity under the sterile drape, only to expose the insertion site.

- *Catheter insertion:*
    - Giving skin traction, insert the needle to about 0.5 cm distal to the vein, at a low-lying angle of 15–30°, and move slightly ahead.
    - Once the back flow is visible, forward the needle to about 0.5 cm at a low angle. Remove the needle from the peel away introducer and advance the introducer ahead. Continued blood flow through it shows that the introducer is within the vein.
    - Hold the catheter with a non-toothed forceps and place it in the introducer, advancing it ahead slowly and threading it ahead to the calculated distance.
    - When the catheter has reached the predetermined distance, slowly withdraw the introducer after stabilizing the catheter by putting firm pressure slightly proximal to insertion site. Once the introducer is out, peel it by holding on to the wings.
    - In case there is resistance in advancing the catheter, massage the vein in proximal direction gently, or intermittently flushing with saline, or extension of shoulder joint along with repositioning of head.
    - Check for blood return by aspirating, and flush with heparinized saline.
    - Keep a gentle pressure at the insertion site with a sterile gauze till complete hemostasis is achieved.
    - Fix the catheter with a sterile tape at the insertion and apply transparent dressing over the insertion site, making it fully visible. Confirm the position of catheter tip using bedside X-ray.

Peripherally inserted central catheter care and maintenance:
- Check for the insertion site and the connections of catheter on a daily basis.
- Utilize aseptic technique when changing tubing.
- Prime volumes should be as low as 0.5 mL. Always use a 5 mL or 10 mL syringe to check for latency of catheter. In case of resistance, do not use force.
- When there is no infusion going through the catheter, place a constant infusion of a slow late, as little as 1 mL/h.

CHAPTER 77: Peripherally Inserted Central Catheter Insertion

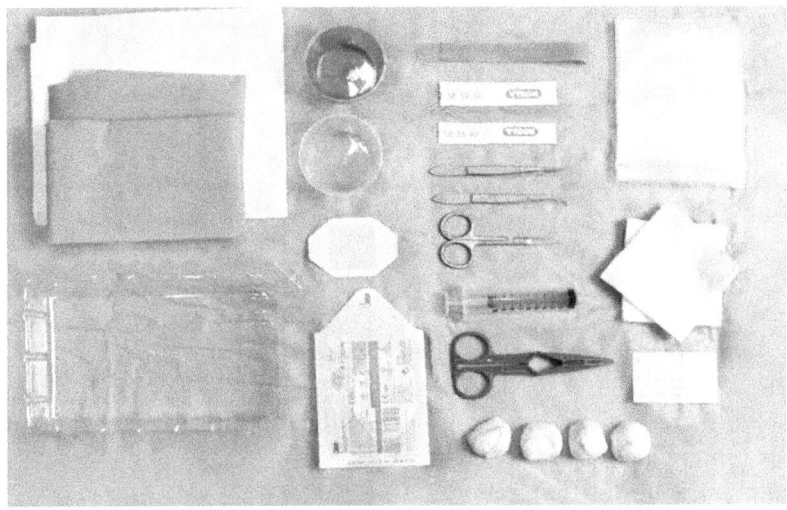

Fig. 1: Equipment required for PICC insertion.

- Do not utilize a small (<2 Fr) PICC for routine blood sampling.
- Packet red blood cell (PRBC) transfusion should preferably be given through peripheral line.
- Keep the catheter in situ only as long as it is medically indicated.

CHAPTER 78: Radial Artery Cannulation

Sanjeev Khera

Indications:
- Frequent sampling (arterial blood gas analysis)—respiratory failure, mechanical ventilation
- Invasive blood pressure monitoring—critically ill child, shock, inotropic support, hypertensive emergencies, and major surgeries.
- Cardiac output monitoring (continuous)

Contraindications:

Absolute	Relative
Poor collateral blood flow (assess Allen or modified Allen test)	Coagulation defects, recent thrombolysis, or anticoagulant therapy
Poorly palpable artery (poor visualization on ultrasonography)	Peripheral vascular disease
Overlying skin infection or abscess	Anatomical anomalies of the artery (congenital or post-traumatic)
Thrombosed artery or arteriovenous fistula (dialysis)	Surgical intervention or grafting at the site of cannulation
Burns (full thickness)	

Equipment:
- Universal precautions—sterile gown, gloves, mask, and cap
- Asepsis—skin disinfectant (povidone iodine/chlorhexidine gluconate), sterile drape, sterile gauze pieces (2 × 2 inch or 4 × 4 inch)
- Intravenous (IV) cannula or radial artery cannula (appropriate size)
- Arm board (neonate or pediatric)
- Syringes (5 mL, 2 mL) with heparinized flush
- Pressure tubing, pressure transducer kit or integrated arterial pressure line.
- Local anesthetic [lignocaine or lidocaine without adrenaline or topical eutectic mixture—EMLA (eutectic mixture of local anesthetics)]
- Ultrasound for guidance if available
- Suture (nonabsorbable, 3-0 or 4-0, silk or nylon)
- Needle holder

- 3-way connector
- Sterile clear dressing (Tegaderm)

Procedure:
- Select and assess the site for adequacy of insertion (check for collateral circulation and any contraindications).
- Localization of radial artery—medial to head of radius and lateral to tendon of flexor carpi radialis near wrist over the anterolateral aspect.
- Positioning of limb—place the hand and forearm over the arm board with wrist slightly extended to make the radial pulse prominent and secure the forearm with tape.
- Examine the cannulation equipment for manufacturing defects and assemble the arterial pressure monitoring kit.
- Apply topical anesthetic or infiltrate local anesthesia at the site.
- Sterilize the site using surface disinfectant and secure it with sterile drapes to ensure asepsis.

Insertion technique:
- Locate artery by palpating with the non-dominant hand to guide insertion.
- At an angle of 30-45° to the skin with the bevel of the needle up, insert the arterial canula using the dominant hand approximately 1 cm proximal to radial head advancing in a cephalad direction.
- Observe while advancing the needle for flash of blood into the barrel or reservoir of the canula indicating entry of needle tip into arterial lumen. Advance the canula further by 1-2 mm.
- Stabilize and hold the canula. Observe for pulsatile backflow of blood in reservoir or by placing a gauze under the hub of canula.
- Two methods of placement of canula—catheter over wire technique or angiocatheter method.
- *Angiocatheter:* At an angle of 30° introduce the catheter further into the lumen by 2 mm. With the hub held firmly, advance the catheter completely into the lumen till the catheter hub.
- *Catheter over wire:* A guidewire is threaded through the needle and with the needle hub held firmly, the catheter is inserted over the needle and guide wire with gentle twisting motion.
- Guide wire or needle (or both) are withdrawn as per the procedure followed.
- Avoid attempting to advance catheter or guidewire if met with resistance.
- Occlude the artery proximally to avoid blood loss till pre-flushed pressure transducer or arterial pressure line is connected.
- Check the waveform on monitor after connecting the pressure line.
- Secure catheter with sterile dressing and tape.

Complications:
- Hematoma, hemorrhage

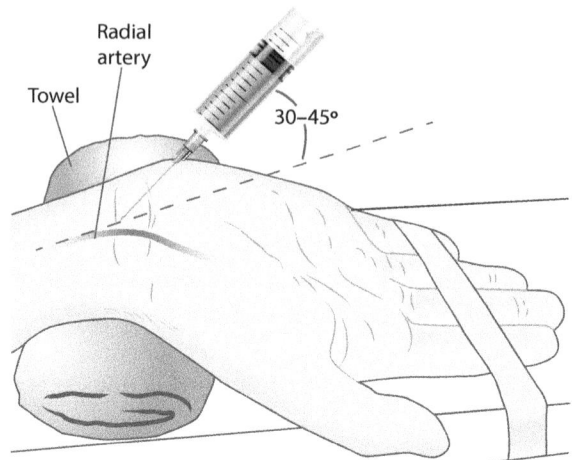

Fig. 1: Technique of radial artery puncture and cannulation.
Source: Chapter 57. Arterial puncture and cannulation. In: Reichman EF (Ed). Emergency Medicine Procedures, 2nd edition. The McGraw-Hill Companies; 2013, Figure 57-5.

- Vasospasm (arterial obstruction)—ischemic damage
- Infections
- Thrombotic or embolic events
- Arteriovenous fistula
- Pseudoaneurysm formation
- Retained guidewire

CHAPTER 79: Umbilical Vein Catheterization

Sanjeev Khera, Gaurav Ray

A safe and effective route for administering fluid and medicines intravenously during and post resuscitation in a newborn using the exposed umbilical stump. The umbilical cord comprises two umbilical arteries and a single umbilical vein.

Indications:
- Vascular access during neonatal resuscitation
- Partial or double volume exchange transfusion
- Requirement of long-term venous access (extreme and very low birth weight, preterm, and sick neonates)
- Anticipated frequent blood sampling

Contraindications:
- Abdominal wall defects (gastroschisis and omphalocele)
- Infections (omphalitis, necrotizing enterocolitis, and peritonitis)

Equipment:
- Euthermia—radiant warmer
- Asepsis/sterile field—povidone iodine/alcohol-based disinfectant, procedure tray, swabs, sterile drape, catheter fixing tape, cord tape/tie.
- Umbilical vein catheter—single/double or triple lumen with/without three-way connectors
  - <1.5 kg–3.5 F
  - >1.5 kg–4 or 5 F
- Universal precautions—surgical gown, sterile gloves (two pairs), surgical mask and cap
- Three-way connectors
- Measuring tape
- Sterile blade (with handle)—No. 11 or 15
- Forceps (non-toothed)
- Syringes—5 mL, 10 mL
- Fluids and medications
- Vacutainers for sample [ethylenediaminetetraacetic acid (EDTA), sterile, heparinized syringe for venous blood gas (VBG)]
- Suture material—silk (2-0, 3-0) with needle
- Needle holder
- Suture cutting scissors/blade

Prerequisite:
- Selection of adequate size catheter

- Measure depth of insertion/length of placement
  - Two-thirds of the distance measured from shoulder to umbilicus or use nomograms modified from Dunn PM. Localization of umbilical catheter by postmortem measurements.
  - Use formula [(birth weight (kg) × 3) + 9]/2 for length of insertion required.

Note: Umbilical vein catheterization (UVC) during emergency procedures/resuscitation to be placed at length when spontaneous backflow of blood is noted in catheter.

- *Team:* Neonatologist/pediatrician/resident and nursing staff.

Procedure:
- *Site preparation:*
  - Clean the cord stump and surrounding area using surface disinfectants. Apply povidone iodine solution and allow to dry for at least 30 seconds.
  - Create a sterile field using surgical drapes.
  - Place a cord tie using a single knot at the base of the cord stump.
- Ensure change of gloves after cleaning, before catheter preparation and insertion
- *Catheter preparation:*
  - Flush the sterile catheter with saline after connecting a three-way connector and turn the knob in closed position.
  - Follow unit protocol.
- Cut the cord horizontally using a straight blade in a single motion leaving approximately 1–1.5 cm of cord stump from skin.
- *Catheter insertion:*
  - Identify umbilical vein usually seen as a large, thin-walled vessel with a collapsed lumen, mostly at 12 o'clock position close to the periphery of stump.
  - Hold the cord stump with forceps or non-dominant hand and apply gentle traction.
  - Insert catheter into the lumen and with gentle pressure slide the vein cephalad.
  - If resistance is observed, slightly loosen the cord tape, and attempt re-insertion.
  - Insert the catheter to the measured length plus the length of stump or the point of backflow of blood as per the requirement of procedure.
  - Turn the hub of three-way connector to open and apply gentle suction to look for backflow of blood.
- *Anticipated difficulties:*
  - Passage of catheter through ductus venosus may present with resistance. The catheter may be pulled back to approximately 4 cm and reinserted while rotating in a clockwise direction.
- Once the position of catheter is confirmed, catheter may be fixed by any of the following techniques:
  - Create a tape bridge between catheter and abdomen.
  - Secure by purse string sutures over the cord stump.
  - Sterile transparent tape over the abdomen and umbilical catheter.
- Cover the catheter hub using povidone iodine-soaked gauze/swab for maintaining sterility.
- Confirm central position of the catheter just above the diaphragm by a radiograph kidigram [anterior-posterior (AP) view].

Precautions:
- Avoid keeping catheters in situ beyond 10 days of age (ideally to be removed by day 7).
- Avoid transfusing hypertonic fluids keeping in mind the possibility of tissue necrosis in case of extravasation.
- Avoid frequent positioning and manipulation of the catheter.
- Ensure to "scrub the hub" with disinfectants before and after change of IV sets to prevent catheter associated infections.
- Prevent accidental air embolus by checking fluids and tubings for air columns before administration.

Complications:
- Infections
- Thromboembolic event
- Uncontrolled bleeding
- *Intracardiac positioning of catheter:*
  - Pericardial effusion/cardiac tamponade
  - Cardiac arrhythmias
  - Left atrial thrombus
- *Catheter malpositioned in portal system causing:*
  - Hepatomegaly
  - Hepatic necrosis, ascites
  - Necrotizing enterocolitis
  - Perforation of colon
- *Others:*
  - Perforation of peritoneum
  - Parenteral nutrition fluid extravasation
  - Portal hypertension
- Catheter breakage/fracture during removal (migration/embolization of broken segments)

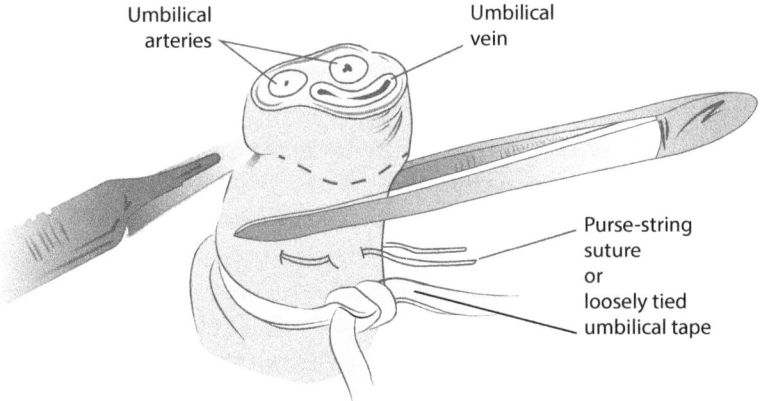

Fig. 1: Umbilical vein catheterization.
Source: aneskey.com

CHAPTER 80
Intercostal Drainage Tube Insertion

Mithlesh Kumar Tiwari

Indications:
- Pneumothorax
- Hemopneumothorax
- Parapneumonic effusion or empyema
- Chylothorax
- Postoperative care (e.g., thoracotomy or lobectomy)

Relative contraindications:
- Coagulopathy and thrombocytopenia
- Pulmonary bullae
- Skin infection over the chest tube insertion site

Materials:
- Universal precautions materials
- Skin prep solution
- Sterile draping
- 1 or 2% lidocaine with epinephrine for local anesthesia or eutectic mixture of local anesthetics (EMLA)
- Scalpel with size 11
- Artery forceps
- 10 mL and 20 mL syringes
- Age-appropriate chest tube or trocar
- Suturing material/Tegaderm/tape
- Under water seal
- Airway, breathing, and circulation (ABC) monitoring and resuscitation kit

Procedure:
- *Classical surgical method of intercostal drainage tube insertion* (**Fig. 1**)
  - Obtain informed written consent.
  - *Monitoring:* Place patient on continuous cardiac monitoring and pulse oximetry
  - *Positioning:*
    - Position the patient in the supine position.
    - Locate area of insertion, i.e., "triangle of safety" (anterior border of latissimus dorsi, lateral border of pectoralis major, a line superior to the horizontal level of the nipple, and apex below the axilla) which is approximated by 4th–5th intercostal space in the anterior axillary line.
    - Mark the insertion point with a pen or back of the needle.

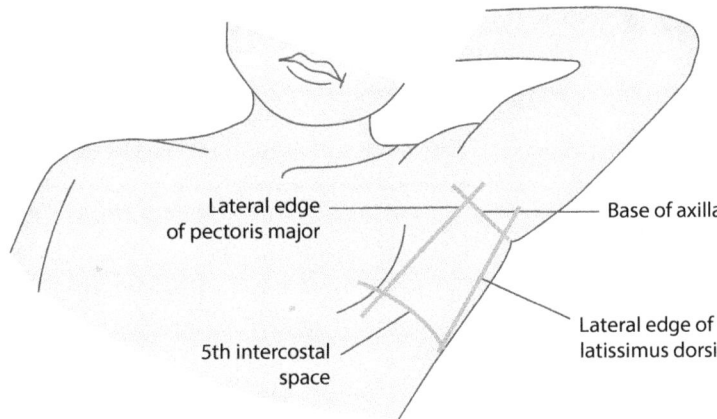

Fig. 1: Intercostal drainage tube (ICDT) insertion site—triangle of safety.

- Use universal precaution and sterile technique to drape the patient.
- Give local anesthesia in the skin and deeper structure using lignocaine.
- Make a small incision parallel to the rib and cut through the subcutaneous layers and intercostal muscles using artery forceps. Insert the clamped chest tube through the incision and advance it manually. Keep the chest tube upward in case of pneumothorax and downward for drainage of fluid.
- Secure the tube with mattress/interrupted sutures.
- Connect the distal end of the tube to underwater seal. Once the tube is connected. unclamped the chest tube and look for column movement.
- Do a chest X-ray (CXR) to confirm the position of the tube.

Complications:
- Bleeding and hemothorax
- Subcutaneous emphysema
- Perforation of underlying lung, heart, and diaphragm
- Infection of the drainage site.

CHAPTER 81

Thoracocentesis: Needle Aspiration of Pneumothorax

Sanjeev Khera

Indications:
- Primary spontaneous pneumothorax
- Tension pneumothorax

Relative contraindications:
- Spontaneous pneumothorax in patients with underlying lung disease
- Traumatic pneumothorax without tension

Materials:
- Universal precautions materials
- Skin prep solution
- Sterile draping
- 1% or 2% lidocaine with epinephrine for local anesthesia or eutectic mixture of local anesthetics (EMLA)
- 18-gauge needle (smaller if child is small)
- IV tubing set
- Three-way stopcock
- 50-mL syringe, 5-mL syringe
- Suturing material/Tegaderm/tape
- Under water seal
- Airway, breathing, and circulation (ABC) monitoring and resuscitation kit

Procedure (Fig. 1):
- *Analgesia:* Oral or parenteral analgesia pre- and postprocedure
- *Anesthesia:* Use local anesthetic or EMLA
- *Monitoring:* Place patient on continuous cardiac monitoring and pulse oximetry
- *Position:* Trauma patient—head up supine; all other: 45°, sitting position
- Puncture site—upper border of the 3rd rib in the second intercostal space along the midclavicular line.
- Attach a 5-mL syringe to the catheter device.
- Puncture the skin at the level of above landmark through upper border of 3rd rib.
- Carefully insert the needle into the pleural space while aspirating the syringe.
- In tension pneumothorax, often you will hear a pop or feel a give away.
- Withdraw the needle while gently advancing the cannula downwards into position.
- Secure cannula with tape/Tegaderm/sutures.
- Attach three-way stopcock and 50-mL syringe.

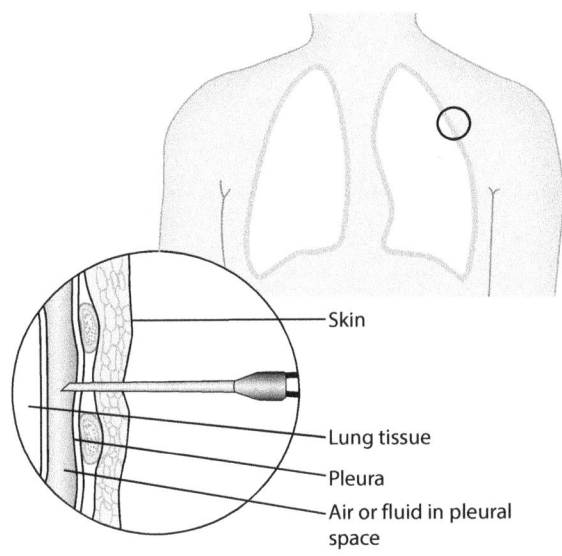

Fig. 1: Puncture site for needle aspiration of pneumothorax.

- Drain until no further drainage.
- Drain can be placed in underwater seal if prolonged drainage is required.
- Post-procedure—consider analgesia and plan for chest tube insertion while monitoring, obtain chest X-ray (CXR).

Complications, prevention, and management:

Complication	Prevention	Management
Air does not flow with opening of clamp	Check position of insertion and depth of insertion	Adjust depth of insertion
Fluid is bloody	Avoid insertion over veins; could be associated hemothorax	Withdraw needle
Cardiovascular deterioration during procedure	ABC monitoring throughout	Suitable resuscitative measures while completing the procedure as procedure itself may relieve cardiovascular deterioration

(ABC: airway, breathing, and circulation)

Documentation in the medical record:
- Consent
- Indications and contraindications for procedure
- Procedure, including preparation, anesthetic, analgesia, and needle size
- Any complications or "none"
- Pre- and postprocedure vital signs.

CHAPTER 82: Abdominal Paracentesis

Sanjeev Khera

Indications:
- Diagnostic
  - Unexplained ascites
  - Spontaneous or secondary bacterial peritonitis
- Therapeutic
  - Large symptomatic ascites
  - Abdominal compartment syndrome

Contraindications:
- Coagulopathy or severe thrombocytopenia
- History of abdominal surgery (possible adhesions)
- Dilated bowel loops
- Local infection at the procedure site
- Acute surgical abdomen

Materials:
- Universal precautions (gloves, mask, surgical cap, and surgical gown)
- Disinfectant (chlorhexidine, povidone iodine)
- Sterile drape
- Local anesthetic (1% lidocaine)
- Paracentesis needle (18G or smaller)
- IV tubing set
- Three-way connector
- Syringes (5 mL, 10 mL)
- Sample collecting bottles
- Ascitic fluid collection bag
- Ultrasound (if available)

Procedure:
- Obtain history relevant to identifying cause/indication (malignancy, chronic liver disease, and portal hypertension) of procedure and confirm presence of fluid both on examination and ultrasound (if available). Also assess the hemodynamic status of the patient.
- Explain the procedure to the parents/patient and take written informed consent.
- Ultrasound guidance will provide a more controlled setting for procedure and can be useful in reducing the chances of a failure or complications.
- Ask patient to micturate prior to procedure (empty urinary bladder).
- *Position:* Ask the patient to lay supine with trunk elevated at 20–30° or place the patient in the lateral decubitus position.

- *Site:*
  - In the midline, at a point midway between the umbilicus and symphysis pubis (approximately 3–4 cm below umbilicus)
  - Point between umbilicus and anterior superior iliac spine in either of the lower abdominal quadrants.
  - Mark the site in insertion of needle.
- Administer local anesthesia to the puncture site using 1% lidocaine.
- Hold the 18G needle connected to IV tubing and three-way connector perpendicular to the skin, insert gradually using the Z-technique and feel for sudden loss of resistance and flow of ascitic fluid in the tubing. Remove the trocar and secure the catheter with adhesive tape.
- Close the three-way connector and connect the tubing to a collection bag.
- On completion of the paracentesis, remove the catheter and secure the puncture site with a sterile dressing.
- Monitor the patient for any complications post-procedure (hypotension, bleed, abdominal pain, or distress)

Complications:
- *Hypotension:* Restrict removal of ascitic fluid (10% body weight)
  - Manage with IV fluid. From the
    - *Blood stained ascitic fluid:* Insert needle from marked site avoiding visible superficial abdominal veins.
    - *Fecal contents in fluid:* Ultrasound-guided insertion of needle can prevent inadvertent rupture of bowel. Monitor patient for any signs of peritonitis and take surgical consult if needed.
    - *Inadequate flow from catheter:* Check and adjust depth of the inserted catheter or reposition patient.

Documentation:
- Written consent duly signed by patient/guardian and the physician.
- Procedure note (date and time of procedure, team details, site, steps of procedure, fluid volume, pre- and postprocedure vitals, and complications if any)

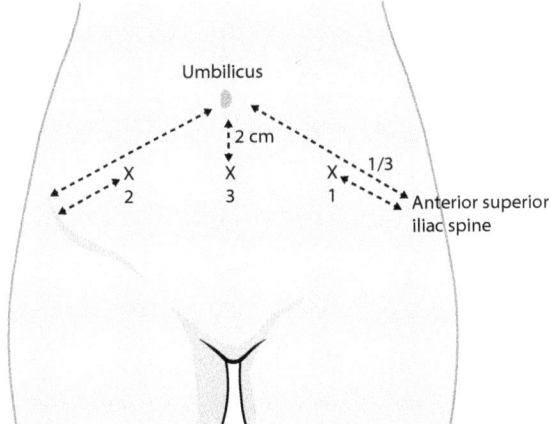

Fig. 1: Sites for abdominal paracentesis.
Source: Harvey JJ, Prentice R, George J. Diagnostic and therapeutic abdominal paracentesis. Med J Aust. 2023;218(1):18-21.

SECTION 13

Charts and Scales

Section Editors: *Vinod Dagar, Abhishek Pandey, Sarvesh Kohli, Ajay Beriwal, Bhaskar Bharadwaj*

- Pediatric Advanced Life Support Algorithms
- Pediatric Early Warning Score
- Triage
- Ventilator Illustration
- Noninvasive Ventilation Illustration
- Sedation Withdrawal
- Rapid-sequence Intubation
- Maintenance Intravenous Fluids in Children
- Total Parenteral Nutrition and Enteral Nutrition
- Edema in Nephrotic Syndrome
- Coma and Pain Scales
- Catheter and Tube Sizes
- Blood Component Replacement
- Abnormal Sodium
- Transudate versus Exudate
- Steroids and Efficacy
- Emergency Drug Preparation
- Important Formulae
- Glucose-6-phosphate Dehydrogenase and Drugs
- Drug Levels
- Electrocardiogram Values
- Intravenous Compatibility Charts
- Sample Collection
- Laboratory Values
- Computed Tomography Scan and Lesions
- Common Pediatric Applications
- Pediatric Neuroimaging Primer
- Pediatric Neurology Charts

CHAPTER 83

Pediatric Advanced Life Support Algorithms

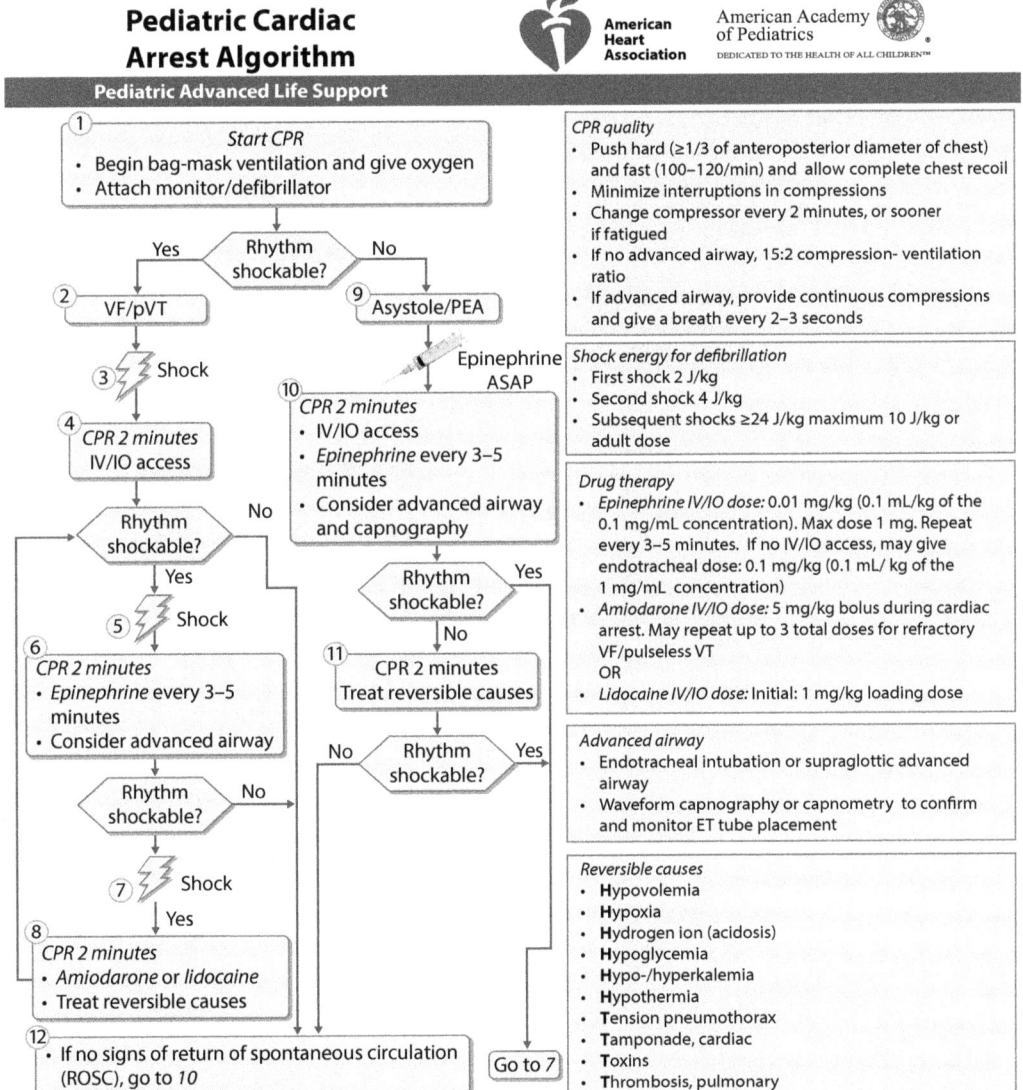

(CPR: cardiopulmonary resuscitation; ET: endotracheal tube; IO: intraosseous; IV: intravenous; PEA: pulseless electrical activity; pVT: pulseless ventricular tachycardia; VF: ventricular fibrillation; VT: ventricular tachycardia)

Pediatric Bradycardia with a Pulse Algorithm

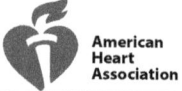 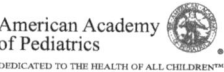

Pediatric Advanced Life Support

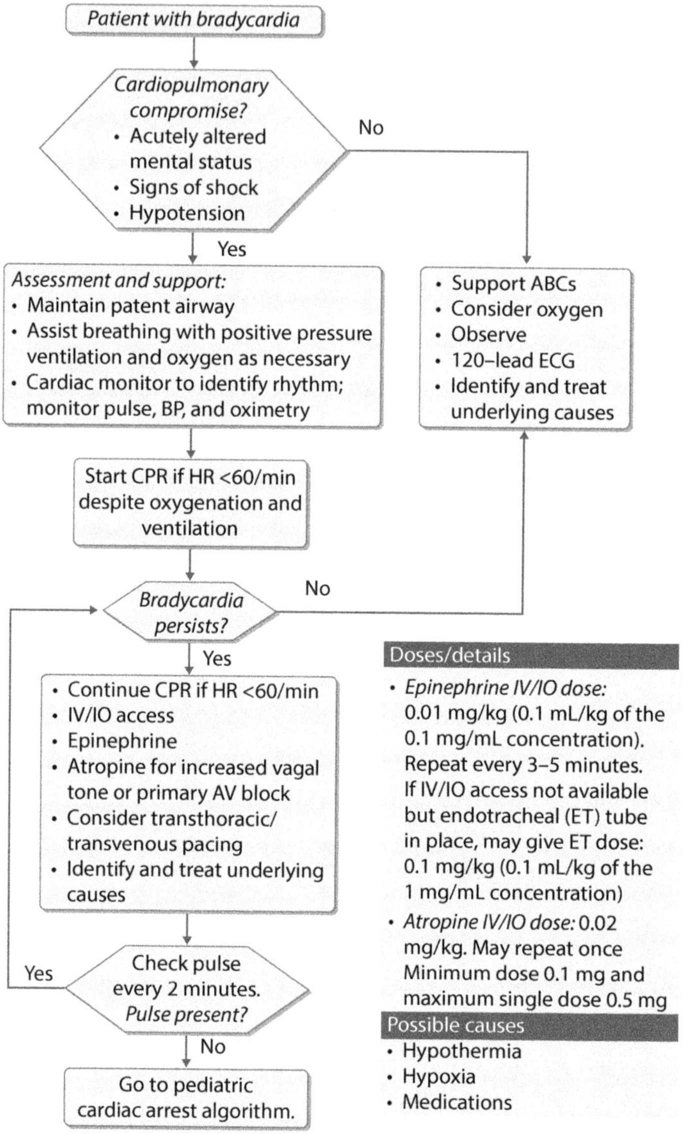

Patient with bradycardia
↓
Cardiopulmonary compromise?
- Acutely altered mental status
- Signs of shock
- Hypotension

No →
- Support ABCs
- Consider oxygen
- Observe
- 120-lead ECG
- Identify and treat underlying causes

Yes ↓

Assessment and support:
- Maintain patent airway
- Assist breathing with positive pressure ventilation and oxygen as necessary
- Cardiac monitor to identify rhythm; monitor pulse, BP, and oximetry

↓

Start CPR if HR <60/min despite oxygenation and ventilation

↓

Bradycardia persists? — **No** →

Yes ↓

- Continue CPR if HR <60/min
- IV/IO access
- Epinephrine
- Atropine for increased vagal tone or primary AV block
- Consider transthoracic/transvenous pacing
- Identify and treat underlying causes

↓

Check pulse every 2 minutes. Pulse present?
— **Yes** → (loop back)
— **No** ↓

Go to pediatric cardiac arrest algorithm.

Doses/details
- *Epinephrine IV/IO dose:* 0.01 mg/kg (0.1 mL/kg of the 0.1 mg/mL concentration). Repeat every 3–5 minutes. If IV/IO access not available but endotracheal (ET) tube in place, may give ET dose: 0.1 mg/kg (0.1 mL/kg of the 1 mg/mL concentration)
- *Atropine IV/IO dose:* 0.02 mg/kg. May repeat once Minimum dose 0.1 mg and maximum single dose 0.5 mg

Possible causes
- Hypothermia
- Hypoxia
- Medications

(ABC: airway, breathing, circulation; AV: atrioventricular; BP: blood pressure; CPR: cardiopulmonary resuscitation; ECG: electrocardiogram; HR: heart rate; IO: intraosseous; IV: intravenous)

CHAPTER 83: Pediatric Advanced Life Support Algorithms

Pediatric Tachycardia with a Pulse Algorithm

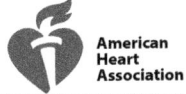
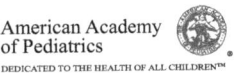

Pediatric Advanced Life Support

Initial assessment and support:
- Maintain patent airway; assist breathing as necessary
- Administer oxygen
- Cardiac monitor to identify rhythm; monitor pulse, blood pressure, and oximetry
- IV/IO access
- 12-Lead ECG if available

Doses/details

Synchronized cardioversion:
Begin with 0.5-1 J/kg; if not effective, increase to 2 J/kg. Sedate if needed, but do not delay cardioversion.

Drug therapy

Adenosine IV/IO dose:
- *First dose:* 0.1 mg/kg rapid bolus (maximum: 6 mg)
- *Second dose:* 0.2 mg/kg rapid bolus (maximum second dose: 12 mg)

↓

Evaluate rhythm with 12-lead ECG or monitor

Probable sinus tachycardia if:
- P waves present/normal
- Variable RR interval
- Infant rate usually <220/min
- Child rate usually <180/min

→ Search for and treat cause

Cardiopulmonary compromise?
- Acutely altered mental status
- Signs of shock
- Hypotension

Yes → Evaluate QRS duration
- Narrow (≤0.09 sec): **Probable supraventricular tachycardia:**
  - P waves absent/abnormal
  - RR interval not variable
  - Infant rate usually ≥220/min
  - Child rate usually ≥180/min
  - History of abrupt rate change

  → If IV/IO access is present, give *adenosine* or
  If IV/IO access is not available, or if adenosine is ineffective, perform synchronized cardioversion

- Wide (>0.09 sec): **Possible ventricular tachycardia**

  Synchronized cardioversion: Expert consultation is advised before additional drug therapies

No → Evaluate QRS duration
- Narrow (≤0.09 sec): **Probable supraventricular tachycardia:**
  - P waves absent/abnormal
  - RR interval not variable
  - Infant rate usually ≥220/min
  - Child rate usually ≥180/min
  - History of abrupt rate change

  → Consider vagal maneuvers
  → If IV/IO access is present, give *adenosine*

- Wide (>0.09 sec): **Possible ventricular tachycardia**

  If rhythm is *regular* and QRS *monomorphic*, consider adenosine

  Expert consultation is recommended

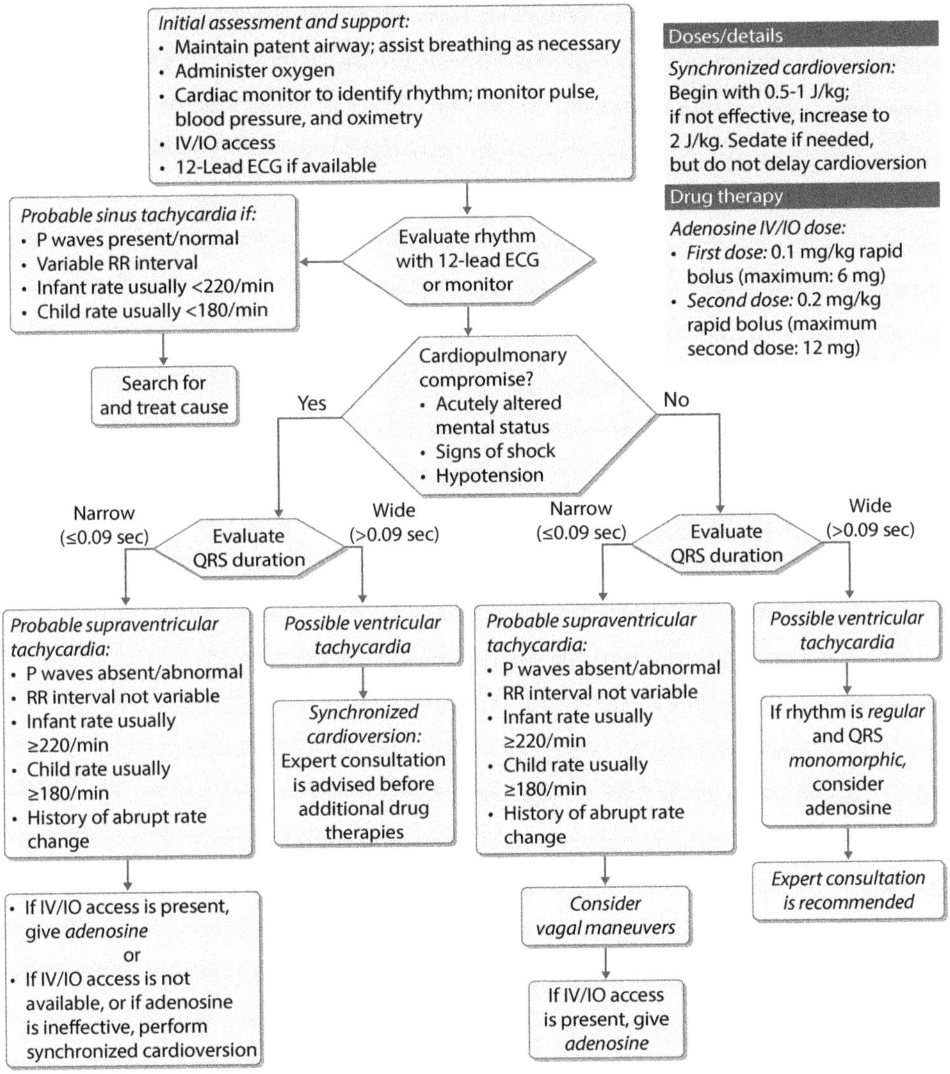

(ECG: electrocardiogram; HR: heart rate; IO: intraosseous; IV: intravenous; RR: respiratory rate)

Pediatric Septic Shock Algorithm

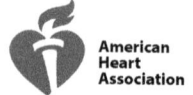 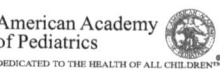

Pediatric Advanced Life Support

1. Identify signs of septic shock
- Altered *mental status* (irritability or decreased level of consciousness)
- Altered *heart rate* (tachycardia or, less commonly, bradycardia)
- Altered *temperature* (fever or hypothermia)
- Altered *perfusion* (prolonged or "flash" capillary refill; cool or very warm extremities; plethoric appearance, mottled color or pallor; possible ecchymosis or purpura; decreased urine output)
- *Hypotension:* May or may not be present

Immediate (10–15 minutes)

2. Initial stabilization
- Support A-B-Cs
- Monitor heart rate, blood pressure, and pulse oximetry
- Establish IV/IO access
- *Fluid boluses:* Give 10–20 mL/kg isotonic crystalloid boluses (10 mL/kg for neonates and those with pre-existing cardiovascular compromise)
- Assess carefully after each bolus

3. Within first hour
- Draw blood for culture and additional laboratory studies, including glucose and calcium—do not delay antibiotic or fluid therapy
- *Antibiotics:* Give broad-spectrum antibiotics
- Assess carefully after each bolus. Repeat fluid boluses as needed to treat shock. Stop if rales, respiratory distress, or hepatomegaly develops
- Give antipyretics if needed
- *Goals of therapy:* Improved mental status, normalization of heart rate and temperature, adequate systolic and diastolic blood pressure, improved perfusion (see 1)

4. Do signs of shock persist after 40–60 mL/kg total fluid administration or evidence of fluid overload?

No → 5. Consider critical care consultation

Yes → 6.
- Obtain critical care consultation
- Initiate and titrate epinephrine *or* norepinephrine

Initial stabilization

7.
- Establish central venous and intra-arterial pressure monitoring
- Continue epinephrine/norepinephrine (as above) and bolus fluid therapy as needed to treat shock
- Verify adequate airway, oxygenation, and ventilation
  Consider stress-dose hydrocortisone if hemodynamics remain inadequate despite adequate fluid resuscitation and vasoactive drug therapy

(A-B-C: airway, breathing, circulation; IO: intraosseous; IV: intravenous)

Source:
1. Brierley J, Carcillo JA, Choong K, Cornell T, Decaen A, Deymann A, et al. Clinical practice parameters for hemodynamic support of pediatric and neonatal septic shock: 2007 update from the American College of Critical Care Medicine. Crit Care Med. 2009;37(2):666-88.
2. Kissoon N, Orr RA, Carcillo JA. Updated American College of Critical Care Medicine—pediatric advanced life support guidelines for management of pediatric and neonatal septic shock: relevance to the emergency care clinician. Pediatr Emerg Care. 2010;26(11):867-9.

Management of Shock After ROSC Algorithm

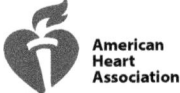 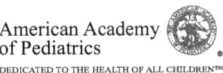

Pediatric Advanced Life Support

Optimize ventilation and oxygenation
- Titrate FiO_2 to maintain oxyhemoglobin saturation 94–99% (or as appropriate to the patient's condition); if possible, wean FiO_2 if saturation is 100%
- Consider advanced airway placement and waveform capnography
- If possible, target a pCO_2 that is appropriate for the patient's condition and limit exposure to severe hypercapnia or hypocapnia

---

Assess for and treat persistent shock
- Identify and treat contributing factors
- Consider 20 mL/kg IV/IO boluses of isotonic crystalloid. Consider smaller boluses (e.g., 10 mL/kg) if poor cardiac function suspected
- Consider the need for inotropic and/or vasopressor support for fluid-refractory shock

Possible contributing factors
- **H**ypovolemia
- **H**ypoxia
- **H**ydrogen ion (acidosis)
- **H**ypoglycemia
- **H**ypo-/hyperkalemia
- **H**ypothermia
- **T**ension pneumothorax
- **T**amponade, cardiac
- **T**oxins
- **T**hrombosis, pulmonary
- **T**hrombosis, coronary
- **T**rauma

Hypotensive shock:
- Epinephrine
- Norepinephrine

Normotensive shock:
- Epinephrine
- Milrinone*

- Monitor for and treat agitation and seizures
- Monitor for and treat hypoglycemia
- Assess blood gas, serum electrolytes, and calcium
- If patient remains comatose after resuscitation from cardiac arrest, maintain targeted temperature management, including aggressive treatment of fever
- Consider consultation and patient transport to tertiary care center

---

Estimation of maintenance fluid requirements
- *Infants <10 kg:* 4 mL/kg per hour
  Example: For an 8-kg infant, estimated maintenance fluid rate
  = 4 mL/kg per hour × 8 kg
  = 32 mL per hour
- *Children 10–20 kg:* 4 mL/kg per hour for the first 10 kg + 2 mL/kg per hour for each kg above 10 kg
  Example: For a 15-kg child, estimated maintenance fluid rate
  = (4 mL/kg per hour × 10 kg)
  + (2 mL/kg per hour × 5 kg)
  = 40 mL/hour + 10 mL/hour
  = 50 mL/hour
- *Children >20 kg:* 4 mL/kg per hour for the first 10 kg + 2 mL/kg per hour for 11–20 kg + 1 mL/kg per hour for each kg above 20 kg
  Example: For a 28-kg child, estimated maintenance fluid rate
  = (4 mL/kg per hour × 10 kg)
  + (2 mL/kg per hour × 10 kg)
  + (1 mL/kg per hour × 8 kg)
  = 40 mL per hour + 20 mL per hour
  + 8 mL per hour
  = 68 mL per hour

After initial stabilization, adjust the rate and composition of intravenous fluids based on the patient's clinical condition and state of hydration. In general, provide a continuous infusion of a dextrose-containing solution for infants. Avoid hypotonic solutions in critically ill children; for most patients use isotonic fluid such as normal saline (0.9% NaCl) or lactated, Ringer's solution with or without dextrose, based on the child's clinical status

---

*Milrinone can cause hypotension, so use and initiation of it should generally be reserved for those experienced with its use, initiation, and side eects (e.g., ICU personnel).
(FiO_2: fraction of inspired oxygen; ICU: intensive care unit; pCO_2: partial pressure of carbon dioxide)

Pediatric Color-coded Length-based Resuscitation Tape

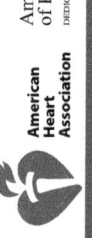

Pediatric Advanced Life Support

Zone	3 kg	4 kg	5 kg	Pink	Red	Purple	Yellow	White	Blue	Orange	Green
ETT uncuffed (mm)	3.5	3.5	3.5	3.5	3.5	4.0	4.5	5.0	5.5	N/A	N/A
ETT cuffed (mm)	3.0	3.0	3.0	3.0	3.0	3.5	4.0	4.5	5.0	5.5	6.0
Lip-tip (cm)	9–9.5	9.5–10	10–10.5	10–10.5	10.5–11	11–12	12.5–13.5	14–15	15.5–16.5	17–18	18.5–19.5
Suction (F)	8	8	8	8	8	8	10	10	10	10	12
L-scope blade	1 straight	1 straight	1 straight	1 straight	1 straight	1–1.5 straight	2 straight/curved	2 straight/curved	2 straight/curved	2–3 straight/curved	2–3 straight/curved
Stylet	6 F	6 F	6 F	6 F	6 F	6 F	10 F	10 F	10 F	14 F	14 F
OPA (mm)	50	50	50	50	50	60	60	60	70	80	80
NPA (F)	14	14	14	14	14	18	20	22	24	26	26
Bag-mask device (minimum mL)	450	450	450	450	450	450	450	450–750	750–1,000	750–1,000	1,000
ETCO$_2$ detector	Ped	Ped	Ped	Ped	Ped	Ped	Ped	Adult	Adult	Adult	Adult
LMA	1	1	1	1.5	1.5	2	2	2	2–2.5	2.5	3
Tidal volume (mL)	20–30	24–40	30–50	40–65	50–85	65–105	80–130	100–165	125–210	160–265	200–330
Frequency	20–25/min	20–25/min	20–25/min	20–25/min	20–25/min	15–25/min	15–25/min	15–25/min	12–20/min	12–20/min	12–20/min

(ETT: endotracheal tube; ETCO$_2$: end-tidal carbon dioxide; F: French; LMA: laryngeal mask airway; NPA: nasopharyngeal airway; OPA: oropharyngeal airway; Ped: pediatric)

Source: Used with permission from The Broselow-Luten System Point of Care Guide is © 2020 Vyaire Medical, Inc.

PALS Systematic Approach Algorithm

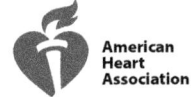
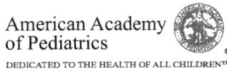

Pediatric Advanced Life Support

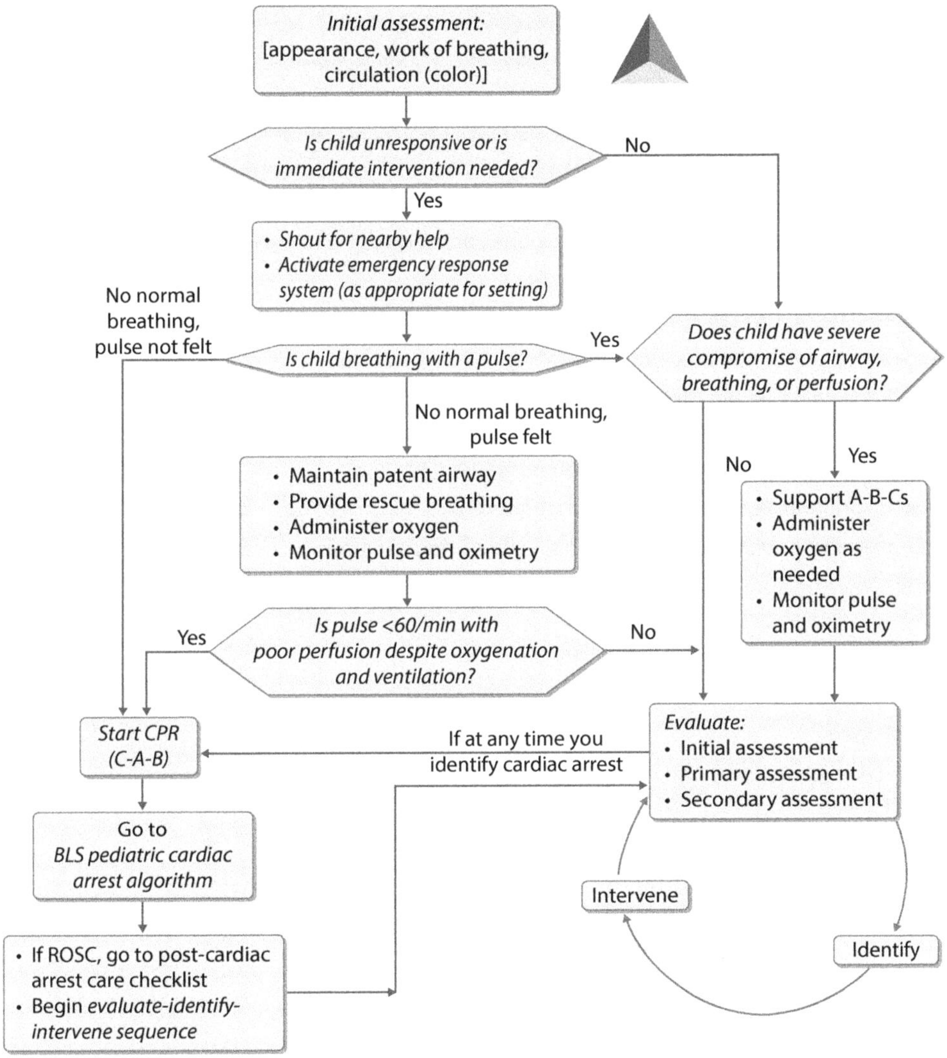

Initial assessment: [appearance, work of breathing, circulation (color)]

Is child unresponsive or is immediate intervention needed?
- No → Does child have severe compromise of airway, breathing, or perfusion?
- Yes →
  - Shout for nearby help
  - Activate emergency response system (as appropriate for setting)

Is child breathing with a pulse?
- No normal breathing, pulse not felt → Start CPR (C-A-B)
- No normal breathing, pulse felt →
  - Maintain patent airway
  - Provide rescue breathing
  - Administer oxygen
  - Monitor pulse and oximetry
- Yes → Does child have severe compromise of airway, breathing, or perfusion?

Does child have severe compromise of airway, breathing, or perfusion?
- No → Evaluate
- Yes →
  - Support A-B-Cs
  - Administer oxygen as needed
  - Monitor pulse and oximetry

Is pulse <60/min with poor perfusion despite oxygenation and ventilation?
- Yes → Start CPR (C-A-B)
- No → Evaluate

Start CPR (C-A-B) → Go to *BLS pediatric cardiac arrest algorithm*
- If ROSC, go to post-cardiac arrest care checklist
- Begin *evaluate-identify-intervene sequence*

If at any time you identify cardiac arrest

Evaluate:
- Initial assessment
- Primary assessment
- Secondary assessment

→ Intervene → Identify → (cycle)

(A-B-C: airway, breathing, circulation; BLS: basic life support; C-A-B: chest compressions, airway, breathing; CPR: cardiopulmonary resuscitation; IO: intraosseous; IV: intravenous; ROSC: return of spontaneous circulation)

Components of Postcardiac Arrest Care

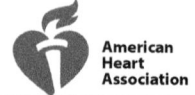 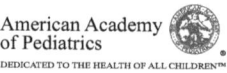

Pediatric Advanced Life Support

	Check
Oxygenation and ventilation	
Measure oxygenation and target normoxemia 94–99% (or child's normal/appropriate oxygen saturation)	☐
Measure and target PaCO$_2$, appropriate to the patient's underlying condition and limit exposure to severe hypercapnia or hypocapnia	☐
Hemodynamic monitoring	
Set specific hemodynamic goals during post-cardiac arrest care and review daily	☐
Monitor with cardiac telemetry	☐
Monitor arterial blood pressure	☐
Monitor serum lactate, urine output, and central venous oxygen saturation to help guide therapies	☐
Use parenteral fluid bolus with or without inotropes or vasopressors to maintain a systolic blood pressure greater than the fifth percentile for age and sex	☐
Targeted temperature management (TTM)	
Measure and continuously monitor core temperature	☐
Prevent and treat fever immediately after arrest and during rewarming	☐
If patient is comatose apply TTM (32°C–34°C) followed by (36°C–37.5°C) or only TTM (36°C–37.5°C)	☐
Prevent shivering	☐
Monitor blood pressure and treat hypotension during rewarming	☐
Neuromonitoring	
If patient has encephalopathy and resources are available, monitor with continuous electroencephalogram	☐
Treat seizures	☐
Consider early brain imaging to diagnose treatable causes of cardiac arrest	☐
Electrolytes and glucose	
Measure blood glucose and avoid hypoglycemia	☐
Maintain electrolytes within normal ranges to avoid possible life-threatening arrhythmias	☐
Sedation	
Treat with sedatives and anxiolytics	☐
Prognosis	
Always consider multiple modalities (clinical and other) over any single predictive factor	☐
Remember that assessments may be modified by TTM or induced hypothermia	☐
Consider electroencephalogram in conjunction with other factors within the first 7 days after cardiac arrest	☐
Consider neuroimaging such as magnetic resonance imaging during the first 7 days	☐

(PaCO$_2$: partial pressure of arterial carbon dioxide)

CHAPTER 84: Pediatric Early Warning Score

	0	1	2	3
Behavior	Playing/appropriate OR Sleeping comfortably	Irritable and consolable	Irritable and NOT consolable	Lethargic, confused OR Reduced response to pain
Cardiovascular	Pink or capillary refill time <12 seconds	Pale OR Capillary refill time 3 seconds	Gray or capillary refill time 4 seconds OR Heart rate 20 above OR Below normal rate for age	Gray and mottled OR Capillary refill time >4 seconds OR Heart rate 30 above OR Below normal heart rate for age
Respiratory	Within normal rate, no retractions AND SpO_2 98–100% on RA	RR >10 above normal limits OR SpO_2 98–100% on any O_2 device OR SpO_2 94–97% on RA, OR Using accessory muscles	RR >20 above normal limits OR SpO_2 90–93% OR Retractions	RR 5 below normal OR SpO_2 <90% OR Retractions and/OR Grunting
Output	Reaching target urine output goal of 0.5–1 mL/kg/h (over the last 4 hours) AND 0–1 BMs/emesis events in the last 12 hours	2 BMs/emesis events in the last 12 hours	3 BMs/emesis events in the last 12 hours	<0.5 mL/kg/h of urine output (over the last 4 hours) OR >3 BMs/emesis events in the last 12 hours

Score	Action
0–3 (green)	No action needed, reassess as per order
4–6 (yellow)	Notify charge nurse, call junior resident, and notify staff physician
7 (red)	Call the rapid response team, call staff physician, and junior resident

In case a single "3" in any category, immediate notification is given to the junior resident and staff MD

(BMs: bowel movements; RA: room air; RR: respiratory rate; SpO_2: peripheral oxygen saturation)

CHAPTER 85

Triage

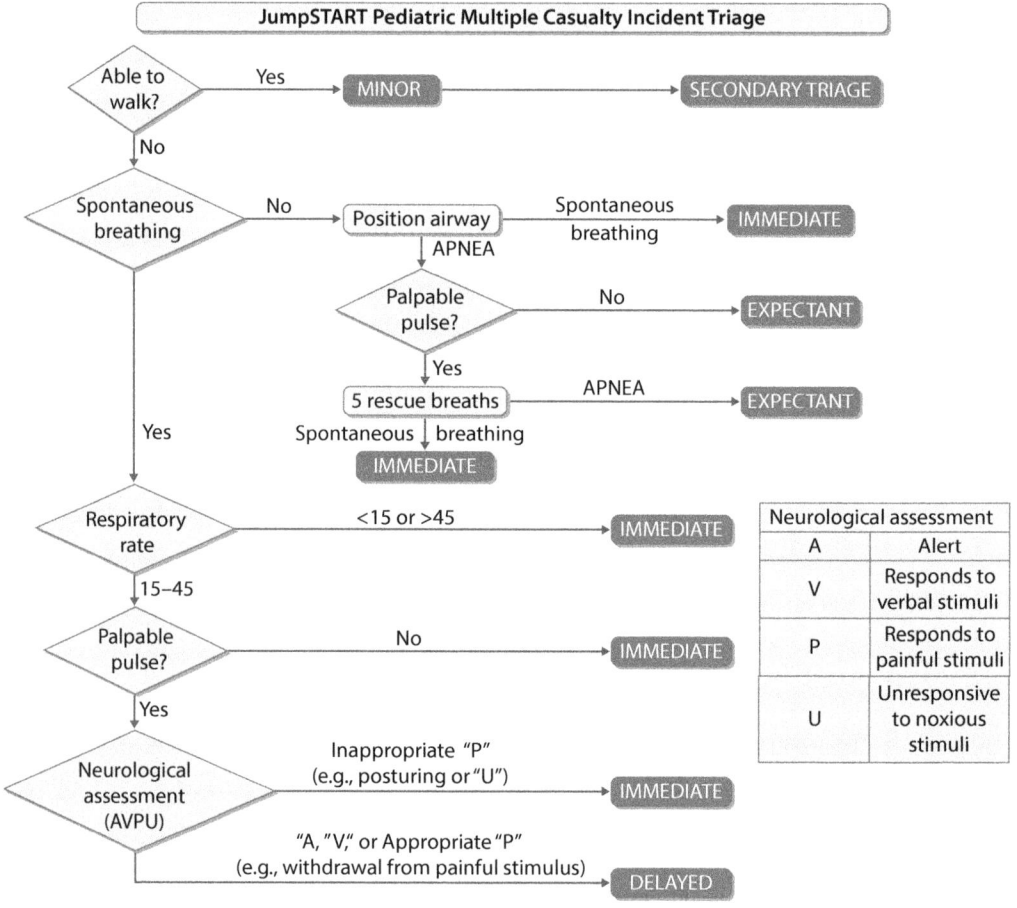

Use jumpSTART if the patient appears to be a child.
Use an adult system, such as START, if the patient appears to be a young adult.

Contd...

Contd...

Triage categories

EXPECTANT — Black Triage Tag Color
- Victim unlikely to survive given severity of injuries, level of available care, or both
- Palliative care and pain relief should be provided

DELAYED — Yellow Triage Tag Color
- Victim's transport can be delayed
- Includes serious and potentially life-threatening injuries, but status not expected to deteriorate significantly over several hours

IMMEDIATE — Red Triage Tag Color
- Victim can be helped by immediate intervention and transport
- Requires medical attention within minutes for survival (up to 60)
- Includes compromises to patient's airway, breathing, circulation

MINOR — Green Triage Tag Color
- Victim with relatively minor injuries
- Status unlikely to deteriorate over days
- May be able to assist in own care: "Walking Wounded"

Source: Adapted from http://www.jumpstarttriage.com/

CHAPTER 86

Ventilator Illustration

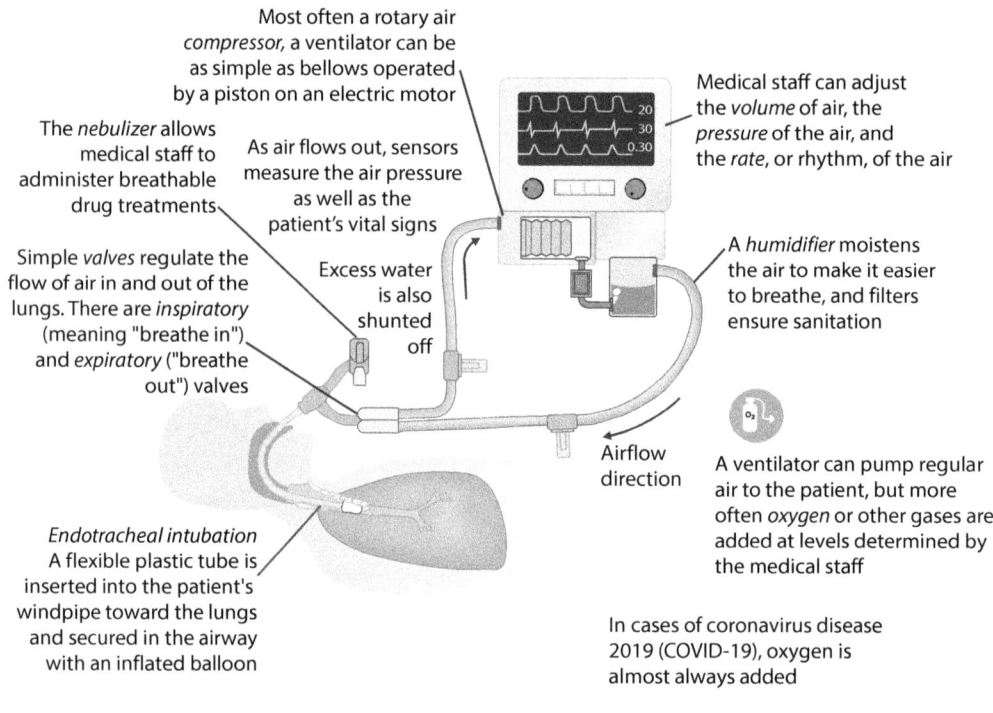

CHAPTER 87: Noninvasive Ventilation Illustration

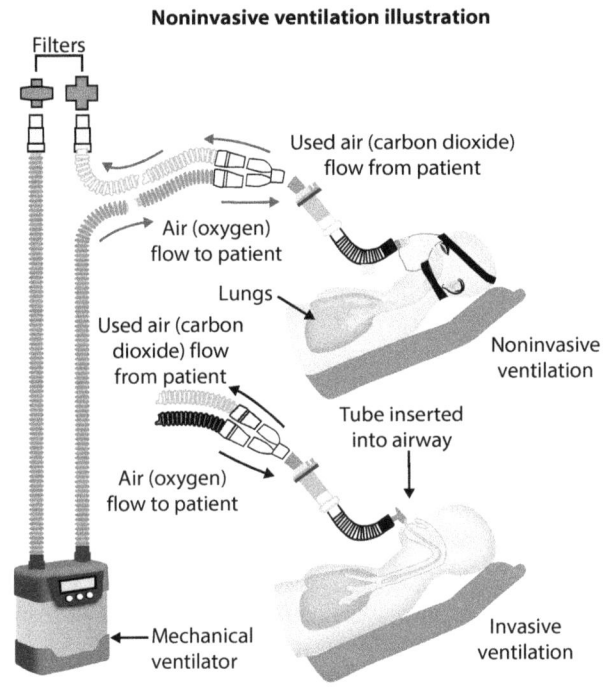

Noninvasive ventilation illustration

CHAPTER 88: Sedation Withdrawal

- *Conversion strategy for weaning from commonly used sedatives and analgesics*:

Transitioning from continuous IV sedation to an intermittent enteral regimen.	
IV to enteral opioid	
Step 1	Start enteral opioid agent at dose calculated conversion from IV to enteral opioid
Step 2	Wean opioid infusion by 50% 30 minutes after the second enteral opioid dose
Step 3	Turn opioid infusion off 30 minutes after the third enteral opioid dose
IV to enteral benzodiazepine	
Step 1	Start enteral benzodiazepine agent at dose calculated conversion from IV to enteral benzodiazepines
Step 2	Wean benzodiazepine infusion by 50% 30 minutes after the first enteral benzodiazepine dose
Step 3	Turn benzodiazepine infusion off 30 minutes after the second enteral benzodiazepine dose

- *Procedure for calculating opioid dose conversions*:

Converting IV to enteral opioids—calculating the enteral dose.			
Continuous medication infusion		**Enteral agent**	**Typical maximum dose**
Fentanyl 2.5 µg/kg/h	• Morphine • Hydromorphone • Oxycodone	• 0.45 mg/kg/dose every 4 hours • 0.07 mg/kg/dose every 4 hours • 0.3 mg/kg/dose every 4 hours	• 15 mg/dose • 5 mg/dose • 10 mg/dose
Fentanyl <2.5 µg/kg/h	• *Step 1*: Calculate enteral morphine equivalent fentanyl __ µg/kg/h × __ kg × 0.18 = __ mg enteral morphine/dose A calculated dose should be given every 4 hours • *Step 2*: Convert to the desired enteral agent if not enteral morphine enteral morphine to enteral hydromorphone __ mg enteral morphine/dose × 0.15 = __ mg enteral hydromorphone/dose A calculated dose should be given every 4 hours • Enteral morphine to enteral oxycodone: __ mg enteral morphine/dose × 0.67 = __ mg enteral oxycodone/dose A calculated dose should be given every 4 hours		
Note: When considering enteral conversion for patients >50 kg wean continuous infusion until the threshold for maximum enteral dose is reached.			

- *Evaluation of IV to enteral benzodiazepine conversion calculations*:

Converting IV to enteral benzodiazepines—calculating the enteral dose.			
Continuous medication infusion	**Enteral agent**		**Typical maximum dose**
Midazolam 0.15 mg/kg/h	• Diazepam • Lorazepam	• 0.27 mg/kg/dose every 6 hours • 0.18 mg/kg/dose every 4 hours	• 10 mg/dose • 5 mg/dose

Midazolam <0.15 mg/kg/h	• *Calculate enteral diazepam equivalent:*
	  Midazolam__mg/kg/h × __kg × 1.8 = __mg enteral diazepam/dose
	  A calculated dose should be given every 6 hours
	• *Calculate enteral lorazepam equivalent:*
	  Midazolam__mg/kg/h × __kg × 1.2 = __mg enteral lorazepam/dose
	  A calculated dose should be given every 4 hours		

Note: When considering enteral conversion for patients >50 kg wean continuous infusion until the threshold for maximum enteral dose is reached.

- *IV wean plans for patients unable to tolerate enteral sedation*:
  - *5-9 days (consider for high risk <5 days):*
    - Calculate 10% of the maximum dose(s) after extubation
    - Wean opioid infusion by the calculated dose every 12 hours
    - Wean benzodiazepine infusion by the calculated dose every 12 hours
    - For patients on opioid and benzodiazepine infusions, wean every 6 hours in an alternating fashion
  - *10-21 days (consider for high risk 5-9 days):*
    - Calculate 10% of the maximum dose(s) after extubation
    - Wean opioid infusion by the calculated dose every 24 hours
    - Wean benzodiazepine infusion by the calculated dose every 24 hours
    - For patients on opioid and benzodiazepine infusions, wean every 12 hours in an alternating fashion

CHAPTER 89: Rapid-sequence Intubation

- *Rapid-sequence intubation—drugs:*

Drug	Dose	Comments
First (adjuncts)		
Atropine	• 0.01–0.02 mg/kg • Minimum 0.1 mg • Maximum 1 mg	Prevents bradycardia and prevents oral secretions
Sedative—hypnotic (second)		
Thiopental	1–5 mg/kg	• Contraindicated in asthmatics • Decreases BP • Avoid in hypotensive child
Ketamine	1–4 mg/kg	May increase BP, ICP, HR, and oral secretions, causing bronchodilatation
Midazolam	0.05–0.1 mg/kg	• May decrease BP and HR • Respiratory depression
Fentanyl	1–5 µg/kg	• Fewest hemodynamic effects • Chest wall rigidity
Etomidate	0.2–0.3 mg/kg	Does not cause hypotension or increased ICP
Paralytic (third)		
Rocuronium	0.6–1.2 mg/kg	• Onset 30 seconds, duration 30–60 minutes • Minimal effect on hemodynamics • Flush line before and after use
Vecuronium	0.1–0.2 mg/kg	• Onset: 70–120 seconds, duration 30–90 minutes, minimal effect on BP/HR • Reversal of effect with atropine or neostigmine within 30 minutes
Succinylcholine	1–2 mg/kg	Onset: 30–60 seconds, duration 3–10 minutes, increases ICP, contraindicated in burns, massive trauma, neuromuscular disorder, malignant hyperthermia, and pseudocholinesterase deficiency

(BP: blood pressure; HR: heart rate; ICP: intracranial pressure)

- *Treatment algorithm for intubation (A) and sedation options (B):*

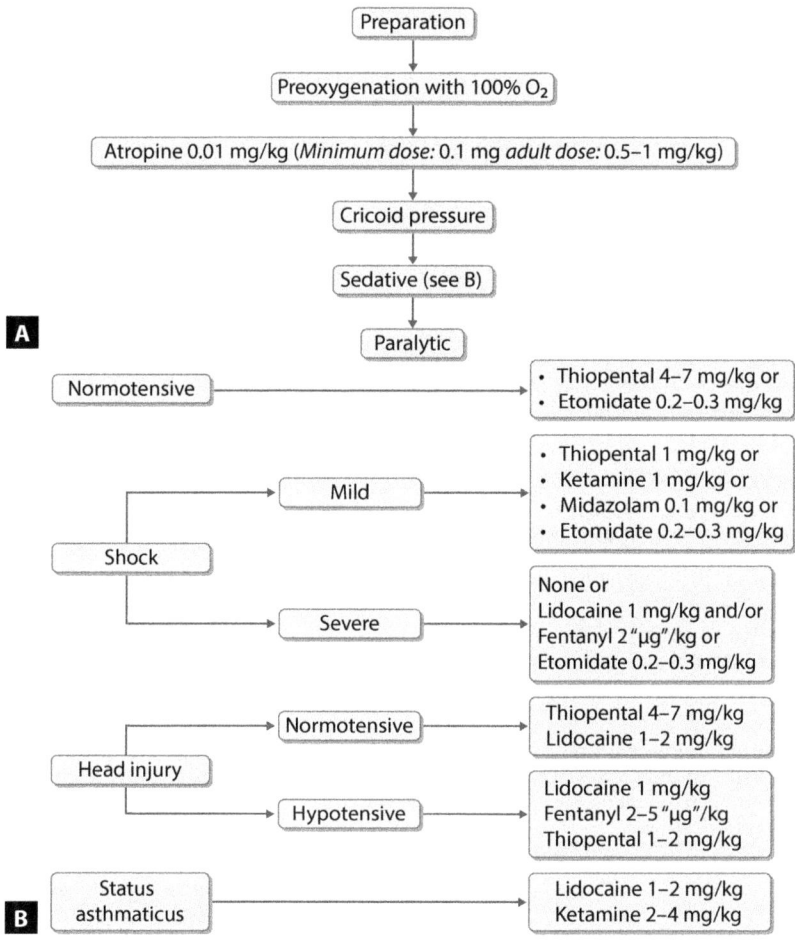

Note: (A) Treatment algorithm for intubation and (B) Sedation options.

CHAPTER 90

Maintenance Intravenous Fluids in Children

Routine maintenance:

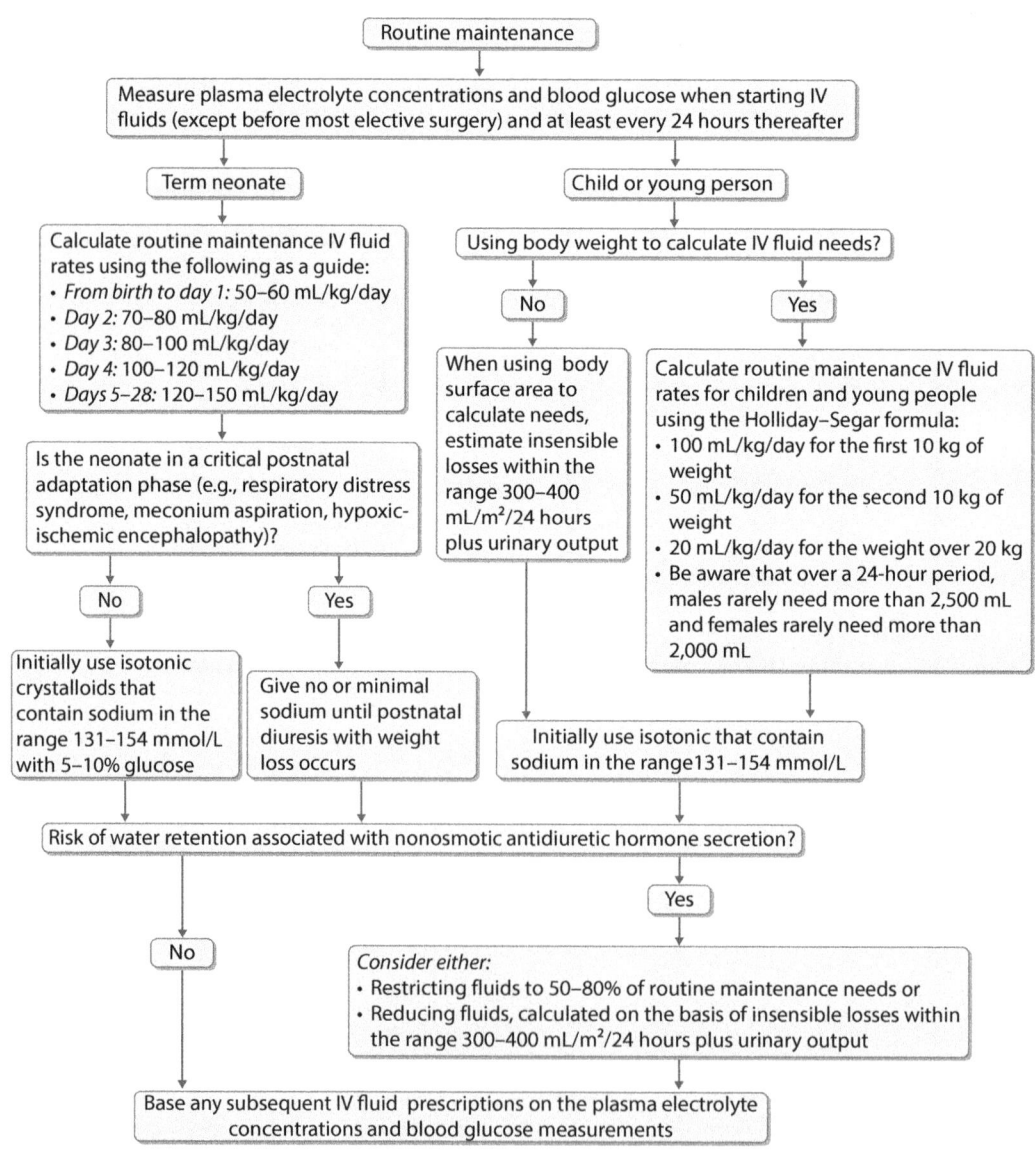

CHAPTER 91: Total Parenteral Nutrition and Enteral Nutrition

- *Approximate requirement of parenteral nutrition in children:*

	Total fluid (mL/kg/day)	Amino acids (g/kg/day)			Dextrose (g/kg/day)			Fat intralipids (g/kg/day)				Total calories needed/day
		1	2	3+	1	2	3+	1	2	3	4+	
Neonate	100	1.5	2	2	10	10–15	15–20	1	2	3	3	100/kg
<10 kg	100	1.5	2	2	10	10	15–20	1	2	3	3	100/kg
10–15	90	1	1.5	2	5	10	15	1	2	3	3	1,000 + 50/kg over 10 kg
15–20	80	1	1.5	1.5–2	5	10	10–15	1	2	2	3	1,000 + 50/kg over 10 kg
20–30	65	1	1	1–2	5	10	10–15	1	1.5	2	2.5	1,500 + 20/kg over 20 kg
>30	50	1	1	1–2	5	5–10	10	1	1.5	1.5	2	1,500 + 20/kg over 20 kg

Note: Total calories/kg/day equals g/kg/day of (amino acids × 4) + (dextrose × 4) + (intralipids × 10).

The number of calories required (kcal/kg/day) is equal to the amount of water required in mL/kg/day

- *Nutritional calculations:*

$$\text{Body mass index (BMI)} = \frac{\text{Weight (kg)}}{[\text{Height (cm)}]^2}$$

- *Caloric content of food:*

Food type	kcal/g
Carbohydrate	3.4
Proteins	4.0
Fat	9.1

- Respiratory quotient (RQ) = CO_2 production (mL/min)/O_2 consumption (mL/min)

Fuel	RQ
Ketones	<0.6
Fat	0.7
Carbohydrates	1
Lipogenesis	>1.1

Harris–Benedict equation of resting energy expenditure (kcal/day)
Males = 66 + [13.7 × weight (kg)] + [5 × height (cm)] − (6.8 × age)
Females = 65.5 + [9.6 × weight (kg)] + [1.8 × height (cm)] − [4.7 × age]

- *Composition and properties of common IV fluids:*

Solution	Na	Cl	K	Ca	Lactate	kcal/L	mOsm
D5W	0	0	0	0	0	170	252
D10W	0	0	0	0	0	240	505
D50W	0	0	0	0	0	1,700	2,530
½ NS	77	77	0	0	0	0	154
NS	154	154	0	0	0	0	308
3% NaCl	513	513	0	0	0	0	1,026
RL	130	109	4	3	28	0	308
20% Mannitol	0	0	0	0	0	0	1,098

- *Enteral nutrition calculation*: Resting energy expenditure calculation:
  - Schofield-HW (weight-based equation)—calculated in kcal/day:

Age	Male	Female
<3 years	60.9 × weight (kg) − 54	61.0 × weight (kg) − 51
3–10 years	22.7 × weight (kg) + 495	22.5 × weight (kg) + 499
10–18 years	17.5 × weight (kg) + 651	12.2 × weight (kg) + 746

  - Schofield-HW equation (weight- and height-based)—calculated in kcal/day:

Age	Male	Female
<3 years	0.167 × weight + 15.174 × height (cm) − 617.6	16.252 × weight + 10.232 × height (cm) − 413.5
3–10 years	19.59 × weight + 1.303 × height (cm) + 414.9	16.969 × weight + 1.618 × height (cm) + 371.2
10–18 years	16.25 × weight + 1.372 × height (cm) + 515.5	8.365 × weight + 4.65 × height (cm) + 200

- *Pediatric intensive care unit (PICU) nutrition guidelines:*

Energy requirements		Protein requirements	
Age	kcal/kg/day	Age	g/kg/day
<1 year	51–54	<1 year	2–3
1–3 years	56–57	1–2 years	2–3
3–5 years	45–57	2–3 years	1.5–2
6–12 years	33–45	3–12	1.5–2
>13 years	26–29	>13 years	1.5
Schofield			

Note: Do not exceed g/kg/day American Society for Parenteral and Enteral Nutrition (ASPEN) guideline.

CHAPTER 91: Total Parenteral Nutrition and Enteral Nutrition

- *Advancing enteral feedings:*

Age	Weight (kg)	Initial infusion	Advance	Goal (mL/h*)
Continuous				
<1 year	<10	1–2 mL/kg/h	1–2 mL/kg q4 or 8 hours	30
1–6 years	10–20	1 mL/kg/h	1 mL/kg q4 or 8 hours	53
7–13 years	20–50	1 mL/kg/h	1 mL/kg q4 or 8 hours	70
>14 years	>50	25–50 mL/h	25–50 mL q4 or 8 hours	100
Bolus/intermittent				
<1 year	<10	5 mL/kg	1–2 mL/kg q4 or 8 hours	20–30
1–6 years	10–20	5 mL/kg	1 mL/kg q4 or 8 hours	15–20
7–13 years	20–50	2–4 mL/kg	2–4 mL/kg q4 or 8 hours	10–15
>14 years	>50	2–4 mL/kg	2–4 mL/kg q4 or 8 hours	10

*Goal rate in nonfluid restricted hemodynamically stable patents. It feeds are tolerated but stopped at any time, restart at the previous rate If significant residuals (>2 × hourly rate if continuous or >50% of bolus feed), hold feedings for 2 hours, recheck residual, then restart at the previous rate and recheck residuals in 2 hours. Consider prokinetics.

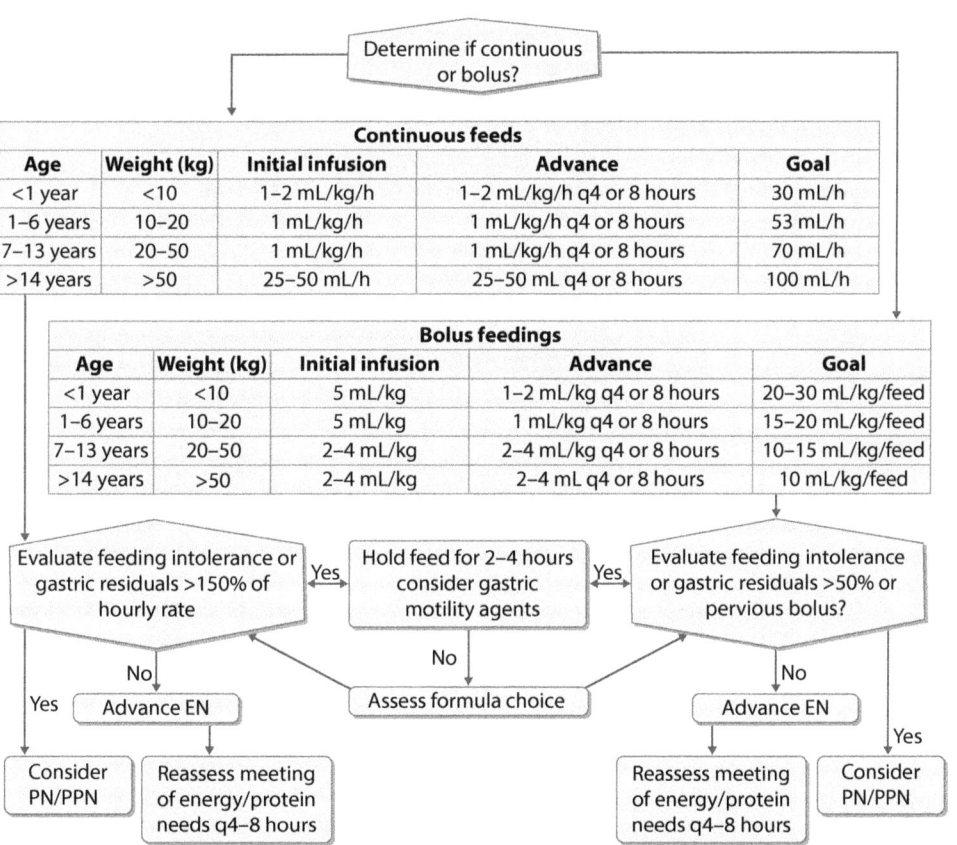

(EN: enteral nutrition; PN: parenteral nutrition; PPN: partial parenteral nutrition)

SECTION 13: Charts and Scales

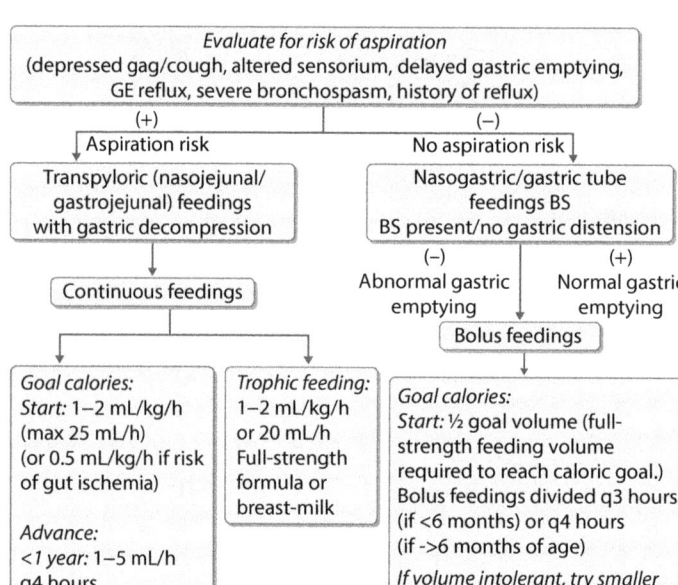

Constipation:
(For age>1 month / non-neutropenic)
No stool after 48 hours of EN

Day # 1
Prune juice

Day # 2
Glycerin supp.

Docusate:
(<3 years: PO 10 mg BID)
(3–6 years: PO 20 mg BID)
(6–12 years: PO 50 mg BID)
(≥12 years: PO100 mg BID)

Senna: (discontinue after 2 normal stools)
(1 month-2 years: PO 2.5 mL BID)
(2–5 years: PO 3.75 mL BID)
(5–12 years: PO 7.5 mL BID)
(≥12 years: PO 1 tab BID)

Fleet enema (for age >2 years)
- Pediatric fleets enema: 2–12 years (66 mL/bottle) 1 enema
- Adult fleet enema: ≥12 years

Diarrhea:
(>4 loose stools/24 hours)

Discontinue laxatives (senna) and stool softeners (docusate)

Discontinue any sorbitol-containing medication

Review osmolarity of formula

Consider withdrawal from opiates

Consider change in formula, or hold tube feedings until diarrhea resolves

Stool viral studies/*Clostridia (C.) difficile*

Stool *C. difficile* toxin and culture (if on antimicrobials)

Enteral feeding intolerance:
Gastric residual volumes (GRV) recorded prior to each bolus feed or q4 hours in patients on continuous gastric feedings with abdominal discomfort, distension or emesis.

If GRV >150 mL; or 5 mL/kg, or >½ volume of previous feeding; or > total 2 hourly infusion rate in patients on continuous feeding–hold feedings and repeat GRV after 2 hours. if repeat GRV is elevated, hold feedings and monitor GRV of 4 hours

If abdominal distension (abdominal girth increased for 2 consecutive measurements) or abdominal discomfort or emesis x2–hold feedings for 4 hours and reassess.

(BS: bowel syndrome: EN: enteral nutrition; GE: gastroesophageal)

CHAPTER 92: Edema in Nephrotic Syndrome

- *Edema in nephrotic syndrome:*
  - Edema is the most common initial presenting complaint in children with nephrotic syndrome.
  - It can present either at the disease onset or at relapse.
  - It can be empirically classified based on clinical appearance and percentage weight gain from baseline, as mild (≤7% increase), moderate (8–15%), and severe (>15% increase).
  - The occurrence of more than mild edema is unusual if urine protein is carefully monitored.
  - Moderate-to-severe edema can however present with marked hypoalbuminemia along with ascites or anasarca which may interfere with daily activities.
  - Children with moderate-to-severe edema can commonly develop intravascular volume depletion, assessment of the intravascular volume status is the key before initiating therapy with diuretics.
  - Assessment of intravascular volume status can be determined by various clinical and biochemical parameters:

Features suggestive of intravascular volume depletion:
- *Clinical:*
  - Pain abdomen, vomiting, dizziness, and lethargy
  - Tachycardia, low volume pulse, and cold extremities
  - Prolonged capillary refill time, postural hypotension or rarely shock
- *Biochemical parameters:*
  - Increased hematocrit
  - Blood urea to creatinine ratio (mg/dL) >100
  - Fractional excretion of sodium (FeNa) <0.5%
  - Urinary potassium index (urine K^+/urine $Na^+ + K^+$) >0.6
  - *USG:* Decreased IVC diameter/increased collapsibility index
- *Plasma loss:*
  - Burns
  - *Capillary leak syndromes:* Sepsis and anaphylaxis
  - *Protein losing syndromes:* Nephritic syndrome and intestinal obstruction

(IVC: inferior vena cava; USG: ultrasonography)

- *Features of hypervolemia*: Refractory anasarca, hypertension, and dyspnea.
- *Management of edema in nephrotic syndrome*:

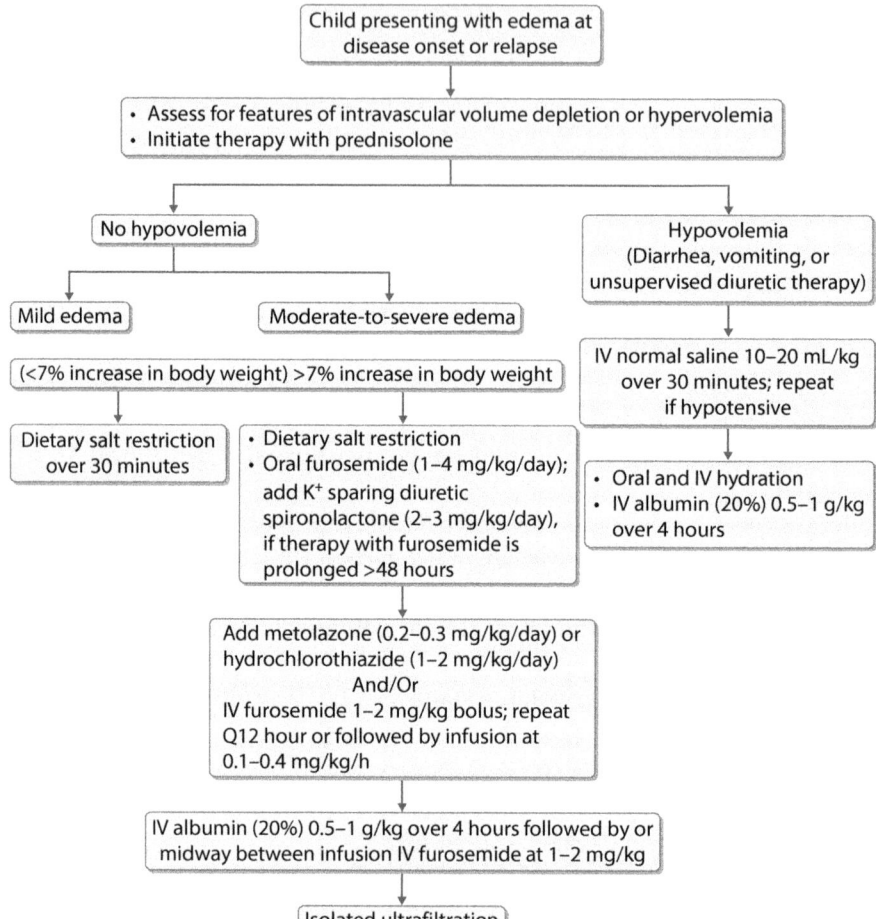

Source: Sinha A, Bagga A, Banerjee S, Mishra K, Mehta A, Agarwal I, et al. Steroid sensitive nephrotic syndrome: Revised guidelines. Indian Pediatr. 2021;58(5):461-1.

CHAPTER 93: Coma and Pain Scales

- *Child's Glasgow Coma Scale:*

	>5 years	<5 years
Eye opening		
E4	Spontaneous	
E3	To voice	
E2	To pain	
E1	None	
C	Unable to open eyes (swelling, ptosis)	
Verbal		
V5	Orientated	Alert, babbles, coos, words, or sentences—normal for age
V4	Confused	Less than usual ability, irritable cry
V3	Inappropriate words	Cries to pain
V2	Incomprehensible sounds	Moans to pain
V1	No response to pain	
T	Child is intubated	
Motor		
M6	Obeys commands	Normal spontaneous movements
M5	Localizes to supraorbital pain (>9 months)	Withdraws to touch (<9 months)
M4	Withdraws from nailbed pain	
M3	Flexion to supraorbital pain	
M2	Extension to supraorbital pain	
M1	No response to supraorbital pain	
P	Child is paralyzed—muscle relaxants or spinal injury	

Notes:
- For children >5 years, the responses are similar to the adult Glasgow Coma Scale.
- Pain should be made by pressing hard on the supraorbital notch (beneath medial end of eyebrow) with your thumb, except for motor score 4, which is tested by pressing hard on the flat fingernail surface with the barrel of a pencil.
- If there is facial trauma or swelling that prevents you from using the supraorbital ridge or there is doubt about the response to the supraorbital stimulus, then pinch the earlobe as an alternative stimulus.
- Score the best response if unclear or asymmetrical. If in doubt repeat after 5 minutes and ask for a second opinion.
- Score as usual in the presence of possibly sedating drugs.
- Plot scores over time on a suitable chart.

- *Revised trauma score:*

Revised trauma score	Glasgow Coma Scale score	Systolic pressure (mm Hg)	Respiratory rate (breaths/min)
4	13–15	>89	10–20
3	9–12	76–89	>29
2	6–8	50–75	6–9
1	4–5	1–49	1–5
0	3	0	0

Note: A score of 0–4 is given for each variable, then scores are added (range 1–12). A total score ≤11 indicates potentially important trauma.

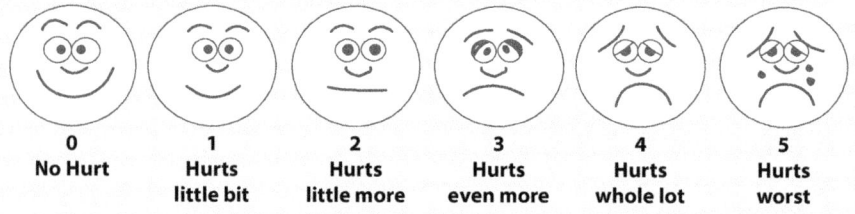

0	1	2	3	4	5
No Hurt	Hurts little bit	Hurts little more	Hurts even more	Hurts whole lot	Hurts worst

Consists of six cartoon faces ranging from a smiling face for "no pain" to a tearful face for "worst pain."

Recommended age: Children as young as 3 years.

Fig. 1: Wong-Baker FACES® Pain Rating Scale.
Source: Retrieved [05 July 2024] with permission from http://www.WongBakerFACES.org. Originally published in Whaley & Wong's Nursing Care of Infants and Children. © Elsevier Inc.

- *Face, Legs, Activity, Cry, Consolability (FLACC) scale:*

Category	Scoring		
	1	2	3
Face	No particular expression or smile	Occasional grimace or frown, withdrawn, disinterested	Frequent to constant quivering chin, clenched jaw
Legs	Normal position or relaxed	Uneasy, restless, and tense	Kicking, or legs drawn up
Activity	Lying quietly, normal position, moves easily	Squirming, shifting back and forth, and tense	Arched, rigid, or jerking
Cry	No cry (awake or asleep)	Moans or whimpers; occasional complaint	Crying steadily, screams or sobs, and frequent complaints
Consolability	Content and relaxed	Reassured by occasional touching, hugging or being talked to, and distractible	Difficult to console or comfort

Note: Each of the five categories (F) Face; (L) Legs; (A) Activity; (C) Cry; (C) Consolability is scored from 0 to 2, which results in a total score between 0 and 10.

CHAPTER 94: Catheter and Tube Sizes

- *Dialysis catheters:*

<3 kg	5F UAC, 8F UVC, and 7F double lumen	10, 15, and 20 cm
3–10 kg	7F/8F/9F double lumen	10, 15, and 20 cm
11–30 kg	9F/10F double lumen	10, 15, and 20 cm
>30 kg	11.5–12.5 F	12–20 cm

  (UAC: umbilical arterial catheter; UVC: umbilical venous catheter)

  Source:
  1. In: Lameire N, Mehta R (Eds). Complications of dialysis, 1st edition. New Delhi: CRC Press; 2000.
  2. In: Maher JF (Ed). Replacement of renal function by dialysis. A Textbook of Dialysis, 3rd edition. Philadelphia: Springer; 1989. pp. 1188.
  3. In: Hörl WH, Koch RM, Lindsay RM, Ronco C, Winchester JF (Eds). Replacement of renal function by dialysis. A Textbook of Dialysis, 5th edition. Philadelphia: Springer; 2004. pp. 1606.

- *Catheter sizes for pediatric patients:*

			Average catheter length (cm)		
Age	Average weight (kg)	Average height (cm)	IJ	SC	Fem
1 month	4.2	55	6.0	5.5	15.7
3 months	5.8	61	6.6	6.0	17.3
6 months	7.8	68	7.3	6.6	19.1
9 months	9.2	72	7.6	6.9	20.1
1 year	10.2	76	8.0	7.3	21.1
1.5 year	11.5	83	8.7	7.9	22.9
2 years	12.8	88	9.2	8.3	24.2
4 years	16.5	103	10.6	9.6	28.1
6 years	20.5	116	11.8	10.7	31.4
8 years	26	127	12.9	11.7	34.2
10 years	31	137	13.8	12.5	36.8
12 years	39	149	15.0	13.5	39.9
14 years	50	165	16.5	14.9	44.0
16 years	62.5	174	17.3	15.7	46.3

  (Fem: femoral; IJ: internal jugular; SC: subclavian)

- *Catheter diameters for pediatric patients:*

Age	IJ	Catheter diameter (French) SC*	Fem
0–6 months	3	3	3
6 months to 2 years	3	3	3–4
3–6 years	4	4	4
7–12 years	4–5	4–5	4–5

*For infants and younger children, the subclavian approach should only be performed by highly experienced operators.
(Fem: femoral; IJ: internal jugular; SC: subclavian)

- *Endotracheal tube:*

Age	Weight (kg)	Internal diameter	External diameter	At lip (cm)	At nose (cm)	Suction catheter (FG)
Newborn	<0.7	2.0	2.9	5.0	6.0	6
Newborn	<1	2.5	3.6	5.5	7	6
Newborn	1	3.0	4.3	6	7.5	7
Newborn	2	3	4.3	7	9	7
Newborn	3	3	4.3	8.5	10.5	7
Newborn	3.5	3.5	4.9	9	11	8
3 months	6	3.5	4.9	10	12	8
1 year	10	4	5.6	11	14	8
2 years	12	4.5	6.2	12	15	8
3 years	14	4.5	6.2	13	16	8
4 years	16	5	6.9	14	17	10
6 years	20	5.5	7.5	15	19	10
8 years	24	6	8.2	16	20	10
10 years	30	6.5	8.9	17	21	12
12 years	38	7	9.5	18	22	12
14 years	50	7.5	10.2	19	23	12
Adult	60	8	10.8	20	24	12
Adult	70	9	12.1	21	25	12

Note:
- ETT size (uncuffed) = Age/4 + 4 (Internal diameter)
- ETT size (cuffed) = Age/4 + 3 (Internal diameter)

- Length (cm at lip) = 12 + Age/2, at nose = 15 + Age/2
- *Tracheostomy sizes tube:*

	Portex			Shiley		
	ID (mm)	OD (mm)	Length (mm)	ID (mm)	OD (mm)	Length (mm)
Term	3	4.2	26	3	4.5	30/39
<6 months	3.5	4.9	28	3.5	5.2	32/40
1 year	4	5.5	29	4	5.9	34/41
2–3 years	4.5	6.2	31	4.5	6.5	36/42
4–5 years	5	6.9	33	5	7.1	44/50
6 years	—	—	—	5.5	7.7	46/52
8 years	6	8.3	38	6	8.3	54
12 years	7	9.7	45	6.5	9	56
14 years	7.5	10.4	49	—	—	—
Adults	8	11	53	—	—	—
Adult	9	12.4	16	8.5	12	71
Adult	10	13.7	68	9	13	71

- *Laryngeal mask airway sizes:*

Size 1	<5 kg	Size 3	30–50 kg
Size 1.5	5–10 kg	Size 4	50–70 kg
Size 2	10–20 kg	Size 5	70–100 kg
Size 2.5	20–30 kg	Size 6	>100 kg

- *Laryngoscope blade types and sizes:*

Age	Miller	Macintosh	Wis-Hippel
Premature neonate	0	—	—
Term neonate	0–1	—	—
1–12 months	1	—	1
1–2 years	1	2	1.5
2–6 years	2	2	—
6–12 years	2	3	—

- *Needle and catheter gauges:*

Ext diameter	Needle SWG	Catheter FG, FR, CH	External diameter	Needle SWG	Catheter FG, FR, CH
0.32	30	1	3	—	9
0.42	27	—	3.3	—	10
0.51	25	—	4	8	12
0.61	23	—	4.7	6	14
0.67	—	2	5.3	—	16
0.81	21	—	6	4	18
0.91	20	—	6.7	—	20
1	—	3	7	2	—
1.3	18	4	7.3	—	22
1.6	16	5	8	1/0	24
2	14	6	8.7	2/0	26
2.3	—	7	9.3	3/0	28
2.7	12	8	10.0	—	30

[SWG: Standard wire Gauge = British Imperial Gauge = 20–20 (log of external diameter) approximately
FG = FR = French = Charrière (CH) = 3 × external diameter]

CHAPTER 95 Blood Component Replacement

- *Estimated blood volume (EBV):*

Age	Total volume of blood (mL/kg)
Preterm infants	90–105
Term newborn	78–86
1–12 months	73–78
1–3 years	74–82
4–6 years	80–86
7–18 years	83–90
Adults	68–88

- *Packed red blood cells (PRBCs):*
  - Unless rapid replacement is required for acute blood loss or shock, infuse no faster than 2–3 mL/kg/h (generally 10–15 mL/kg aliquots over 4 hours) to avoid congestive heart failure.
  - A rule of thumb in severe compensated anemia is to give an X mL/kg aliquot, where X = patient Hb (g/dL); for example, if Hb = 5 g/dL, transfuse 5 mL/kg over 4 hours
  - To calculate the volume of PRBC to achieve a desired hematocrit (Hct), use the following equation:

$$\text{Volume of PRBC (mL)} = \frac{\text{EBV (mL)} \times (\text{desired Hct} - \text{actual Hct})}{\text{Hct of PRBCs}}$$

  - EBV is the estimated blood volume (age-specific EBV) and the HcT of PRBCs is usually 55–70%.
  - To calculate the volume of PRBC needed for a double-volume exchange, use the following equation:

$$\frac{\text{EBV (mL)} \times \text{patient Hct} \times 2}{\text{Hct of PRBC}}$$

- *Platelets:* Should not be refrigerated because this promotes premature platelet
  - Activation and clumping. Usually give 4 U/m^2, or approximately 10 mL/kg of normally
  - Concentrated platelet product. The platelet count is raised by 10,000–15,000/µL by giving 1 U/m^2. For infants and children, 10 mL/kg will increase the platelet count by approximately 50,000/µL. Usually, 1 unit = 50 mL after processing, ≥5.5 × 10^{11} platelet/unit.

- *Fresh frozen plasma (FFP):* Contains all clotting factors except platelets. 1 mL of FFP is expected to provide 1 unit of activity of all factors except labile factors V and VIII. The usual amount is 10–15 mL/kg; repeat doses as needed. In acquired thrombotic thrombocytopenic purpura (TTP), plasma exchange is the treatment of choice. Usually, 1 unit = 250–300 mL after processing.
- *Cryoprecipitate:* Enriched for factor VIII (5–10 U/mL), von Willebrand factor (vWF), and fibrinogen. Usually, 1 unit = 10–15 mL after processing (80 units factor VIII and 250 mg fibrinogen).
- Units of factor VIII = Weight (kg) × desired % replacement × 0.5
- Units of factor IX = Weight (kg) × desired % replacement.
- *Desired factor replacement in hemophilia:*

Joint or simple hematoma	20–70
Simple dental extraction	50
Major soft tissue bleed	80–100
Serious oral bleeding	80–100
Head injury	100
Major surgery (dental, orthopedic, other)	100

CHAPTER 96

Abnormal Sodium

Laboratory findings in patients with abnormal sodium:

	Serum			Urine			Specify gravity	BUN/ UUN	FeNa (%)	Urine volume
	Na	K	Osm	Na	K	Osm				
Hypernatremic dehydration	↑	↔	↑	<40	↔	>500	>1.030	>1:10	<1	↓
ATN	V	V	V	>40	↔	= serum	= 1.010	<1:10	>3	↑ Or ↓
SIADH	↓	↔	↓	>40	↑	>300	>1.020	>1:20	>1, <3	↓
Central DI	↑	↔	↑	<10	↓	<100	<1.005	<1:5	<1	↓
Salt poisoning	↑	↔	↑	>50	↔	>300	↔ or ↑	V	>3	↔
Factitious hyponatremia (e.g., hyperglycemia)	↓	↑ or ↓	↑	V	↑	>250	↔ or ↑	V	>1	↑ or ↔
Pseudohyponatremia (hyperlipidemia)	↓	↔	↔	↔	↔	↔	↔	V	<1	↔
Adrenal insufficiency	↓	↑	↓	>40	↓	↔	↔	↔	>1	V

(ATN: acute tubular necrosis; BUN: blood urea nitrogen; DI: diabetes insipidus; FeNa: fractional excretion of sodium; SIADH: syndrome of inappropriate antidiuretic hormone; UUN: urine urea nitrogen; V: variable)

Factitious hyponatremia:
- *Hyperlipidemia:* Na decreased by $0.002 \times$ lipid (mg/dL)
- *Hyperproteinemia:* Na decreased by $0.25 \times$ [protein (g/dL) – 8]
- *Hyperglycemia:* Na decreased 1.6 mEq/L for each 100 mg/dL rise in glucose

Syndrome of inappropriate antidiuretic hormone (SIADH) versus cerebral salt wasting (CSW)

	SIADH	CSW
Trigger	Multifactorial and more common in critically ill children	Usually after CNS insult
Clinical feature	Mild edema or euvolemia	Hypovolemia
Urine output	Normal to low	High volume
Urine sodium	>20 mEq/L	>>20 mEq/L
BP	Normal	Normal to low
Course	Benign	Intravascular volume depletion leading to hypoperfusion and hypotension
Treatment	• Volume restriction • Increased salt intake • Diuretics	Replace salt and water loss

(BP: blood pressure; CNS: central nervous system)

CHAPTER 97: Transudate versus Exudate

Evaluation of transudate versus exudates (pleural, pericardial, or peritoneal fluid):

Measurement	Transudate	Exudates
Specific gravity	<1.016	>1.016
Protein (g/dL)	<3	>3
Fluid: Serum protein ratio	<0.5	≥0.5
LDH (IU)	<200	≥200
LDH fluid: Serum ratio	<0.6	≥0.6
WBC	<10,000/µL	>10,000/µL
RBC	<5,000	>5,000
Glucose	>40	<40
pH	>7.2	<7.2

(LDH: lactate dehydrogenase; RBC: red blood cell; WBC: white blood cell)

CHAPTER 98: Steroids and Efficacy

Relative activity of systemic steroids:

		Compound	Glucocorticoid activity	Mineralocorticoid activity	Equivalent dose (anti-inflammatory)
G L U C O C O R T I C O I D S	Short-acting ($t\frac{1}{2}$ <12 hours/0	Hydrocortisone	1	1	20 mg
	Intermediate-acting ($t\frac{1}{2}$ 12–36 hours)	• Prednisolone • Methylprednisolone • Triamcinolone	4 5 5	0.8 0.5 0	5 4 4
	Long-acting ($t\frac{1}{2}$ >36 hours)	• Dexamethasone • Betamethasone	25 25	0 0	0.75 0.75
M I N E R A L O C O R T I C O I D S		• Desoxycorticosterone acetate	0	100	• Equivalent salt-retaining dose 2.5 mg
		• Fludrocortisone • Aldosterone	10 0.3	150 3,000	• 0.2 mg • Not used clinically

CHAPTER 99: Emergency Drug Preparation

Commonly used intravenous (IV) infusions:

Medication	Usual doses	Dilute in 50 mL normal saline (NS) or 5% dextrose (5% D)	1 mL/h will deliver
Adrenaline	0.05–1 µg/kg/min	0.3 mg/kg	0.1 µg/kg/min
Dobutamine	5–20 µg/kg/min	15 mg/kg	5 µg/kg/min
Dopamine	5–20 µg/kg/min	15 mg/kg	5 µg/kg/min
Milrinone	0.25–0.75 µg/kg/min	1.5 mg/kg	0.5 µg/kg/min
Noradrenaline	0.05–1 µg/kg/min	0.3 mg/kg (in 5% D only)	0.1 µg/kg/min
Nitroglycerine	0.5–10 µg/kg/min	3 mg/kg	1 µg/kg/min
Nitroprusside	0.5–10 µg/kg/min	3 mg/kg	1 µg/kg/min
Midazolam	1–10 µg/kg/min	3 mg/kg	1 µg/kg/min
Fentanyl	1–10 µg/kg/h	50 µg/kg	1 µg/kg/h
Morphine	10–60 µg/kg/h	1 mg/kg	20 µg/kg/h
Aminophylline	0.2–1 mg/kg/h	25 mg/kg	0.5 mg/kg/h
Terbutaline	0.1–0.4 µg/kg/min	0.5 mg/kg in 40 mL NS	0.1 µg/kg/min @ 0.5 mL/h

CHAPTER 100: Important Formulae

Plasma osmolality	2 (Na) + Glucose/18 + BUN/2.8
Osmolar gap	Measured osmolality – Calculated osmolality
Anion gap	(Serum Na + K) – (Cl + HCO_3)
Alveolar oxygen tension	PAO_2 = (FiO_2 × (Pb – 47)) – $PaCO_2$/0.8
A-a gradient	$AaDO_2 = PAO_2 - PaO_2$
Shunt fraction	Qs/Qt = ($CcO_2 - CaO_2$)/($CcO_2 - CvO_2$)
Arterial oxygen content	CaO_2 = (Hb × 1.34 × SaO_2) + (PaO_2 × 0.003)
Mixed venous oxygen content (CvO_2)	CvO_2 = (Hb × 1.34 × SvO_2) + (PvO_2 × 0.003)
End capillary oxygen content	CcO_2 (Hb × 1.34 × SaO_2) + (PAO_2 × 0.003)
Cardiac index	Cardiac output (CO)/body surface area
Mean arterial pressure (MAP)	(Systolic × 2 diastolic)/3
Systemic vascular resistance (SVR)	SVR = (MAP – CVP or mean RAP) × 80/CO
Pulmonary vascular resistance (PVR)	PVR = (mean PA – PCWP) × 80/CO
QT duration (corrected)	QTc = QT (s)/square root RR interval
Creatinine clearance	• K × height (cm)/serum creatinine or (140 – age) (weight in kg)/72 × serum creatinine • K = 0.45 in term neonates, 0.35 in preterm, 0.55 in children and in adult females, 0.7 in adolescent and adult males
Renal failure index	Urine Na × plasma creatinine/urine creatinine × 100
Winter formula for determining adequacy of respiratory compensation for metabolic acidosis	pCO_2 = 1.5 (HCO_3) + 8 + 2 or delta 10 mm Hg pCO_2 = delta × 0.08 pH
Fractional excretion of Na (FENa)	• FENa = Urine Na × plasma creatinine/urine creatinine × plasma Na • <1% in prerenal, >1% in renal failure
Body surface area	(4 × weight in kg + 7)/(weight + 90) or weight in kg × height in cm/3,600
Insensible water losses	400 mL/m²/day
Correction for sodium for hyperglycemia	Na + (glucose – 100) × 0.016
Corrected calcium	[0.8 × (normal albumin – patient albumin)] + total Ca^+
Centigrade	°C = (F – 32)/5/9

Contd...

Contd...

Fahrenheit (F)	°F = °C × 9/5 + 32
Urinary bladder capacity in children	
• <2 years old	• (Weight in kg × 7) mL
• >2 years old	• [(age in years + 2) × 30] mL
Mentzer index (MCV/RBC)	>13.5 – Thalassemia; <11.5 – iron deficiency anemia
Corrected reticulocyte count (CRC)	• %Reticulocyte × [patient hematocrit (Hct)]/(normal Hct)
	• 1.5 suggest hemolysis due to blood loss or hemolysis

($AaDO_2$: alveolar–arterial oxygen pressure difference; BUN: blood urea nitrogen; CaO_2: arterial oxygen content; CcO_2: pulmonary end-capillary oxygen content; CVP: central venous pressure; Hb: hemoglobin; MCV: mean corpuscular volume; PA: pulmonary arterial pressure; $PaCO_2$ partial pressure of arterial carbon dioxide; PAO_2: partial pressure of alveolar oxygen; PaO_2: partial pressure of arterial oxygen; Pb: barometric pressure; pCO_2: partial pressure of carbon dioxide; PCWP: pulmonary capillary wedge pressure; PvO_2: mixed venous oxygen tension; RAP: right atrial pressure; RBC: red blood cell; SaO_2: arterial oxygen saturation; SvO_2: mixed venous oxygen saturation)

CHAPTER 101: Glucose-6-phosphate Dehydrogenase and Drugs

Oxidizing agents and glucose-6-phosphate dehydrogenase (G6PD) deficiency:

- Para-aminosalicylic acid
- Acetaminophen
- Acetylsalicylic acid
- Aniline dye
- Antipyrine
- Ascorbic acid
- Chloramphenicol
- Dapsone
- Fava beans
- Furazolidone
- Henna
- Naphthalene
- Nitrofurantoin
- Primaquine
- Probenecid
- Sulfasalazine
- Sulfacetamide
- Sulfanilamide
- Sulfisoxazole
- Sulfoxone
- Vitamin K (water-soluble analog)
- Methylene blue

CHAPTER 102: Drug Levels

Drug	Indication	Therapeutic range	Critical value	Comments
Acetaminophen	Analgesic	5–20 µg/mL	>200 µg/mL drawn 4 hours after ingestion	Determination if a concentration is toxic is dependent upon when it is drawn in relation to the time of ingestion of the dose; multiple serum concentrations will be needed to monitor improvement and removal of drug
Amikacin	Antimicrobial	• *Peak*: 15–30 µg/mL • *Trough*: 4–8 µg/mL	>10 µg/mL	• *Peak*: 30 minutes; after end of infusion • *Trough*: Before next dose
Amiodarone	Antiarrhythmic	0.5–2 µg/mL	>2.5 µg/mL	• Trough concentration • Serum amiodarone levels >2.5 µg/mL had a positive predictive value of 76% for adverse drug events
Amitriptyline	Antidepressant/analgesic (neuropathic pain)	125–250 ng/mL	>500 ng/mL	• Trough concentration • Life threatening cardiac toxicity and/or seizures with concentration >1,000 ng/mL
Carbamazepine	Antiepileptic/mood stabilizer	4–12 µg/mL	>20 µg/mL	• Trough concentrations preferred • Correlate serum concentration with clinical presentation
Cyclosporine	Immunosuppressant	100–400 µg/mL	>500 µg/mL	• Specific goal concentration dependent upon clinical situation • For concentrations drawn with intravenous (IV) therapy, blood should be drawn from site other than that where drug is infusing (cyclosporine adheres to plastic); TDM levels are dependent on transplant type

Contd...

Contd...

Drug	Indication	Therapeutic range	Critical value	Comments
				• Blood concentrations can be method (immunoassay or mass spectrometry) dependent
Digoxin	Inotrope, AV node blocker	0.8–1.2 ng/mL* (immunoassay)	>2.5 ng/mL	• Concentrations should be drawn >8 hours after last dose • *Concentrations >1.5 in heart failure patients may be associated with higher mortality • Consult assay instructions for potential interfering factors
Doxepin	Antidepressant	110–250 ng/mL	>500 ng/mL	Trough concentration
Ethosuximide	Antiepileptic	40–100 µg/mL	>200 µg/mL	Trough concentration
Flecainide	Antiarrhythmic	0.2–1.0 µg/mL	>1.0 µg/mL	• Midpoint or trough concentration • Monitoring recommended when given concurrently with medications that may decrease metabolism (increase concentrations)
Flucytosine	Antifungal	25–50 µg/mL	>100–200 µg/mL	Concentration should be a peak drawn 2 hours post dose
Gentamicin	Antimicrobial	• Peak 5–10 µg/mL • Trough <2 µg/mL	• Peak >12 µg/mL • Trough >2 µg/mL	Monitoring of serum levels is suggested in patients with height and weight that are much different from normal; peak: 1 hour after infusion *Trough:* Before next dose
Imipramine	Antidepressant	>180–240 ng/mL	(>500 ng/mL)	Concentration = imipramine + desipramine (metabolite)
Lamotrigine	Antiepileptic/ mood stabilizer	1–4 µg/mL	>20 µg/mL	• Trough concentration • High concentrations generally associated with increased somnolence/confusion
Lidocaine	Antiarrhythmic	1.5–5 µg/mL	>6 µg/mL	Concentration can be drawn at any point (from separate IV line)
Lithium	Mood stabilizer	*Acute:* 1–1.6 mEq/L *Chronic:* 0.6–1.2 mEq/L	• >2.0 mEq/L • >5 mEq/L potentially fatal	• Serum concentrations may increase in presence of hyponatremia • *Concentration:* 12 hours after dose

Contd...

Contd...

Drug	Indication	Therapeutic range	Critical value	Comments
Nortriptyline	Antidepressant/analgesic (neuropathic pain)	50–150 ng/mL	>500 ng/mL	Trough concentration
Phenobarbital	Antiepileptic	15–40 µg/mL	>60 µg/mL	Trough or midinterval concentration
Phenytoin	Antiepileptic	10–20 µg/mL	>40 µg/mL	• Toxic >20 µg/mL • Toxicity may occur at lower concentrations in presence of hypoalbuminemia; consider free phenytoin
Primidone	Antiepileptic	5–12 µg/mL	>15 µg/mL	Metabolized to phenobarbital
Procainamide (PA) (metabolite: NAPA)	Antiarrhythmic	PA: 4–8 µg/mL (NAPA: 10–20 µg/mL)	• >10 µg/mL • (>40 µg/mL)	Midpoint or trough concentration; PA monitoring is particularly important in patients who might be fast acetylators (60–70% of northern Europeans and 50% of black and white Americans) and in patients with renal impairment; PA and N-acetylprocainamide (NAPA) levels always should be measured on the same sample
Protriptyline	Antidepressant	70–250 ng/mL	>500 ng/mL	Trough concentration
Quinidine	Antiarrhythmic	2–5 µg/mL	>6 µg/mL	Midpoint or trough concentration
Salicylate	Analgesic/anti-inflammatory	10–30 mg/dL	>40 mg/dL	Serum concentration should be used in conjunction with clinical presentation to make decision on therapy; multiple serum concentrations will be necessary to monitor improvement and removal of drug
Sirolimus	Immunosuppressant	5–15 ng/mL	>20 µg/mL	• Trough concentration • Whole blood samples • Therapeutic levels can be lower when used in combination with other immunosuppresants; blood concentrations can be method (immunoassay or mass spectrometry dependent)

Contd...

Contd...

Drug	Indication	Therapeutic range	Critical value	Comments
Tacrolimus	Immuno-suppressant	5–20 ng/mL	>25 ng/mL	• *Trough:* 12 hours after given dose • Whole blood samples • Therapeutic levels can be lower when used in combination with other immunosuppressants
Theophylline	Bronchodilator	5–20 µg/mL	>25 µg/mL	• Pulmonary literature suggest that concentrations 5–15 mg/L may be as efficacious with less toxicity • Trough or midinterval concentration depending upon drug formulation
Tobramycin	*Peaks:* • 4–8 µg/mL—standard • 8–12 µg/mL—once daily *Trough:* • <1.0 µg/mL—standard • <0.5 µg/mL—once daily			• Goal concentration (peak and trough) dependent upon dosing method • *Peak:* 1 hour after end of infusion • *Trough:* Before next dose
Valproic acid	Antiepileptic/mood stabilizer	50–125 µg/mL	>200 µg/mL	Toxicity may occur at lower concentrations in presence of hypoalbuminemia; consider free valproic acid; trough concentration preferred
Vancomycin	Antimicrobial	Trough concentrations: • *General:* 10–15 µg/mL • *Pneumonia:* 15–20 µg/mL	Trough >30 µg/mL	• Monitoring of peaks no longer recommended • Goal trough concentration dependent upon indication • *Trough*: Before next dose
Voriconazole	Antifungal	>0.25–1,000 µg/mL	>6 µg/mL	Trough concentration preferred; steady state achieved after 7 days of therapy

Note:
- Ranges are approximate and may vary with laboratory and/or assay.
- Proper interpretation of therapeutic drug concentrations requires that the specimen be drawn at an appropriate time in relation to drug administration.

(AV: atrioventricular; TDM: therapeutic drug monitoring)

CHAPTER 103: Electrocardiogram Values

Pulse, blood pressure (BP), and body surface area (BSA) ranges:

Age	Weight (kg)	Surface area (m²)	Pulse 95% range	Mean BP 95% range
Term	3.5	0.23	95–145	40–60
3 months	6	0.31	110–175	45–75
6 months	7.5	0.38	110–175	50–90
1 year	10	0.47	105–170	50–100
3 years	14	0.61	82–140	50–100
7 years	22	0.86	70–120	60–90
10 years	30	1.10	60–110	60–90
12 years	38	1.30	60–100	65–95
14 years	50	1.50	60–100	65–95
Adult	60	1.65	65–115	95–125
Adult	70	1.80	65–115	95–125

Age <9 years: Weight (kg) approximately = (2 × age) + 9
Age >9 years: Weight (kg) approximately = 3 × age
Surface area (m²) = (4W + 7)/(W + 90)

Normal pediatric electrocardiogram (ECG) parameters:

Age	Heart rate (bpm)	QRS axis*	PR interval (seconds)*	QRS duration (seconds)†
0–7 days	95–160 (125)	+30 to 180 (110)	0.08–0.12 (0.10)	0.05 (0.07)
1–3 weeks	105–180 (145)	+30 to 180 (110)	0.08–0.12 (0.10)	0.05 (0.07)
1–6 months	110–180 (145)	+10 to +125 (+70)	0.08–0.13 (0.11)	0.05 (0.07)
6–12 months	110–170 (135)	+10 to +125 (+60)	0.10–0.14 (0.12)	0.05 (0.07)
1–3 years	90–150 (120)	+10 to +125 (+60)	0.10–0.14 (0.12)	0.06 (0.07)
4–5 years	65–135 (110)	0 to +110 (+60)	0.11–0.15 (0.13)	0.07 (0.08)

Contd...

Contd...

Age	Heart rate (bpm)	QRS axis*	PR interval (seconds)*	QRS duration (seconds)†
6–8 years	60–130 (100)	−15 to +110 (+60)	0.12–0.16 (0.14)	0.07 (0.08)
9–11 years	60–110 (85)	−15 to +110 (+60)	0.12–0.17 (0.14)	0.07 (0.09)
12–16 years	60–110 (85)	−15 to +110 (+60)	0.12–0.17 (0.15)	0.07 (0.10)
Above 16 years	60–100 (80)	−15 to +110 (+60)	0.12–0.20 (0.15)	0.08 (0.10)

*Normal range and (mean).
†Mean and (98th percentile).

Ventricular hypertrophy criteria:
- *Right ventricular hypertrophy (RVH) criteria*

Must have at least one of the following:
- Upright T wave in lead V1 after 3 days of age to adolescence
- Presence of Q wave in V1 (QR or QRS pattern)
- *Increased right and anterior QRS voltage (with normal QRS duration):*
  - R in lead V1, ≥98th percentile for age
  - S in lead V6, ≥98th percentile for age
- Right ventricle strain (associated with inverted T wave in V1 with tall R wave)

- *Left ventricular hypertrophy (LVH) criteria*

Left ventricle strain (associated with inverted T wave in leads V6, I, and/or aVF)
Supplemental criteria:
- Left axis deviation (LAD) for patient's age
- Volume overload (associated with Q wave >5 mm and tall T waves in V5 or V6)
- *Increased QRS voltage in left leads (with normal QRS duration):*
  - R in lead V6 (and I, aVL, V5), >98th percentile for age
  - S in lead V1, >98th percentile for age

CHAPTER 104

Intravenous Compatibility Charts

Cisatracurium (Nimbex)	
Acyclovir	**
Albumin	?
Ampicillin	**
Calcium chloride	?
Calcium gluconate	YES
Ceftriaxone	YES
Clindamycin	YES
Dexamethasone (Decadron)	YES
Dexmedetomidine	YES
Diazepam (Valium)	**
Dobutamine	YES
Dopamine	YES
Epinephrine	YES
Famotidine	YES
Fentanyl	YES
Fosphenytoin	?
Furosemide/chlorothiazide	?
Furosemide (Lasix)	**
Gentamicin	YES
Heparin	**
Insulin, regular	?
Ketamine	?
Magnesium sulfate	YES
Meropenem	?
Methadone	?
Methylprednisolone	**

Dexmedetomidine (Precedex)	
Acyclovir	?
Albumin	?
Ampicillin	YES
Calcium chloride	?
Calcium gluconate	YES
Ceftriaxone	YES
Cisatracurium	YES
Clindamycin	YES
Dexamethasone (Decadron)	YES
Diazepam (Valium)	NO
Dobutamine	YES
Dopamine	YES
Epinephrine	YES
Famotidine	YES
Fentanyl	YES
Fosphenytoin	?
Furosemide/chlorothiazide	?
Furosemide (Lasix)	YES
Gentamicin	YES
Heparin	YES
Insulin, regular	?
Ketamine	?
Magnesium sulfate	YES
Meropenem	?
Methadone	?
Methylprednisolone	YES

Dobutamine	
Acyclovir	NO
Albumin	?
Ampicillin	?
Calcium chloride	**
Calcium gluconate	**
Ceftriaxone (Rocephin)	?
Cisatracurium (Nimbex)	YES
Clindamycin	?
Dexamethasone (Decadron)	?
Dexmedetomidine (Precedex)	YES
Diazepam (Valium)	**
Dopamine	YES
Epinephrine	YES
Famotidine (Pepcid)	YES
Fentanyl	YES
Fosphenytoin (Cerebyx)	?
Furosemide/chlorothiazide	NO
Furosemide (Lasix)	NO
Gentamicin	?
Heparin	**
Insulin, regular	**
Ketamine	?
Magnesium sulfate	**
Meropenem (Merrem)	YES
Methadone	?
Methylprednisolone (Solu-Medrol)	?

Contd...

Contd...

Cisatracurium (Nimbex)		Dexmedetomidine (Precedex)		Dobutamine	
Metronidazole (Flagyl)	YES	Metronidazole (Flagyl)	YES	Metronidazole (Flagyl)	?
Midazolam	YES	Midazolam	YES	Midazolam (Versed)	**
Milrinone	?	Milrinone	YES	Milrinone (Primacor)	YES
Morphine	YES	Morphine	YES	Morphine	YES
Nafcillin	?	Nafcillin	?	Nafcillin	NO
Norepinephrine	YES	Norepinephrine	YES	Norepinephrine (Levophed)	YES
Phenylephrine	YES	Phenylephrine	YES	Phenylephrine (Neo-synephrine)	YES
Potassium chloride	YES	Potassium chloride	YES	Potassium chloride	**
Ranitidine	YES	Ranitidine	YES	Ranitidine (Zantac)	YES
Sodium bicarbonate	**	Sodium bicarbonate	YES	Sodium bicarbonate	NO
Terbutaline	?	Terbutaline	?	Terbutaline	?
TPN + Lipids	?	TPN + Lipids	?	TPN + Lipids	YES
Vancomycin	YES	Vancomycin	YES	Vancomycin	?
Vasopressin	?	Vasopressin	?	Vasopressin	YES
Vecuronium	?	Vecuronium	YES	Vecuronium	YES

(YES: compatible at y-site; NO: incompatible; ?: no compatibility information available; **: conflicting data, contact pharmacy)

Dopamine		Epinephrine		Fentanyl	
Acyclovir	NO	Acyclovir	?	Acyclovir	?
Albumin	?	Albumin	?	Albumin	?
Ampicillin	**	Ampicillin	NO	Ampicillin	YES
Calcium Chloride	YES	Calcium chloride	**	Calcium chloride	?
Calcium Gluconate	?	Calcium gluconate	**	Calcium gluconate	YES
Ceftriaxone	?	Ceftriaxone	?	Ceftriaxone (Rocephin)	?
Cisatracurium	YES	Cisatracurium	YES	Cisatracurium (Nimbex)	YES
Clindamycin	?	Clindamycin	?	Clindamycin	YES
Dexamethasone (Decadron)	?	Dexamethasone (Decadron)	?	Dexamethasone (Decadron)	YES
Dexmedetomidine	YES	Dexmedetomidine	YES	Dexmedetomidine (Precedex)	?
Diazepam (Valium)	?	Diazepam (Valium)	**	Diazepam (Valium)	YES
Dobutamine	YES	Dobutamine	YES	Dobutamine	YES
Epinephrine	YES	Dopamine	YES	Dopamine	YES
Famotidine	YES	Famotidine	YES	Epinephrine	YES

Contd...

Contd...

Dopamine		Epinephrine		Fentanyl	
Fentanyl	YES	Fentanyl	YES	Famotidine (Pepcid)	?
Fosphenytoin	?	Fosphenytoin	?	Fosphenytoin (Cerebyx)	?
Furosemide/chlorothiazide	?	Furosemide/chlorothiazide	?	Furosemide/chlorothiazide	?
Furosemide (Lasix)	**	Furosemide (Lasix)	**	Furosemide (Lasix)	YES
Gentamicin	**	Gentamicin	?	Gentamicin	YES
Heparin	YES	Heparin	YES	Heparin	YES
Insulin, regular	NO	Insulin, regular	?	Insulin, regular	?
Ketamine	?	Ketamine	?	Ketamine	YES
Magnesium sulfate	?	Magnesium sulfate	?	Magnesium sulfate	?
Meropenem	YES	Meropenem	?	Meropenem (Merrem)	?
Methadone	?	Methadone	?	Methadone	?
Methylprednisolone	YES	Methylprednisolone	?	Methylprednisolone (Solu-Medrol)	?
Metronidazole (Flagyl)	**	Metronidazole (Flagyl)	?	Metronidazole (Flagyl)	YES
Midazolam	YES	Midazolam	YES	Midazolam (Versed)	YES
Milrinone	YES	Milrinone	YES	Milrinone (Primacor)	YES
Morphine	YES	Morphine	YES	Morphine	YES
Nafcillin	?	Nafcillin	?	Nafcillin	YES
Norepinephrine	YES	Norepinephrine	**	Norepinephrine (Levophed)	YES
Phenylephrine	?	Phenylephrine	?	Phenylephrine (Neo-synephrine)	?
Potassium chloride	YES	Potassium chloride	YES	Potassium chloride	YES
Ranitidine (Zantac)	YES	Ranitidine	YES	Ranitidine (Zantac)	YES
Sodium bicarbonate	NO	Sodium bicarbonate	?	Sodium bicarbonate	YES
Terbutaline	?	Terbutaline	?	Terbutaline	?
TPN + Lipids	**	TPN + Lipids	?	TPN + Lipids	YES
Vancomycin	?	Vancomycin	NO	Vancomycin	YES
Vasopressin	YES	Vasopressin	YES	Vasopressin	?
Vecuronium	YES	Vecuronium	YES	Vecuronium	YES

(YES: compatible at y-site; NO: incompatible; ?: no compatibility information available; **: conflicting data, contact pharmacy)

Furosemide (Lasix)		Furo/chlorothiazide		Heparin	
Acyclovir	?	Acyclovir	?	Acyclovir	YES
Albumin	YES	Albumin	?	Albumin	?
Ampicillin	?	Ampicillin	?	Ampicillin	**
Calcium chloride	?	Calcium chloride	?	Calcium chloride	?
Calcium gluconate	?	Calcium gluconate	?	Calcium gluconate	YES

Contd...

Contd...

Furosemide (Lasix)		Furo/chlorothiazide		Heparin	
Ceftriaxone	?	Ceftriaxone	?	Ceftriaxone (Rocephin)	YES
Cisatracurium	**	Cisatracurium	?	Cisatracurium (Nimbex)	**
Clindamycin	?	Clindamycin	?	Clindamycin	YES
Dexamethasone (Decadron)	?	Dexamethasone (Decadron)	?	Dexamethasone (Decadron)	YES
Dexmedetomidine	YES	Dexmedetomidine	?	Dexmedetomidine (Precedex)	YES
Diazepam (Valium)	NO	Diazepam (Valium)	NO	Diazepam (Valium)	NO
Dobutamine	**	Dobutamine	NO	Dobutamine	**
Dopamine	**	Dopamine	NO	Dopamine	YES
Epinephrine	YES	Epinephrine	?	Epinephrine	YES
Famotidine	**	Famotidine	?	Famotidine (Pepcid)	YES
Fentanyl	YES	Fentanyl	?	Fentanyl	YES
Fosphenytoin (Cerebyx)	?	Fosphenytoin	?	Fosphenytoin (Cerebyx)	?
Furosemide/chlorothiazide	?	Furosemide (Lasix)	YES	Furosemide/chlorothiazide	?
Gentamicin	NO	Gentamicin	NO	Furosemide (Lasix)	YES
Heparin	YES	Heparin	?	Gentamicin	**
Insulin, regular	?	Insulin, regular	NO	Insulin, Regular	**
Ketamine	?	Ketamine	?	Ketamine	?
Magnesium sulfate	?	Magnesium sulfate	?	Magnesium sulfate	YES
Meropenem	YES	Meropenem	?	Meropenem (Merrem)	YES
Methadone	?	Methadone	NO	Methadone	?
Methylprednisolone	?	Methylprednisolone	?	Methylprednisolone (Solu-Medrol)	**
Metronidazole	?	Metronidazole	?	Metronidazole (Flagyl)	YES
Midazolam	NO	Midazolam	NO	Midazolam (Versed)	YES
Milrinone	NO	Milrinone	NO	Milrinone (Primacor)	YES
Morphine	**	Morphine	NO	Morphine	YES
Nafcillin	?	Nafcillin	?	Nafcillin	YES
Norepinephrine	YES	Norepinephrine	NO	Norepinephrine (Levophed)	**
Phenylephrine	?	Phenylephrine	?	Phenylephrine (Neo-synephrine)	YES
Potassium chloride	**	Potassium chloride	NO	Potassium chloride	YES
Ranitidine	YES	Ranitidine	YES	Ranitidine (Zantac)	YES
Sodium bicarbonate	YES	Sodium bicarbonate	?	Sodium bicarbonate	YES
Terbutaline	?	Terbutaline	?	Terbutaline	?
TPN + Lipids	YES	TPN + Lipids	NO	TPN + Lipids	**
Vancomycin	?	Vancomycin	NO	Vancomycin	**
Vasopressin	?	Vasopressin	?	Vasopressin	YES
Vecuronium	NO	Vecuronium	NO	Vecuronium	YES

(YES: compatible at y-site; NO: incompatible; ?: no compatibility information available; **: conflicting data, contact pharmacy)

Insulin, regular		Ketamine		Midazolam (Versed)	
Acyclovir	?	Acyclovir	?	Acyclovir	?
Albumin	?	Albumin	?	Albumin	NO
Ampicillin	YES	Ampicillin	?	Ampicillin	NO
Calcium chloride	?	Calcium chloride	?	Calcium chloride	?
Calcium gluconate	?	Calcium gluconate	?	Calcium gluconate	YES
Ceftriaxone	?	Ceftriaxone	?	Ceftriaxone (Rocephin)	?
Cisatracurium	?	Cisatracurium	?	Cisatracurium (Nimbex)	YES
Clindamycin	?	Clindamycin	?	Clindamycin	YES
Dexamethasone (Decadron)	?	Dexamethasone (Decadron)	?	Dexamethasone (Decadron)	NO
Dexmedetomidine	?	Dexmedetomidine	?	Dexmedetomidine (Precedex)	?
Diazepam (Valium)	?	Diazepam (Valium)	NO	Diazepam (Valium)	?
Dobutamine	**	Dobutamine	?	Dobutamine	**
Dopamine	NO	Dopamine	?	Dopamine	YES
Epinephrine	?	Epinephrine	?	Epinephrine	YES
Famotidine	YES	Famotidine	?	Famotidine (Pepcid)	YES
Fentanyl	?	Fentanyl	YES	Fentanyl	YES
Fosphenytoin (Cerebyx)	?	Fosphenytoin	?	Fosphenytoin (Cerebyx)	NO
Furosemide/chlorothiazide	NO	Furosemide/chlorothiazide	?	Furosemide/chlorothiazide	NO
Furosemide (Lasix)	?	Furosemide (Lasix)	?	Furosemide (Lasix)	NO
Gentamicin	YES	Gentamicin	?	Gentamicin	YES
Heparin	YES	Heparin	?	Heparin	YES
Ketamine	?	Insulin, regular	?	Insulin, regular	YES
Magnesium sulfate	YES	Magnesium sulfate	?	Ketamine	YES
Meropenem	YES	Meropenem	?	Magnesium sulfate	?
Methadone	?	Methadone	?	Meropenem (Merrem)	?
Methylprednisolone	NO	Methylprednisolone	?	Methadone	YES
Metronidazole (Flagyl)	?	Metronidazole (Flagyl)	?	Methylprednisolone (Solu-Medrol)	YES
Midazolam	YES	Midazolam	YES	Metronidazole (Flagyl)	YES
Milrinone	YES	Milrinone	?	Milrinone (Primacor)	YES
Morphine	YES	Morphine	YES	Morphine	YES
Nafcillin	NO	Nafcillin	?	Nafcillin	NO
Norepinephrine	NO	Norepinephrine	?	Norepinephrine (Levophed)	YES
Phenylephrine	?	Phenylephrine	?	Phenylephrine (Neosynephrine)	?

Contd...

Contd...

Insulin, regular		Ketamine		Midazolam (Versed)	
Potassium chloride	YES	Potassium chloride	?	Potassium chloride	**
Ranitidine	**	Ranitidine	?	Ranitidine (Zantac)	YES
Sodium bicarbonate	**	Sodium bicarbonate	?	Sodium bicarbonate	NO
Terbutaline	?	Terbutaline	?	Terbutaline	?
TPN + Lipids	YES	TPN + Lipids	?	TPN + Lipids	NO
Vancomycin	YES	Vancomycin	?	Vancomycin	YES
Vasopressin	YES	Vasopressin	?	Vasopressin	?
Vecuronium	?	Vecuronium	?	Vecuronium	YES

(YES: compatible at y-site; NO: incompatible; ?: no compatibility information available; **: conflicting data, contact pharmacy)

Milrinone (Primacor)		Morphine		Norepinephrine (Levophed)	
Acyclovir	YES	Acyclovir	**	Acyclovir	?
Albumin	?	Albumin	?	Albumin	?
Ampicillin	YES	Ampicillin	YES	Ampicillin	NO
Calcium chloride	YES	Calcium chloride	YES	Calcium chloride	YES
Calcium gluconate	YES	Calcium gluconate	?	Calcium gluconate	?
Ceftriaxone	?	Ceftriaxone	YES	Ceftriaxone (Rocephin)	?
Cisatracurium	?	Cisatracurium	YES	Cisatracurium (Nimbex)	YES
Clindamycin	YES	Clindamycin	YES	Clindamycin	?
Dexamethasone (Decadron)	YES	Dexamethasone (Decadron)	YES	Dexamethasone (Decadron)	?
Dexmedetomidine	YES	Dexmedetomidine	?	Dexmedetomidine (Precedex)	YES
Diazepam (Valium)	?	Diazepam (Valium)	YES	Diazepam (Valium)	NO
Dobutamine	YES	Dobutamine	YES	Dobutamine	YES
Dopamine	YES	Dopamine	YES	Dopamine	YES
Epinephrine	YES	Epinephrine	YES	Epinephrine	**
Famotidine	?	Famotidine	YES	Famotidine (Pepcid)	YES
Fentanyl	YES	Fentanyl	YES	Fentanyl	YES
Fosphenytoin	?	Fosphenytoin	?	Fosphenytoin (Cerebyx)	?
Furosemide/chlorothiazide	NO	Furosemide/chlorothiazide	NO	Furosemide/chlorothiazide	NO
Furosemide (Lasix)	NO	Furosemide (Lasix)	**	Furosemide (Lasix)	?
Gentamicin	YES	Gentamicin	YES	Gentamicin	?
Heparin	YES	Heparin	YES	Heparin	**

Contd...

Contd...

Milrinone (Primacor)		Morphine		Norepinephrine (Levophed)	
Insulin, regular	YES	Insulin, regular	YES	Insulin, regular	NO
Ketamine	?	Ketamine	YES	Ketamine	?
Magnesium sulfate	YES	Magnesium sulfate	YES	Magnesium Sulfate	YES
Meropenem	YES	Meropenem	YES	Meropenem (Merrem)	YES
Methadone	?	Methadone	?	Methadone	?
Methylprednisolone	YES	Methylprednisolone	YES	Methylprednisolone (Solu-Medrol)	YES
Metronidazole (Flagyl)	YES	Metronidazole (Flagyl)	YES	Metronidazole (Flagyl)	?
Midazolam	YES	Midazolam	YES	Midazolam (Versed)	YES
Morphine	YES	Milrinone	YES	Milrinone (Primacor)	YES
Nafcillin	?	Nafcillin	YES	Morphine	YES
Norepinephrine	YES	Norepinephrine	YES	Nafcillin	**
Phenylephrine	?	Phenylephrine	?	Phenylephrine (Neo-synephrine)	YES
Potassium chloride	YES	Potassium chloride	YES	Potassium chloride	YES
Ranitidine (Zantac)	YES	Ranitidine	YES	Ranitidine (Zantac)	YES
Sodium bicarbonate	YES	Sodium bicarbonate	**	Sodium bicarbonate	NO
Terbutaline	?	Terbutaline	?	Terbutaline	?
TPN + Lipids	YES	TPN + Lipids	**	TPN + Lipids	YES
Vancomycin	YES	Vancomycin	YES	Vancomycin	?
Vasopressin	YES	Vasopressin	?	Vasopressin	YES
Vecuronium	YES	Vecuronium	YES	Vecuronium	YES

(YES: compatible at y-site; NO: incompatible; ?: no compatibility information available; **: conflicting data, contact pharmacy)

Terbutaline		Vasopressin		Vecuronium	
Acyclovir	?	Acyclovir	?	Acyclovir	?
Albumin	?	Albumin	?	Albumin	?
Ampicillin	?	Ampicillin	?	Ampicillin	?
Calcium chloride	?	Calcium chloride	?	Calcium chloride	?
Calcium gluconate	?	Calcium gluconate	?	Calcium gluconate	?
Ceftriaxone	?	Ceftriaxone	?	Ceftriaxone (Rocephin)	?
Cisatracurium	?	Cisatracurium	?	Cisatracurium (Nimbex)	?
Clindamycin	?	Clindamycin	?	Clindamycin	?
Dexamethasone (Decadron)	?	Dexamethasone (Decadron)	?	Dexamethasone (Decadron)	?

Contd...

Contd...

Terbutaline		Vasopressin		Vecuronium	
Dexmedetomidine	?	Dexmedetomidine	?	Dexmedetomidine (Precedex)	?
Diazepam (Valium)	?	Diazepam (Valium)	?	Diazepam (Valium)	NO
Dobutamine	?	Dobutamine	YES	Dobutamine	YES
Dopamine	?	Dopamine	YES	Dopamine	YES
Epinephrine	?	Epinephrine	YES	Epinephrine	YES
Famotidine	?	Famotidine	?	Famotidine (Pepcid)	?
Fentanyl	?	Fentanyl	?	Fentanyl	YES
Fosphenytoin	?	Fosphenytoin	?	Fosphenytoin (Cerebyx)	?
Furosemide/chlorothiazide	?	Furosemide/chlorothiazide	?	Furosemide/chlorothiazide	NO
Furosemide (Lasix)	?	Furosemide (Lasix)	?	Furosemide (Lasix)	NO
Gentamicin	?	Gentamicin	YES	Gentamicin	YES
Heparin	?	Heparin	YES	Heparin	YES
Insulin, regular	YES	Insulin, regular	YES	Insulin, regular	?
Ketamine	?	Ketamine	?	Ketamine	?
Magnesium sulfate	?	Magnesium sulfate	?	Magnesium sulfate	?
Meropenem	?	Meropenem	YES	Meropenem (Merrem)	?
Methadone	?	Methadone	?	Methadone	?
Methylprednisolone	?	Methylprednisolone	?	Methylprednisolone (Solu-Medrol)	?
Metronidazole (Flagyl)	?	Metronidazole (Flagyl)	YES	Metronidazole (Flagyl)	?
Midazolam	?	Midazolam	?	Midazolam (Versed)	YES
Milrinone	?	Milrinone	YES	Milrinone (Primacor)	YES
Morphine	?	Morphine	?	Morphine	YES
Nafcillin	?	Nafcillin	?	Nafcillin	?
Norepinephrine	?	Norepinephrine	YES	Norepinephrine (Levophed)	YES
Phenylephrine	?	Phenylephrine	YES	Phenylephrine (Neo-synephrine)	?
Potassium chloride	?	Potassium chloride	?	Potassium chloride	?
Ranitidine	?	Ranitidine (Zantac)	?	Ranitidine (Zantac)	YES
Sodium bicarbonate	?	Sodium bicarbonate	YES	Sodium bicarbonate	?
TPN + Lipids	?	Terbutaline	?	Terbutaline	?
Vancomycin	?	TPN + Lipids	?	TPN + Lipids	?
Vasopressin	?	Vancomycin	?	Vancomycin	YES
Vecuronium	?	Vecuronium	?	Vasopressin	?

(YES: compatible at y-site; NO: incompatible; ?: no compatibility information available)

CHAPTER 105

Sample Collection

Special sample collection:

Specimen	Volume (mL)	Tube	Handling
Plasma ammonia	1–3	Green, purple	On ice, immediate transfer to laboratory, levels rise rapidly on standing
Plasma amino acids (obtain after 3 hours fast)	1–3	Green top	On ice, if must store, then spin down, separate plasma and freeze
Plasma carnitine acylcarnitine profile	1–3 blotting paper	Green top	• On ice • Dry and mail to reference laboratory
Lactate	3	Gray top	On ice
Karyotyping	3	Green top	Room temperature
Very long chain fatty acids	3	Purple top	Room temperature
White blood cells for enzyme/deoxyribonucleic acid (DNA)	3	Purple top	Room temperature
Urine organic acids	5–10	–	Deliver immediately or freeze
Urine amino acids	5–10	–	Deliver immediately or freeze
Serology and immunohematology	5	Red top	Room temperature
Skin biopsy		Tissue culture media or patient's plasma	Refrigerate, do not freeze

Purple: ethylenediaminetetraacetic acid (EDTA) bottle; Green: heparin/lithium bottle; Gray: potassium oxalate and sodium fluoride bottle

CHAPTER 106: Laboratory Values

- *Alanine aminotransferase (ALT):*
  - *Major sources:* Liver, skeletal muscle, and myocardium

	Conventional units	International System of Units (SI)
12–13 years:		
• Female	10–30 U/L	10–30 U/L
• Male	10–55 U/L	10–55 U/L
14–15 years:		
• Female	5–30 U/L	5–30 U/L
• Male	10–45 U/L	10–45 U/L
>16 years:		
• Female	5–35 U/L	5–35 U/L
• Male	10–40 U/L	10–40 U/L

- *Aldolase:*
  - *Major sources:* Skeletal muscle and myocardium

10–24 months	3.4–11.8 U/L	3.4–11.8 U/L
2–16 years	1.2–8.8 U/L	1.2–8.8 U/L
Adult	1.7–4.9 U/L	1.7–4.9 U/L

- *Alkaline phosphate:*
  - *Major sources:* Liver, bone, intestinal mucosa, placenta, and kidney

Infant	150–420 U/L	150–420 U/L
2–10 years	100–320 U/L	100–320 U/L
Adolescent male	100–390 U/L	100–390 U/L
Adolescent female	100–320 U/L	100–320 U/L
Adult	30–120 U/L	30–120 U/L

- *Ammonia:*
  - Heparinized venous specimen on ice analyzed within 30 minutes

Newborn	90–150 µg/dL	64–107 µmol/L
0–2 weeks	79–129 µg/dL	56–92 µmol/L
Infant/child	29–70 µg/dL	21–50 µmol/L
Adult	15–45 µg/dL	11–32 µmol/L

- *Amylase:*
  - Major sources: Pancreas, salivary glands, and ovaries

0–3 months	0–30 U/L	0–30 U/L
3–6 months	0–50 U/L	0–50 U/L
6–12 months	0–80 U/L	0–80 U/L
>1 year	30–100 U/L	30–100 U/L

- *Antinuclear antibody (ANA):*
  - Negative   <1:40
  - Patterns with clinical correlation
  - *Centromere*: CREST
  - *Nucleolar*: Scleroderma
  - *Homogeneous*: SLE

  (CREST: calcinosis, Raynaud phenomenon, esophageal dysmotility, sclerodactyly, and telangiectasia; SLE: systemic lupus erythematosus)

- *Antistreptolysin O titer:*
  - A fourfold rise in paired serial specimens is significant

Newborn	**Similar to the mother's value**
6–24 months	≤50 Todd units/mL
2–4 year	≤160 Todd units/mL
≥5 years	≤330 Todd units/mL

- *Aspartate aminotransferase (AST):*
  - Major sources: Liver, skeletal muscle, kidney, myocardium, and erythrocytes

0–10 days	47–150 U/L	47–150 U/L
10 days to 24 months	9–80 U/L	9–80 U/L
>24 months		
Female	13–35 U/L	13–35 U/L
Male	15–40 U/L	15–40 U/L

- *Bicarbonate:*

Newborn	17–24 mEq/L	17–24 mmol/L
Infant	19–24 mEq/L	19–24 mmol/L
2 months to 2 years	16–24 mEq/L	16–24 mmol/L
>2 years	22–26 mEq/L	22–26 mmol/L

- *Blood gas, arterial (breathing room air):*

	pH	PaO_2 (mm Hg)	$PaCO_2$ (mm Hg)	HCO_3^- (mEq/L)
Cord blood	7.28 ± 0.05	18.0 ± 6.2	49.2 ± 8.4	14–22
Newborn (birth)	7.11–7.36	8–24	27–40	13–22
5–10 minutes	7.09–7.30	33–75	27–40	13–22
30 minutes	7.21–7.38	31–85	27–40	13–22
60 minutes	7.26–7.49	55–80	27–40	13–22
1 day	7.29–7.45	54–95	27–40	13–22
Child/adult	7.35–7.45	83–108	32–48	20–28

- *Calcium (total):*

  - Premature neonate   6.2–11 mg/dL   1.55–2.75 mmol/L
  - 0–10 days   7.6–10.4 mg/dL   1.9–2.6 mmol/L
  - 10 days to 24 months   9–11 mg/dL   2.25–2.75 mmol/L
  - 24 months to 12 years   8.8–10.8 mg/dL   2.2–2.7 mmol/L
  - 12–18 years   8.4–10.2 mg/dL   2.1–2.55 mmol/L

- *Calcium (ionized):*

  - 0–1 months   3.9–6.0 mg/dL   1.0–1.5 mmol/L
  - 1–6 months   3.7–5.9 mg/dL   0.95–1.5 mmol/L
  - 1–18 years   4.9–5.5 mg/dL   1.22–1.37 mmol/L
  - Adult   4.75–5.3 mg/dL   1.18–1.32 mmol/L

- *Chloride:*

  - 0–6 months   97–108 mEq/L   97–108 mmol/L
  - 6–12 months   97–106 mEq/L   97–106 mmol/L
  - Child/adult   97–107 mEq/L   97–107 mmol/L

- *Creatine kinase (creatine phosphokinase):*
  - *Major sources:* Myocardium, skeletal muscle, smooth muscle, and brain

    - Newborn   145–1,578 U/L   145–1,578 U/L
    - >6 weeks to an adult male   20–200 U/L   20–200 U/L
    - >6 weeks to an adult female   20–180 U/L   20–180 U/L

- *Creatinine (serum):*

  - Cord   0.6–1.2 mg/dL   53–106 µmol/L
  - Newborn   0.3–1.0 mg/dL   27–88 µmol/L
  - Infant   0.2–0.4 mg/dL   18–35 µmol/L
  - Child   0.3–0.7 mg/dL   27–62 µmol/L
  - Adolescent   0.5–1.0 mg/dL   44–88 µmol/L
  - Adult male   0.9–1.3 mg/dL   80–115 µmol/L
  - Adult female   0.6–1.1 mg/dL   53–97 µmol/L

- *Erythrocyte sedimentation rate (ESR):*

  - Child   0–10 mm/h
  - Adult male   0–15 mm/h
  - Adult female   0–20 mm/h

- *Ferritin:*

  - Newborn   25–200 ng/mL   56–450 pmol/L
  - 1 month   200–600 ng/mL   450–1,350 pmol/L
  - 2–5 months   50–200 ng/mL   112–450 pmol/L
  - 6 months to 15 years   7–140 ng/mL   16–315 pmol/L
  - Adult male   20–250 ng/mL   45–562 pmol/L
  - Adult female   10–120 ng/mL   22–270 pmol/L

- *Folate (serum):*

  - Newborn   16–72 ng/mL   16–72 nmol/L
  - Child   4–20 ng/mL   4–20 nmol/L
  - Adult   10–63 ng/mL   10–63 nmol/L

- *Galactose:*

  - Newborn   0–20 mg/dL   0–1.11 mmol/L
  - Older child   <5 mg/dL   <0.28 mmol/L

- *Gamma-glutamyl transferase (GGT):*
  - Major sources: Liver (biliary tree) and kidney

  - Cord   37–193 U/L   37–193 U/L
  - 0–1 month   13–147 U/L   13–147 U/L
  - 1–2 months   12–123 U/L   12–123 U/L
  - 2–4 months   8–90 U/L   8–90 U/L
  - 4 months to 10 years   5–32 U/L   5–32 U/L
  - 10–15 years   5–24 U/L   5–24 U/L
  - Adult male   11–49 U/L   11–49 U/L
  - Adult female   7–32 U/L   7–32 U/L

- *Glucose (serum):*

Preterm	20–60 mg/dL	1.1–3.3 mmol/L
Newborn, <1 day newborn	40–60 mg/dL	2.2–3.3 mmol/L
>1 day	50–90 mg/dL	2.8–5.0 mmol/L
Child	60–100 mg/dL	3.3–5.5 mmol/L
>16 years	70–105 mg/dL	3.9–5.8 mmol/L

- *Haptoglobin:*

  - Newborn   5–48 mg/dL   50–480 mg/L
  - >30 days   26–185 mg/dL   260–1,850 mg/L

- *Hemoglobin A1C:*

  - Normal   4.5–5.6%
  - At risk for diabetes   5.7–6.4%
  - Diabetes mellitus   ≥6.5%

- *Hemoglobin F, % total hemoglobin [mean (SD)]:*

  - 1 day   77.0 (7.3)
  - 5 days to 3 weeks   76.8 (5.8)
  - 6–9 weeks   70.0 (7.3)
  - 3–4 months   52.9 (11)
  - 6 months   23.2 (16)
  - 8–11 months   1.6 (1.0)
  - Adult   <2.0

- *Iron:*

Newborn	100–250 µg/dL	17.9–44.8 µmol/L
Infant	40–100 µg/dL	7.2–17.9 µmol/L
Child	50–120 µg/dL	9.0–21.5 µmol/L
Adult male	65–175 µg/dL	11.6–31.3 µmol/L
Adult female	50–170 µg/dL	9.0–30.4 µmol/L

- *Lactate:*

  Capillary blood:

0–90 days	9–32 mg/dL	1.1–3.5 mmol/L
3–24 months	9–30 mg/dL	1.0–3.3 mmol/L
2–18 years	9–22 mg/dL	1.0–2.4 mmol/L
Venous	4.5–19.8 mg/dL	0.5–2.2 mmol/L
Arterial	4.5–14.4 mg/dL	0.5–1.6 mmol/L

- *Lactate dehydrogenase (at 37°C):*
  - *Major sources:* Myocardium, liver, skeletal muscle, erythrocytes, platelets, and lymph nodes

0–4 days	290–775 U/L
4–10 days	545–2,000 U/L
10 days to 24 months	180–430 U/L
24 months to 12 years	110–295 U/L
>12 years	100–190 U/L

- *Lead:*

Child	<10 µg/dL	<0.48 µmol/L

- *Lipase:*

0–30 days	6–55 U/L
1–6 months	4–29 U/L
6–12 months	4–23 U/L
>1 year	3–32 U/L

Magnesium	1.26–2.1 mEq/L	0.63–1.05 mmol/L
Methemoglobin	0.78% (± 0.37%) of total hemoglobin	
Osmolality	275–295 mOsm/kg	275–295 mmol/kg

- *Phenylalanine:*

Preterm	2.0–7.5 mg/dL	121–454 µmol/L
Newborn	1.2–3.4 mg/dL	73–206 µmol/L
Adult	0.8–1.8 mg/dL	48–109 µmol/L

- *Phosphorus:*

• 0–9 days	4.5–9.0 mg/dL	1.45–2.91 mmol/L
• 10 days to 24 months	4–6.5 mg/dL	1.29–2.10 mmol/L
• 3–9 years	3.2–5.8 mg/dL	1.03–1.87 mmol/L
• 10–15 years	3.3–5.4 mg/dL	1.07–1.74 mmol/L
• >15 years	2.4–4.4 mg/dL	0.78–1.42 mmol/L

- *Potassium:*

• Preterm	3.0–6.0 mEq/L	3.0–6.0 mmol/L
• Newborn	3.7–5.9 mEq/L	3.7–5.9 mmol/L
• Infant	4.1–5.3 mEq/L	4.1–5.3 mmol/L
• Child	3.4–4.7 mEq/L	3.4–4.7 mmol/L
• Adult	3.5–5.1 mEq/L	3.5–5.1 mmol/L

Pyruvate	0.7–1.32 mg/dL	0.08–0.15 mmol/L
Rheumatoid factor	<30 U/mL	
Sodium:		
<1 year	130–145 mEq/L	130–145 mmol/L
>1 year	135–147 mEq/L	135–147 mmol/L

- *Total iron-binding capacity (TIBC):*

• Infant	100–400 µg/dL	17.9–71.6 µmol/L
• Adult	250–425 µg/dL	44.8–76.1 µmol/L

- *Transferrin:*

• Newborn	130–275 mg/dL	1.30–2.75 g/L
• 3 months to 16 years	203–360 mg/dL	2.03–3.6 g/L
• Adult	215–380 mg/dL	2.15–3.8 g/L

- *Troponin-I:*

• 0–30 day	<4.8 µg/L
• 31–90 day	<0.4 µg/L
• 3–6 months	<0.3 µg/L
• 7–12 months	<0.2 µg/L
• 1–18 years	<0.1 µg/L

- *Urea nitrogen:*

• Premature (<1 week) newborn	3–25 mg/dL	1.1–8.9 mmol/L
• Infant/child	2–19 mg/dL	0.7–6.7 mmol/L
• Adult	5–18 mg/dL	1.8–6.4 mmol/L
	6–20 mg/dL	2.1–7.1 mmol/L

- *Uric acid:*

0–30 days	1.0–4.6 mg/dL	0.059–0.271 mmol/L
1–12 months	1.1–5.6 mg/dL	0.065–0.33 mmol/L
1–5 years	1.7–5.8 mg/dL	0.1–0.35 mmol/L
6–11 years	2.2–6.6 mg/dL	0.13–0.39 mmol/L
Male 12–19 years	3.0–7.7 mg/dL	0.18–0.46 mmol/L
Female 12–19 years	2.7–5.7 mg/dL	0.16–0.34 mmol/L

- *Vitamin B_{12} (cobalamin):*

Newborn	160–1,300 pg/mL	118–959 pmol/L
Child/adult	200–835 pg/mL	148–616 pmol/L

- *Vitamin D_3 (1,25-dihydroxy-vitamin D):*

	16–65 pg/mL	42–169 pmol/L
Vitamin C (ascorbic acid)	0.4–2.0 mg/dL	23–114 µmol/L

- *Vitamin A (retinol):*

Preterm	13–46 µg/dL	0.46–1.61 µmol/L
Full term	18–50 µg/dL	0.63–1.75 µmol/L
1–6 years	20–43 µg/dL	0.7–1.5 µmol/L
7–12 years	26–72 µg/dL	0.9–1.7 µmol/L
13–19 years	20–49 µg/dL	0.9–2.5 µmol/L

- *Evaluation of cerebrospinal fluid:*

Age	White blood cell (WBC) count/µL (median)	95th percentile
0–28 days	0–12 (3)	19
29–56 days	0–6 (2)	9
Child	0–7	
Glucose		
Preterm	24–63 mg/dL	1.3–3.5 mmol/L
Term	34–119 mg/dL	1.9–6.6 mmol/L
Child	40–80 mg/dL	2.2–4.4 mmol/L

  Protein cerebrospinal fluid (CSF):

Preterm	65–150 mg/dL	0.65–1.5 g/L
0–14 days	79 (±23) mg/dL	0.79 (±0.23) g/L
15–28 days	69 (±20) mg/dL	0.69 (±0.20) g/L
29–42 days	58 (±17) mg/dL	0.58 (±0.17) g/L
43–56 days	53 (±17) mg/dL	0.53 (±0.17) g/L
Child	5–40 mg/dL	5–40 mg/dL

- *Opening pressure (lateral recumbent position):*

Newborn	8–11 cmH$_2$O
1–18 years	11.5–28 cmH$_2$O
Respiratory variations	0.5–1 cmH$_2$O

CHAPTER 107: Computed Tomography Scan and Lesions

- *Computed tomography (CT) characteristics:*

Bleeding	Absorption of X-rays proportional to the amount of hemoglobin	
	Initial	Isodense
	After hours	Isodense → hyperdense
	During absorption	Hyperdense → isodense → hypodense
	Organization	Isodense → hyperdense → slightly hyperdense
	Calcification	Isodense asymmetrical hyperdense
Effusion	Compare with venous blood	
	Transudate and cyst contents	Hypodense
	Exudates	Hypodense → isodense
Abscess	Compare with surrounding tissues	
	Pus	As for solid tissues
	Fatty degeneration	Isodense → hypodense
	Caseation	Strongly hypodense
	Wall consolidation	Isodense → hyperdense
	Hypodense areas	Smooth/irregular, sharp/ill-defined border, possibly with fluid level, septa, and vesicles
Necrosis	Compare with normal tissues	Hypodense

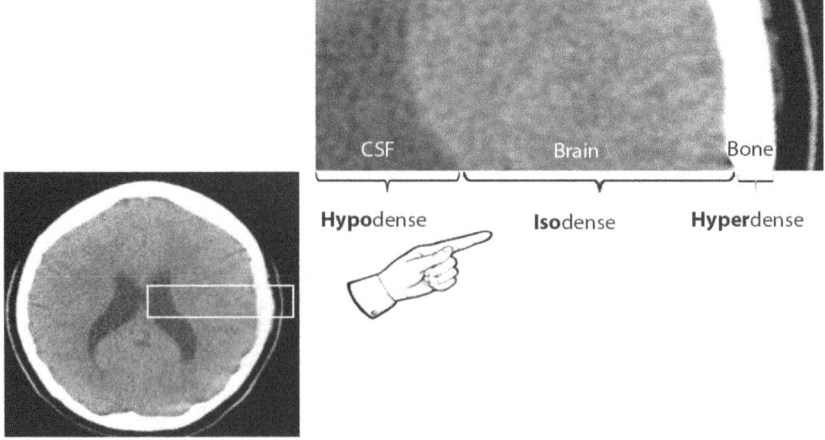

Fig. 1: Classification of density on CT scan.

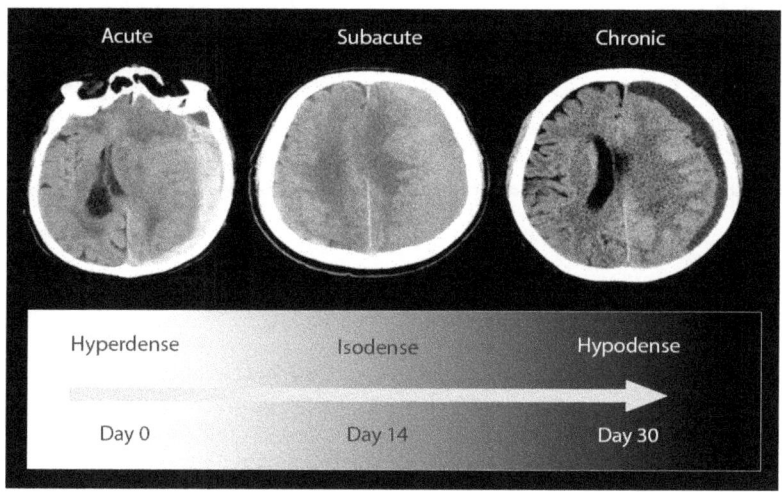

Fig. 2: Evolution of bleeding on CT scan imaging.

CHAPTER 108

Common Pediatric Applications

Pediatric Oncall		Medical Calculator Pediatrics	
IAP growth chart		Peds Cardiology Handbook	
Face2gene		Peds Dose Calc	
Pedi STAT		Bilibuddy	
Pediatrics Central		Pediatric Emergencies	
Nelson Pediatrics Abx 2023		Pediref: Pocket Pediatrics	
AnthroCal		PulseOxTool	
Harriet Lane Handbook			

CHAPTER **109**

Pediatric Neuroimaging Primer

Neuroimaging in pediatrics involves multiple modalities based on the underlying pathology and the hemodynamic stability of the child. The common modalities and the overview of their interpretation are as follows:
- *Cranial ultrasound:*
  - Cranial ultrasound, also known as neurosonography, is an imaging modality primarily used for evaluating the brains of neonates and infants using fontanelles as acoustic windows.
  - The interpretation of cranial ultrasound requires the following considerations:
    - *Symmetry:* Compare both sides of the brain for symmetry.
    - *Echogenicity:* Assess differences in echogenicity, which can indicate various pathologies.
    - *Ventricular size:* Measure and compare ventricular sizes to normal age-related values.
    - *Cystic changes:* Identify any cystic areas, which can suggest chronic changes or cystic anomalies.
  - Common findings and their interpretation are illustrated in **Table 1**.

TABLE 1: Cranial ultrasound: Common findings and their interpretation.

Intracranial hemorrhage	• *Subependymal hemorrhage/germinal matrix hemorrhage (GMH):* Seen as echogenic (bright) areas near the caudothalamic groove • *Intraventricular hemorrhage (IVH):* Blood within the ventricular system appears echogenic • *Parenchymal hemorrhage:* Echogenic areas within the brain parenchyma
Hydrocephalus	• *Enlarged ventricles:* Dilated lateral ventricles with or without transependymal cerebrospinal fluid (CSF) flow • *Third and fourth ventricles:* Assess for dilatation
Periventricular leukomalacia	• *Acute phase:* Increased echogenicity in the periventricular white matter • *Chronic phase:* Cystic changes in the periventricular region
Congenital anomalies	• *Ventriculomegaly:* Abnormally enlarged ventricles • *Holoprosencephaly:* Incomplete separation of cerebral hemispheres, seen as fused midline structures • *Dandy–Walker malformation:* Enlargement of the fourth ventricle, cystic dilatation, and hypoplasia of the cerebellar vermis
Infections	• *Ventriculitis:* Echogenic debris within the ventricles • *Abscesses:* Focal echogenic lesions that may show fluid levels or complex structures

- *Computed tomography CT scan:*
  - CT scan uses X-ray technology to create detailed cross-sectional images of the body's internal structures. CT scans are commonly used in medical practice for a variety of clinical applications due to their quick provision of comprehensive images.
  - The systematic approach for interpreting CT head is shown in **Table 2**.

TABLE 2: Systematic approach to interpret a computed tomography (CT) head and common findings.

Scout view	Examine the scout image for positioning and overall orientation
Check for artifacts	Identify any artifacts that may affect image quality, such as patient movement or metal objects
Assess the brain: Parenchyma	• *Gray matter and white matter differentiation:* Look for any loss of differentiation, which could indicate edema or ischemia 　– *Symmetry:* Compare both sides of the brain for symmetry 　– *Attenuation:* Assess for areas of abnormal attenuation (hyperdense or hypodense areas)
Evaluate the ventricular system	• *Size and shape:* Ensure the ventricles are of normal size and shape • Enlarged ventricles may indicate hydrocephalus • *Midline shift:* Check for any displacement of the midline structures, which could suggest a mass effect
Examine the basal cisterns and sulci	• *Effacement:* Look for effacement (compression) of the cisterns and sulci, which could indicate increased intracranial pressure (ICP) • *Subarachnoid hemorrhage*: Identify any hyperdense areas in the subarachnoid space, which may suggest hemorrhage
Assess for hemorrhage	• *Intra-axial hemorrhage:* Blood within the brain tissue appears hyperdense (bright) • *Extra-axial hemorrhage:* Blood outside the brain tissue, including subdural, epidural, and subarachnoid hemorrhage
Check the bony structures	• *Skull fractures:* Look for any discontinuities in the bone • *Sinuses:* Examine the paranasal sinuses for opacification, which might indicate sinusitis or fracture
Look for signs of stroke	• *Early ischemic changes:* Loss of gray–white matter differentiation, hypoattenuation, and swelling • *Hyperdense vessel sign:* A hyperdense middle cerebral artery (MCA) could indicate a thrombus
Evaluate the soft tissues	• *Orbits:* Check the eyes and surrounding structures • *Scalp and soft tissues:* Look for swelling or hematomas
Common findings and their significance	• *Ischemic stroke:* Hypodense areas corresponding to the affected vascular territory • *Hemorrhagic stroke:* Hyperdense areas within the brain parenchyma • *Subdural hematoma:* Crescent-shaped hyperdense area between the brain and the skull • *Epidural hematoma:* Lentiform (lens-shaped) hyperdense area between the skull and the dura mater • *Hydrocephalus:* Enlarged ventricles with or without transependymal flow of CSF • *Brain tumors:* Mass lesions that may cause a mass effect, edema, and potential calcifications

- On CT scan, the structures which attenuate the radiation the least, appear dark (*hypodense*) and which attenuate the radiation the most, appear bright (*hyperdense*). The attenuation is quantitatively measured in terms of Hounsfield units.
- Contrast medium is administered when looking for infectious, neoplastic, or vascular pathologies and administered in a dose of 2 mL/kg of body weight.
- *Magnetic resonance imaging (MRI):*
  - MRI uses strong magnetic fields and radio waves to create detailed images of the body's organs and tissues. Different MRI sequences can effectively highlight various tissues, structures, and pathologies, providing comprehensive insights for accurate diagnosis and treatment. These are illustrated in **Table 3**.
  - Contraindications of MRI—presence of implanted electronic devices in the body, e.g., cardiac pacemaker, cochlear implant, and metallic devices which are non-MRI compatible like aneurysm clips, metallic stents, etc.

TABLE 3: Various sequences of magnetic resonance imaging (MRI) and their interpretation.

Sequence	Purpose	Appearance	Clinical use
T1-weighted imaging	Provides detailed anatomical information with high spatial resolution	• Tissues with high fat content (like subcutaneous fat and bone marrow) appear bright (*hyperintense*) • Cerebrospinal fluid (CSF) appears dark (*hypointense*)	Excellent for visualizing the anatomy and detecting fat-containing structures and lesions
T2-weighted imaging	Highlights fluid and edema	• CSF, edema, and most pathological fluids appear bright (*hyperintense*) • Fat and most solid tissues appear darker (*hypointense*)	Ideal for identifying edema, inflammation, and detecting tumors, as well as characterizing cystic lesions
Fluid-attenuated inversion recovery (FLAIR)	Suppresses the signal from CSF, making it easier to see periventricular lesions	CSF appears dark (*hypointense*) and areas of edema or gliosis appear bright (*hyperintense*)	Commonly used in brain imaging to detect lesions like multiple sclerosis plaques and other white matter abnormalities
Diffusion-weighted imaging (DWI)	Measures the random Brownian motion of water molecules within tissue	Areas of restricted diffusion, such as acute infarction or high cellularity tumors, appear bright (*hyperintense*)	• Crucial in the early detection of stroke and in identifying highly cellular tumors or abscesses • The diffusion restriction can be seen as early as within an hour of insult, show peak restriction by 48–72 hours and then start to decline to become normal by 7–10 days

Contd...

Contd...

Sequence	Purpose	Appearance	Clinical use
Apparent diffusion coefficient (ADC) imaging	Measures the extent of water molecule diffusion within tissues, differentiating between various tissue types and pathological conditions	• Areas with freely diffusing water (e.g., normal brain tissue, cysts) appear bright (*hyperintense*) • Areas with restricted water diffusion (e.g., acute infarctions, highly cellular tumors) appear dark (*hypointense*)	• *Stroke:* Differentiates acute ischemic stroke (low ADC) from other conditions. ADC maps are essential for early stroke diagnosis • *Tumor characterization:* This helps distinguish between benign and malignant tumors, as malignant tumors often show restricted diffusion (low ADC) • *Infection:* This identifies abscesses (restricted diffusion) versus necrotic or cystic regions (high ADC)
Gradient echo (GRE) imaging (T2 star or T2*)	Sensitive to magnetic susceptibility effects	Blood products, calcium, and other materials with different magnetic properties from surrounding tissues show signal loss	Used for detecting microbleeds, calcifications, and certain vascular malformations
Short tau inversion recovery (STIR)	Suppresses the signal from fat	Fat appears dark, while fluid and most other tissues are bright	Commonly used in musculoskeletal imaging to detect bone marrow edema, muscle injuries, and other soft tissue pathologies
Proton density (PD) imaging	Balances between T1 and T2 weighting, emphasizing the number of hydrogen protons in tissues	Structures with high-proton density appear bright, while those with low-proton density are dark	Useful for imaging joints and assessing cartilage and meniscal abnormalities
MR angiography (MRA)	Visualizes blood vessels	*Techniques:* • *Time-of-flight (TOF) MRA:* Uses the flow of blood to generate contrast • *Phase contrast (PC) MRA:* Encodes the velocity of blood flow	Detecting stenosis, aneurysms, and other vascular abnormalities

Contd...

CHAPTER 109: Pediatric Neuroimaging Primer

Contd...

Sequence	Purpose	Appearance	Clinical use
Magnetic resonance venography (MRV)	To assess the venous system for conditions such as venous thrombosis, venous stenosis, and other vascular anomalies	Techniques: • *TOF MRV:* Exploits the flow of blood to create contrast between veins and surrounding tissues • *PC MRV:* Encodes blood flow velocity to visualize the venous system • *Contrast-enhanced MRV (CE-MRV):* Uses gadolinium-based contrast agents to enhance venous structures	• *Vascular malformations:* Assesses abnormalities such as arteriovenous malformations (AVMs) and venous angiomas • *Presurgical planning:* Provides detailed venous anatomy for planning surgeries, particularly in the brain and spinal cord
Functional MRI (fMRI)	Measures brain activity by detecting changes associated with blood flow	*Technique:* Blood oxygen level-dependent *(BOLD)* contrast	Research and mapping brain functions before epilepsy and tumor surgery

Magnetic resonance spectroscopy (MRS)	• To demonstrate and quantify brain metabolites noninvasively
	• The metabolites detected are N-acetylaspartate (NAA), creatine, choline, lactate, and lipid
		MRS scan requires additional steps as compared to routine MRI
		• Shimming the magnetic field
		• Suppressing the water signal
		• Choosing spectroscopic technique
		  – Single-voxel spectroscopy
		  – Multi-voxel spectroscopy
			• NAA is increased in Canavan disease
			• NAA is decreased in conditions with axonal loss
			• Choline levels are high in proliferative tumors, leukodystrophies
			• Lactate represents anerobic metabolism

CHAPTER 110: Pediatric Neurology Charts

- Glasgow Coma Scale

Activity	Score	Child/adolescent	Score	Infant
Eye opening	4	Spontaneous	4	Spontaneous
	3	To speech	3	To speech/sound
	2	To pain	2	To painful stimuli
	1	None	1	None
Verbal	5	Oriented	5	Coos/babbles
	4	Confused	4	Irritable cry
	3	Inappropriate	3	Cries to pain
	2	Incomprehensible	2	Moans to pain
	1	None	1	None
Motor	6	Obeys commands	6	Normal spontaneous movement
	5	Localizes to pain	5	Withdraws to touch
	4	Withdraws to pain	4	Withdraws to pain
	3	Abnormal flexion	3	Abnormal flexion (decorticate)
	2	Abnormal extension	2	Abnormal extension (decerebrate)
	1	None (flaccid)	1	None (flaccid)

- Modified Ashworth Scale for grading spasticity

Modified Ashworth Scale grade	Descriptor
0	No increase in muscle tone
1	Slight increase in muscle tone, manifested by a catch and release or by minimal resistance at the end of the range of motion when the affected part(s) is(are) moved in flexion or extension
1+	Slight increase in muscle tone, manifested by a catch followed by minimal resistance through the remainder of the range of motion, but the affected part(s) is(are) easily moved
2	More marked increase in muscle tone through most of the range of movement, but the affected part(s) is(are) easily moved
3	Considerable increases in muscle tone; passive movement difficult
4	Affected part(s) is(are) rigid in flexion or extension

- Gross motor function classification system (children aged 6–12 years)

Levels	Descriptor
Level I	Walks without restrictions; limitations in more advanced motor skills
Level II	Walks without assistive devices; limitations walking outdoors and in the community
Level III	Walks with assistive mobility devices; limitations walking outdoors and in the community
Level IV	Self-mobility with limitations; children are transported or use power mobility outdoors and in the community
Level V	Self-mobility is extremely limited even with the use of assistive technology

- Cerebral perfusion pressure

Age	Minimum CPP target	Minimal MAP target if ICP is unknown but is suspected to be elevated
<1 year	40 mm Hg	60 mm Hg
1–2 years	45 mm Hg	65 mm Hg
3–4 years	50 mm Hg	70 mm Hg
5–6 years	55 mm Hg	75 mm Hg
7–10 years	60 mm Hg	80 mm Hg
11–15 years	65 mm Hg	85 mm Hg
>15 years	70 mm Hg	90 mm Hg

Cerebral perfusion pressure (CPP) = Mean arterial pressure (MAP) − Intracranial pressure (ICP)

- Cerebrospinal fluid and lumbar puncture

Age-group	Mean cerebrospinal fluid (CSF) production rate	CSF volume	Safe CSF volume that can be taken while doing lumbar puncture
Adult	22 mL/h	150–170 mL	15–17 mL
Adolescent	18 mL/h	120–170 mL	12–17 mL
Young child	12 mL/h	100–150 mL	10–15 mL
Infant	10 mL/h	60–90 mL	6–9 mL
Term neonate	1 mL/h	20–40 mL	2–4 mL

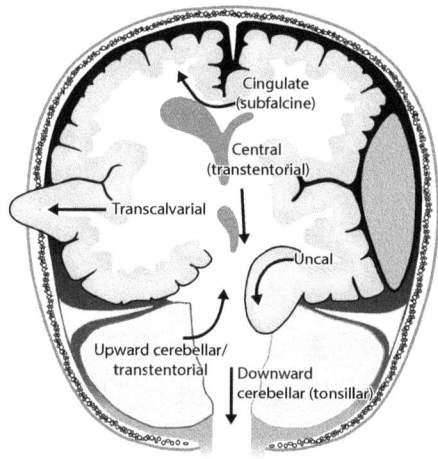

Fig. 1: Types of brain herniation.

Syndrome	Mechanism	Clinical findings	Imaging findings
Transtentorial—descending Unilateral–lateral (uncal)	Medial temporal lobe pushes downward into the posterior fossa through the incisura	• Variable impairment in consciousness • *Earliest sign:* Ipsilateral pupil dilatation • External ophthalmoplegia • Contralateral hemiparesis • Decerebrate posturing	• Widening of contralateral temporal horn, ipsilateral ambient cistern and ipsilateral prepontine cistern • Uncus extending into the suprasellar cistern
Transtentorial—descending bilateral (central)	Downward displacement of the cerebral hemispheres and the basal nuclei compressing and displacing the diencephalon and the midbrain rostrocaudally through the tentorial notch	• Early coma • Medium sized, fixed pupils • Decorticate posturing • Cheyne–Stokes respiration • Diabetes insipidus	• Effacement of sulci • Obliteration of the suprasellar cistern • Compression and posterior displacement of the quadrigeminal cistern
Transtentorial—ascending	Infratentorial mass effect protruding upward compressing the midbrain	• Nausea/vomiting • Progressive stupor	• Spinning top appearance of midbrain • Narrowing of bilateral ambient cisterns • Filling of quadrigeminal cisterns
Tonsillar	Cerebellar tonsils protruding below the foramen magnum compressing the medulla and upper cervical cord	• Hypertension–bradycardia–bradypnea (Cushing reflex) • Coma • Respiratory arrest • Bilateral arm dysesthesia	• Cerebellar tonsils at the level of the dens on axial images • Cerebellar tonsils on sagittal images 7 mm below foramen magnum (5 mm in adult)
Subfalcine—cingulate	Brain tissue extending under the falx in the supratentorial cerebrum	• Small reactive pupils • Headache • Contralateral leg paralysis	• Attenuation of ipsilateral aspect of frontal horn • Asymmetric anterior falx • Obliteration of ipsilateral atrium of lateral ventricle • Septum pellucidum shift

Source: Ramachandran R, Bansal A. Approach and management of children with raised intracranial pressure. J Pediatr Crit Care. 2015;2:13-24.

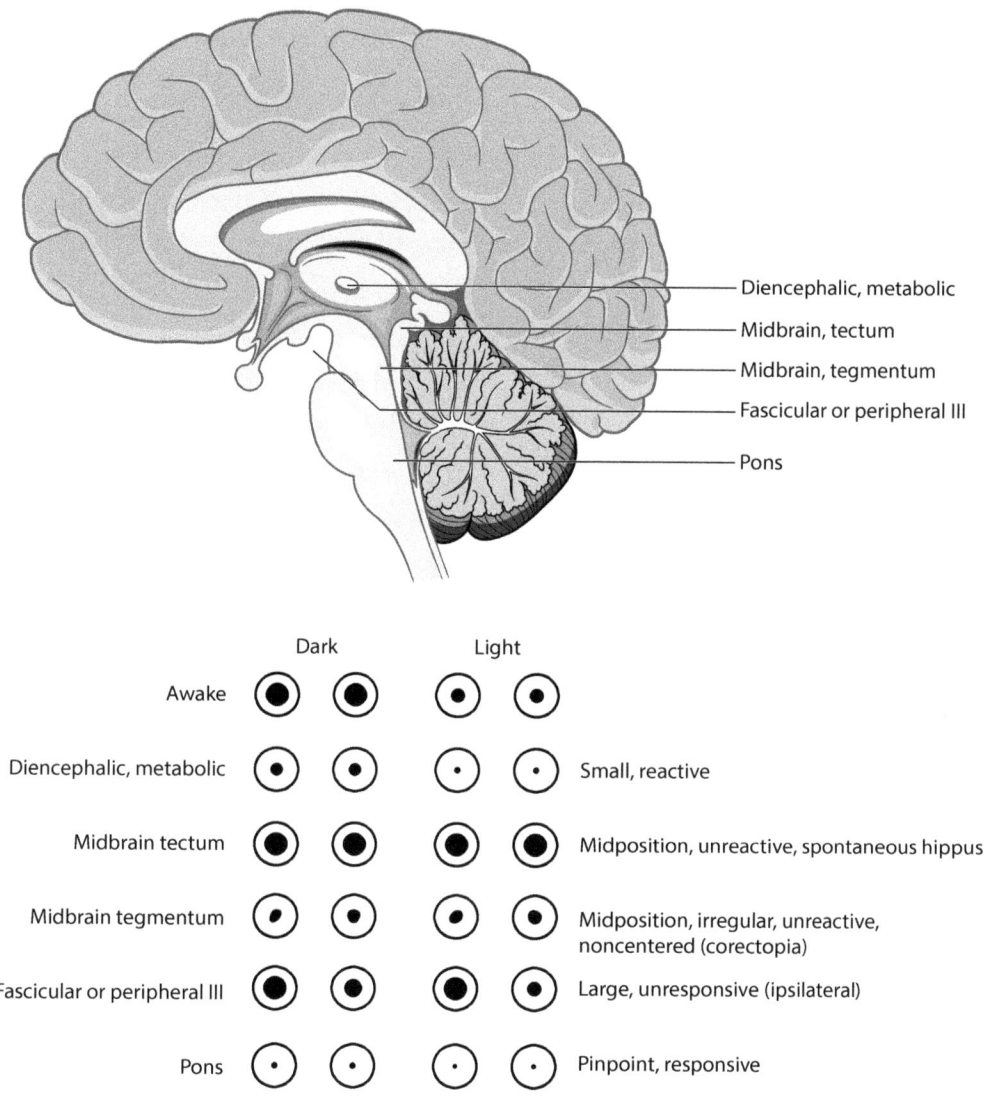

Fig. 2: Pupillary response and localization.
Source: Neupsy Key. The localization of lesions causing coma. [online] Available from https://neupsykey.com/the-localization-of-lesions-causing-coma/ [Last accessed July, 2024].

Suggested Reading

SECTION 1: Supporting a Sick Child

1. American Heart Association. Pediatric Advanced Support Manual (PALS) Provider Manual [AHA, Pediatric Advanced Life Support (PALS) Provider Manual], 1st edition. Kowloon, Hong Kong: American Heart Association Inc; 2020.
2. Custer JW, Rau RE. Johns Hopkins: The Harriet Lane Handbook, 22nd edition. Amsterdam: Elsevier Mosby; 2021.
3. Ghai OP, Paul V, Bagga A. Ghai Essential Pediatrics, 10th edition. New Delhi: CBS Publishers and Distributors Pvt Ltd; 2023.
4. In: Shaffner DH, McCloskey JJ, Hunt EA, Tasker RC (Eds). Rogers' Textbook of Pediatric Intensive Care, 6th edition. Philadelphia: Wolters Kluver Health; 2023.
5. Kliegman RM, St. Geme III JW, Blum NJ, Tasker RC, Wilson KM, Schuh AM, et al. Nelson Textbook of Pediatrics, 22nd edition. Elsevier; 2024.
6. Loscalzo J, Fauci AS, Kasper DL, Hauser SL, Longo D, Jameson JL. Harrison's Principles of Internal Medicine, 21st edition. New York: McGraw-Hill; 2022.
7. Zimmerman JJ, Rotta AT. Fuhrmann and Zimmerman's Pediatric Critical Care, 6th edition. Maryland Heights, United States: Mosby; 2021.

SECTION 2: Respiratory Disorders

1. American Heart Association. Pediatric Advanced Support Manual (PALS) Provider Manual [AHA, Pediatric Advanced Life Support (PALS) Provider Manual], 1st edition. Kowloon, Hong Kong: American Heart Association Inc; 2020.
2. Emeriaud G, López-Fernández YM, Iyer NP, Bembea MM, Agulnik A, Barbaro RP, et al. Executive Summary of the Second International Guidelines for the Diagnosis and Management of Pediatric Acute Respiratory Distress Syndrome (PALICC-2). Pediatr Crit Care Med. 2023;24(2):143-68.
3. Global Initiative for Asthma. (2023). Global Initiative for Asthma: Global strategy for asthma management and prevention. [online] Available from https://ginasthma.org/2023-gina-main-report/ [Last accessed May, 2024].
4. In: Bush A, Deterding RR, Li A, Ratjen F, Sly P, Zar H, et al. Kendig's and Wilmott's disorders of the respiratory tract in children, 10th edition. New Delhi, India: Elsevier-Health Sciences Division; 2023.
5. Kirolos A, Manti S, Blacow R, Tse G, Wilson T, Lister M, et al. A Systematic Review of Clinical Practice Guidelines for the Diagnosis and Management of Bronchiolitis. J Infect Dis. 2020;222(Suppl 7):S672-9.
6. Kliegman RM, St. Geme III JW, Blum NJ, Tasker RC, Wilson KM, Schuh AM, et al. Nelson Textbook of Pediatrics, 22nd edition. Elsevier; 2024.
7. Respiratory Tract Infection- Group Education Module. Indian Academy of Pediatrics consensus for the management of RTI in children, 2010.

SECTION 3: Cardiovascular Disorders

1. Custer JW, Rau RE. Johns Hopkins: The Harriet Lane Handbook, 22nd edition. Amsterdam: Elsevier Mosby; 2021.
2. Ghai OP, Paul V, Bagga A. Ghai Essential Pediatrics, 10th edition. New Delhi: CBS Publishers and Distributors Pvt Ltd; 2023.
3. Kliegman RM, St. Geme III JW, Blum NJ, Tasker RC, Wilson KM, Schuh AM, et al. Nelson Textbook of Pediatrics, 22nd edition. Elsevier; 2024.
4. Loscalzo J, Fauci AS, Kasper DL, Hauser SL, Longo D, Jameson JL. Harrison's Principles of Internal Medicine, 21st edition. New York: McGraw-Hill; 2022.
5. Park MK, Salamat M. Park's pediatric cardiology for practitioners, 7th edition. Amsterdam: Elsevier; 2020.

SECTION 4: Hematological and Oncological Disorders

1. Custer JW, Rau RE. Johns Hopkins: The Harriet Lane Handbook, 22nd edition. Amsterdam: Elsevier Mosby; 2021.
2. Ghai OP, Paul V, Bagga A. Ghai Essential Pediatrics, 10th edition. New Delhi: CBS Publishers and Distributors Pvt Ltd; 2023.
3. In: Lipton JM, Fish JD, Lanzkowsky P (Eds). Lanzkowsky's Manual of Pediatric Hematology and Oncology, 7th edition. Amsterdam: Elsevier 2021.
4. In: Shaffner DH, McCloskey JJ, Hunt EA, Tasker RC (Eds). Rogers' Textbook of Pediatric Intensive Care, 6th edition. Philadelphia: Wolters Kluwer Health; 2023.
5. Kliegman RM, St. Geme III JW, Blum NJ, Tasker RC, Wilson KM, Schuh AM, et al. Nelson Textbook of Pediatrics, 22nd edition. Elsevier; 2024.
6. Zimmerman JJ, Rotta AT. Fuhrmann and Zimmerman's Pediatric Critical Care, 6th edition. Maryland Heights, United States: Mosby; 2021.

SECTION 5: Endocrine Disorders

1. Custer JW, Rau RE. Johns Hopkins: The Harriet Lane Handbook, 22nd edition. Amsterdam: Elsevier Mosby; 2021.
2. Ghai OP, Paul V, Bagga A. Ghai Essential Pediatrics, 10th edition. New Delhi: CBS Publishers and Distributors Pvt Ltd; 2023.
3. In: Shaffner DH, McCloskey JJ, Hunt EA, Tasker RC (Eds). Rogers' Textbook of Pediatric Intensive Care, 6th edition. Philadelphia: Wolters Kluwer Health; 2023.
4. Kliegman RM, St. Geme III JW, Blum NJ, Tasker RC, Wilson KM, Schuh AM, et al. Nelson Textbook of Pediatrics, 22nd edition. Elsevier; 2024.
5. Sperling MA, Majzoub JA, Menon RK, Stratakis CA. Sperling pediatric endocrinology, 5th edition. Amsterdam: Elsevier; 2020.
6. Zimmerman JJ, Rotta AT. Fuhrmann and Zimmerman's Pediatric Critical Care, 6th edition. Maryland Heights, United States: Mosby; 2021.

SECTION 6: Renal Disorders

1. Gülhan B, Özaltın F. Hemolytic Uremic Syndrome in Children. Turk Arch Pediatr. 2021;56(5):415-22.
2. Kliegman RM, St. Geme III JW, Blum NJ, Tasker RC, Wilson KM, Schuh AM, et al. Nelson Textbook of Pediatrics, 22nd edition. Elsevier; 2024.

3. Khandelwal P, McLean N, Menon S. Update on Pediatric Acute Kidney Injury. Pediatr Clin North Am. 2022;69(6):1219-38.
4. Srivastava RN, Bagga A. Pediatric Nephrology, 6th edition. New Delhi: Jaypee Brothers Medical Publishers (P) Ltd; 2016.

SECTION 7: Gastrointestinal and Liver Disorders

1. Custer JW, Rau RE. Johns Hopkins: The Harriet Lane Handbook, 22nd edition. Amsterdam: Elsevier Mosby; 2021.
2. Dhawan A, Guandalini S. Textbook of Pediatric Gastroenterology, Hepatology and Nutrition, 2nd edition. Philadelphia: Springer; 2022.
3. Ghai OP, Paul V, Bagga A. Ghai Essential Pediatrics, 10th edition. New Delhi: CBS Publishers and Distributors Pvt Ltd; 2023.
4. In: Shaffner DH, McCloskey JJ, Hunt EA, Tasker RC (Eds). Rogers' Textbook of Pediatric Intensive Care, 6th edition. Philadelphia: Wolters Kluwer Health; 2023.
5. Kliegman RM, St. Geme III JW, Blum NJ, Tasker RC, Wilson KM, Schuh AM, et al. Nelson Textbook of Pediatrics, 22nd edition. Elsevier; 2024.
6. Zimmerman JJ, Rotta AT. Fuhrmann and Zimmerman's Pediatric Critical Care, 6th edition. Maryland Heights, United States: Mosby; 2021.

SECTION 8: Neurological Disorders

1. Custer JW, Rau RE. Johns Hopkins: The Harriet Lane Handbook, 22nd edition. Amsterdam: Elsevier Mosby; 2021.
2. Ghai OP, Paul V, Bagga A. Ghai Essential Pediatrics, 10th edition. New Delhi: CBS Publishers and Distributors Pvt Ltd; 2023.
3. In: Shaffner DH, McCloskey JJ, Hunt EA, Tasker RC (Eds). Rogers' Textbook of Pediatric Intensive Care, 6th edition. Philadelphia: Wolters Kluwer Health; 2023.
4. Kliegman RM, St. Geme III JW, Blum NJ, Tasker RC, Wilson KM, Schuh AM, et al. Nelson Textbook of Pediatrics, 22nd edition. Elsevier; 2024.
5. Pina-Garza JE, James KC. Fenichel's clinical pediatric neurology, 8th edition. Amsterdam: Elsevier; 2020.
6. Sarnat HB. Guillain-Barré syndrome. Nelson textbook of Pediatrics, 19th edition. Amsterdam: Elsevier; 2011.
7. Winer JB. Treatment of Guillain-Barré syndrome. QJM. 2002;95(11):717-21.
8. Zimmerman JJ, Rotta AT. Fuhrmann and Zimmerman's Pediatric Critical Care, 6th edition. Maryland Heights, United States: Mosby; 2021.

SECTION 9: Neonatal Disorders

1. Custer JW, Rau RE. Johns Hopkins: The Harriet Lane Handbook, 22nd edition. Amsterdam: Elsevier Mosby; 2021.
2. Ghai OP, Paul V, Bagga A. Ghai Essential Pediatrics, 10th edition. New Delhi: CBS Publishers and Distributors Pvt Ltd; 2023.
3. Hansen AR, Martin CR, Stark AR, Eichenwald EC. Cloherty and Stark's Manual of Neonatal Care, 9th edition. Pennsylvania, United States: Wolters Kluwer Health; 2022.
4. Kliegman RM, St. Geme III JW, Blum NJ, Tasker RC, Wilson KM, Schuh AM, et al. Nelson Textbook of Pediatrics, 22nd edition. Elsevier; 2024.

SECTION 10: Infections

1. Ghai OP, Paul V, Bagga A. Ghai Essential Pediatrics, 10th edition. New Delhi: CBS Publishers and Distributors Pvt Ltd; 2023.
2. Kliegman RM, St. Geme III JW, Blum NJ, Tasker RC, Wilson KM, Schuh AM, et al. Nelson Textbook of Pediatrics, 22nd edition. Elsevier; 2024.

SECTION 11: Toxicology and Environmental Hazards

1. American Heart Association. Pediatric Advanced Support Manual (PALS) Provider Manual [AHA, Pediatric Advanced Life Support (PALS) Provider Manual], 1st edition. Kowloon, Hong Kong: American Heart Association Inc; 2020.
2. Custer JW, Rau RE. Johns Hopkins: The Harriet Lane Handbook, 22nd edition. Amsterdam: Elsevier Mosby; 2021.
3. Ghai OP, Paul V, Bagga A. Ghai Essential Pediatrics, 10th edition. New Delhi: CBS Publishers and Distributors Pvt Ltd; 2023.
4. In: Shaffner DH, McCloskey JJ, Hunt EA, Tasker RC (Eds). Rogers' Textbook of Pediatric Intensive Care, 6th edition. Philadelphia: Wolters Kluwer Health; 2023.
5. Kliegman RM, St. Geme III JW, Blum NJ, Tasker RC, Wilson KM, Schuh AM, et al. Nelson Textbook of Pediatrics, 22nd edition. Elsevier; 2024.
6. Loscalzo J, Fauci AS, Kasper DL, Hauser SL, Longo D, Jameson JL. Harrison's Principles of Internal Medicine, 21st edition. New York: McGraw-Hill; 2022.
7. Zimmerman JJ, Rotta AT. Fuhrmann and Zimmerman's Pediatric Critical Care, 6th edition. Maryland Heights, United States: Mosby; 2021.

SECTION 12: Procedures

1. Ghai OP, Paul V, Bagga A. Ghai Essential Pediatrics, 10th edition. New Delhi: CBS Publishers and Distributors Pvt Ltd; 2023.
2. King C, Henretig FM, King BR, Loiselle J, Ruddy RM, Wiley JF. Textbook of Pediatric Emergency Procedures, 2nd edition. Pennsylvania, United States: Wolters Kluwer Health; 2007.

SECTION 13: Charts and Scales

1. American Heart Association. Pediatric Advanced Support Manual (PALS) Provider Manual [AHA, Pediatric Advanced Life Support (PALS) Provider Manual], 1st edition. Kowloon, Hong Kong: American Heart Association Inc; 2020.
2. Custer JW, Rau RE. Johns Hopkins: The Harriet Lane Handbook, 22nd edition. Amsterdam: Elsevier Mosby, 2021.
3. Ghai OP, Paul V, Bagga A. Ghai Essential Pediatrics, 10th edition. New Delhi: CBS Publishers and Distributors Pvt Ltd; 2023.
4. In: Shaffner DH, McCloskey JJ, Hunt EA, Tasker RC (Eds). Rogers' Textbook of Pediatric Intensive Care, 6th edition. Philadelphia: Wolters Kluwer Health; 2023.
5. King C, Henretig FM, King BR, Loiselle J, Ruddy RM, Wiley JF. Textbook of Pediatric Emergency Procedures, 2nd edition. Pennsylvania, United States: Wolters Kluwer Health; 2007.
6. Kliegman RM, St. Geme III JW, Blum NJ, Tasker RC, Wilson KM, Schuh AM, et al. Nelson Textbook of Pediatrics, 22nd edition. Elsevier; 2024.
7. Loscalzo J, Fauci AS, Kasper DL, Hauser SL, Longo D, Jameson JL. Harrison's Principles of Internal Medicine, 21st edition. New York: McGraw-Hill; 2022.
8. Zimmerman JJ, Rotta AT. Fuhrmann and Zimmerman's Pediatric Critical Care, 6th edition. Maryland Heights, United States: Mosby; 2021.

Index

Page numbers followed by *b* refer to box, *f* refer to figure, *fc* refer to flowchart, and *t* refer to table

A

Abdomen 253
Abdominal compartment syndrome 139, 278
Abdominal distension, tense 257
Abdominal examination 85, 141
Abdominal pain
　acute 139
　　management of 142*fc*
　causes of 139*t*
Abdominal paracentesis 278
　sites for 279*f*
Abdominal wall defects 271
Abscess 116, 344, 347, 349
　abdominal 140, 142
　brain 161, 169
　drainage 36
　incision 36
　peritonsillar 47
　retropharyngeal 56
Acetaminophen 156, 217, 224, 243, 321, 322
　intoxication, stages of 224*t*
　poisoning 157, 226, 226*fc*
　toxicity 224
Acetone 217
Acetylsalicylic acid 321
Acidosis 47, 217
　respiratory 30
Acinetobacter 192
Acquired demyelinating disorders 183
Activated partial thromboplastin time 91, 102, 107, 108
Acute respiratory distress syndrome 47, 52, 54, 103
　management 54*fc*
Acyanotic congenital heart disease 61
Acyclovir 182
Addison disease 118
Adrenal crisis 118, 119*fc*
　management of 118
Adrenal insufficiency
　primary 118
　secondary 118
Adrenaline 60
Adrenocorticotropic hormone 119, 205
Air, movement of 65
Air-leak syndromes 190

Airway 3, 4, 7, 190
　breathing, and circulation 16, 19, 21, 23, 48, 51, 76, 78, 83, 87, 92, 97, 100, 103, 105, 171, 223, 229, 232, 277, 284, 286, 289
　management 37, 162
　obstruction 68, 74
Alanine
　aminotransferase 337
　transaminase 226
Aldolase 337
Alkali denaturation test 144
Alkaline phosphatase 29, 337
Alkalosis, respiratory 30, 155
Alpha-amino-3-hydroxy-5-methyl-4-
　　isoxazolepropionic acid receptor 186
Alpha-hydroxylase deficiency 205*fc*
Altitude, high 74
Alveolar arterial oxygen pressure difference 320
Alveolar capillary unit 47
Alveolar hypoventilation 74
Alveolar oxygen
　partial pressure of 320
　tension 319
Amanita poisoning 156
Ambiguous genitalia 202, 203
Ambu bag 257
Amikacin 322
Amino acids 301
Aminoglycosides 24
Aminotransferase 247
Amiodarone 322
Amitriptyline 322
Ammonia 337
Amphotericin 24
Ampicillin 126
Amylase 338
Analgesia 36, 37*t*, 239, 243, 276, 296
Analgesics 37, 296
Anaphylactic shock 16
　management of 16*fc*
Anaphylaxis 9
Anemia 47
Angiocatheter 269
Angiotensin-converting enzyme 12, 83, 83*f*
　inhibitors 26

Angiotensin-receptor neprilysin inhibitor 83
Aniline dye 321
Anion gap 31, 319
    acidosis, normal 32*t*
Antecedent trauma 140
Anticholinergic agents 63
Anticholinesterase 218
Anticipated difficult airway 254, 257, 272
Antidote-N-acetylcysteine 226
Antidotes 220
Antiepileptic drug 167, 198
Antihypertensives, dosing of 86*t*
Antimicrobial therapy, topical 242
Anti-Müllerian hormone 203
Antinuclear antibody 132, 154, 184, 185, 338
Antiphospholipid antibody 132
Antipyrine 321
Antiseizure therapy 165, 166, 167
Antisnake venom 236
Antistreptolysin O titer 338
Antitubercular treatment 163
Antivenom therapy 239
Aorta, coarctation of 79, 84
Aortic stenosis 79
Aortoesophageal fistula 151
Apnea 196
Appendicitis 141
Aquaporin-4 185
Areflexia 175
Argininosuccinic acid 200
Arterial blood gas 5, 6, 10, 12, 15, 30, 63, 64, 73, 105,
       154, 198, 210, 223, 227, 247, 259
    analysis 69, 141, 268
       approach to 30
    changes of 30*t*
    management of 35*fc*
Arterial carbon dioxide, partial pressure of 30, 34,
       157, 290, 320,
Arterial lactate 6, 199
Arterial oxygen
    content 319, 320
       partial pressure of 13, 33, 34, 105, 320
       saturation 34, 320
Arterial pressure monitoring, invasive 6
Arteriovenous fistula 268
Artery forceps 274
Artesunate 182
Ascitic fluid collection bag 278
Ascorbic acid 321
Ashworth scale grade, modified 352
Aspartate aminotransferase 247, 338
Aspirin 217
Assisted ventilation, goals of 67
Asthma, acute severe 62, 64*fc*
Ataxia 175

Atmospheric pressure, decreased 74
Atrial pressure 320
Atrial thrombus 273
Atrioventricular septal defect 79
Atropine 37, 254, 257, 298
    infusion 228
Autoimmune central nervous system disorders 183*fc*
Autoimmune disorder 120, 183, 185, 186*fc*
Autoimmune encephalitis 183, 184
Autoimmune encephalopathy 184*t*
Autoimmune movement disorders 183, 184
    investigations for 185*t*
Autonomic storm 237
Axillary vein 265
Azithromycin 214

B

Bacteria 180
Bacterial diseases 214
Barbiturates 37, 217
Barometric pressure 320
Bartter syndrome 24
Basic life support 289
Benzodiazepine 37, 239, 296, 297
    conversion calculations 297
    reversal 37
Beta-blocker 26, 217
Beta-hydroxylase deficiency 205*fc*
Bicarbonate therapy 111
Bicarbonate
    based solutions 134
    standard and actual 33
Bickerstaff encephalitis 184
Binding agents 220
Biochemical parameter 213, 305
Bleeding 151, 275, 344
    approach to child with 108*fc*
    diathesis 143
    disorders 107, 107*t*
    episodes 99
    prolonged 107
    sites of 99
Blood
    clotting test, whole 236
    component replacement 313
    culture 93, 194
    gas 67
       analysis 199
       arterial 338
    glucose 199
    loss, whole 9
    pressure 8, 10, 12, 83, 87, 105, 171, 210, 217, 223,
       284, 298, 315, 326
       acute 84

device 37
diastolic 86
low 11
monitoring, invasive 268
normal 9
systolic 86
stained ascitic fluid 279
sugar 212
tests 184
transfusions 153
urea nitrogen 116, 141, 227, 247, 315, 320
Blunt injury 245
Blurred vision 228
Body
mass index 43
surface area 319, 326
Bone disease 262
Bowel
distention 139
habits 140
movements 291
obstruction 148
sounds 141
syndrome 304
Bradycardia 85, 217, 228
Brain
herniation, type of 353f
noncontrast computed tomography of 174
perfusion 4
tumor 47, 169
Brainstem evoked response audiometry 185
Breathing 3, 7
assessment of 4
disordered control of 47
room air 338
spontaneously 255
Broad-spectrum intravenous antibiotics 93
Bronchial asthma 60
Bronchiolar narrowing 60
Bronchiolitis, acute 60, 61fc
Bronchodilators 60
Bronchopneumonia 60
Bronchorrhea 228
Bronchospasm 228
Bruxism 212
Bullae, pulmonary 274
Burn 242
care 36
estimation of 244f
injury
early management and resuscitation
of 242
produces 242
intervention 243fc
management of 243

wounds, evaluation of 242
Button battery
ingestion 151
removal, protocol for 152fc

C

Calcinosis 338
Calcitonin 28
Calcium 339
sensing receptor mutation 28
Camphor 217
Campylobacter jejuni 175
Cannulation equipment, examine 269
Capillary filling time 8, 10, 191, 210, 212
Capillary leak syndromes 9, 305
Capnography 5
Captopril 81
Carbamate ingestion 228, 229fc
Carbamazepine 28, 322
Carbamoyl phosphate synthetase 200
Carbohydrates 40, 301
Carbon dioxide
detector 257
elimination 67
partial pressure of 30, 77, 170, 171,
173, 241, 287, 320
Carbon monoxide 219
Cardiac
arrest 245
arrhythmias 273
dysfunction 131
function 251f
index 319
lesions, duct-dependent 18
magnetic resonance imaging 81
output 77
monitoring 268
tamponade 18, 273
Cardiogenic shock 6, 11
etiology of 11
management of 11, 12fc, 82fc
Cardiomyopathy 11
Cardiopulmonary resuscitation 201, 241,
283, 284, 289
Cardiovascular
collapse 258
disorders 71
functions 4
instability, management of 231
status 251
system 28, 85, 237
Carditis 11
Carpopedal spasm 28
Carvedilol 81

Catheter
    diameter 310
    insertion 266
    intracardiac positioning of 273
    over wire 269
    preparation 272
    sizes 309
    suction 257, 310
Ceftriaxone 182
Central cyanosis 73
Central line placement 36
Central nervous system 80, 84, 99, 100, 116, 129, 186, 193, 223, 237, 238, 315
    depression 74
    effects 228
    infections 164
    manifestations 222
Central venous
    catheter kit 259
    oxygen saturation 6, 15
    pressure 10, 154, 251, 320
        monitoring 6
Cephalosporins 126
Cerebral
    edema 169
    herniation, signs of 170
    malaria 181, 212
    perfusion pressure 169, 353
        target, minimum 353
    venous thrombosis 169
Cerebrospinal fluid 105, 163, 174, 176, 179, 181, 182, 184, 185, 185, 212, 353
    evaluation of 343
    parameters, normal 195t
Chest
    compressions 289
    examination 140
    lower 189, 190
    radiograph 93
    syndrome, acute 104
    upper 190
    wall excursion, magnitude of 4
    X-ray 64, 76, 94, 105, 247
Chloramphenicol 214, 321
Chlorhexidine solution 265
Chloride 339
Chlorothiazide 330
Choanal atresia 190
Choroids plexus papilloma 169
Chvostek sign 28
Chylothorax 274
Circulation 8
Cisatracurium 328
Clinically isolated syndrome 183
Clinicopathological syndrome 91

Clitoral reduction surgery 205
Clitoromegaly 204
Clonic seizures 196
Clonidine 87
Clotting factor 99
Coagulation
    disorders of 107, 107t
    parameter 224
Coagulopathy 274, 278
    management of 155, 155t
Cobalamin 343
Cobra 234
Coma 161
    and pain scales 307
    approach to 161, 163fc
    causes of 161
    generalized 161
    induction 167
Compensated shock, management of 210fc
Compensatory response, equation for 31
Complete blood count 10, 15, 76, 85, 94, 96, 105, 132, 141, 144, 146, 163, 184, 199, 227, 236, 247
Computed tomography 19, 100, 149, 163, 172b, 173, 174, 182, 247, 348
    characteristics 344
    head 348t
    lesions 344
Congenital adrenal hyperplasia 204
Congenital diaphragmatic hernia 190
Congenital heart
    disease 11, 12, 76, 79t
    lesions, duct-dependent 18
Congenital pneumonia 190
Congestive cardiac failure 18, 47, 79, 101
    drugs and dosage for management of 81t
    management of 82fc
    onset of 80t
Connective tissue disorders 11
Consanguinity 153
Consciousness 3
    loss of 17, 173, 174
Contactin-associated protein-like 2 186
Continuous ambulatory peritoneal dialysis 136
Continuous cyclic peritoneal dialysis 136
Continuous positive airway pressure 48, 51, 54, 191, 241
Continuous renal replacement therapy 136, 136t
Continuous venovenous hemodialysis 136
Contusion, pulmonary 47
Conventional units 337
Coombs test
    direct 102
    indirect 102
Corpus luteum cyst 140
Corrosive tissue injury 151

Cortisol 114
Coryza 56
Cough 222
Cramps, abdominal 17, 228
Cranial nerve 170
Cranial ultrasound 347, 347t
C-reactive protein 94, 105, 184, 185
Creatine kinase 339
 myoglobin binding 247
Creatine phosphokinase 339
Creatinine 339
 clearance 319
Croup 57fc
Cryoprecipitate 314
Cryptococcus 180
Cryptorchidism
 bilateral 202
 unilateral 202
Current, pathway of 246
Cushing's syndrome 24
Cushing's triad 170
Cyanides 217
Cyanosis 11, 18, 19, 73, 189, 191, 217
 late-onset 73
 management of 76fc
 underlying cause of 74
Cyanotic congenital heart disease 11, 73, 74
Cyanotic heart disease 52
Cyanotic spell 77
 management of 78fc
Cyclosporine 322
Cystic changes 347

D

Dandy-Walker malformation 347
Dapsone 321
Deep sedation 36
Deep vein thrombosis 179
Defecation 77
Dehydroepiandrosterone 205
Delhi Neonatal Infection Study Group 192
Demyelinating disorders 183, 183t
Dengue 180, 209
 based on warning signs, classification of 209fc
 fever 209
 severe 209
Deoxyribonucleic acid 181, 185
Dexmedetomidine 328
Dextrose 41, 111, 134, 232, 301
Diabetes insipidus 23, 120, 315
 central 120
 management of 121fc
 nephrogenic 120
Diabetes mellitus 139

Diabetic ketoacidosis 31, 111, 113fc
 clinical features of 111
 management 111
 mild 112
Diacylglycerol kinase epsilon 130
Dialysis 128, 220
 catheters 309
 indications for 128b, 133
 sustained low efficiency 135, 136
Diaphragm movement 253
Diarrhea 140
Diazepam 297
Diazoxide 87
Diffuse axonal injury 172
Diffusion-weighted imaging 184
Digitalis 217
Digoxin 81, 323
Dihydrotestosterone 203, 205
Dipeptidyl-peptidase-like protein-6 184
Disability 5, 8
Disease-specific ventilation 67
Disseminated encephalomyelitis,
 acute 163, 181, 182, 183
Disseminated intravascular coagulation 91, 94, 102, 103, 108, 131
 causes 91t
 clinical features 91t
 diagnosis 92fc
 laboratory workup of 91t
 management of 92fc
Distal
 air movement 4
 femur 262
 tibia 262
Distended neck veins 18
Distilled water 78, 198
Diuresis 220
Dobutamine 328, 239
Dopamine 329
 2 receptor 184
Downes-Vidyasagar score 191t
Doxepin 323
Doxycycline 214
Dressing adhesives 265
Drowning, management for 241fc
Drugs, hypersensitivity to 126
Duchenne muscular dystrophy 80
Dyspnea 306
Dystonia 183

E

Ecchymoses 107
Eculizumab 131
Edema 305
 origin of 52
 pulmonary 74, 211

Elapid bites 235
Electrical injury 245
    clinical considerations of 247*fc*
    mechanisms of y 246
    type of 245, 245*t*
Electrocardiogram 12, 29, 75, 96, 105, 284, 285, 326
Electrocardiogramprostaglandin E1 19
Electrocardiography 241, 247
Electroencephalography 154, 163, 167, 184, 185, 186
Electrolysis 85, 141, 151
Electrolytes 199, 290
    correction of 204
Electromyography 179
Elemental iron 230
Emergency
    endotracheal intubation 254
    management 58, 201*fc*
Emesis 219
Emission computed tomography, single-photon 184
Empyema 274
Enalapril 81
Encephalitis 116, 169
Encephalopathy 217
    hypertensive 238
    hypoxic ischemic 169, 197
Endocrinal disorder 109, 120
End-organ functions 4
Endoscopic therapy 145
Endoscopy 144
Endotracheal intubation 254, 256*f*
Endotracheal tube 59, 145, 256*f*, 283, 288, 310
    size 68
End-tidal carbon dioxide 288
Energy requirements 302
Enteral feedings, advancing 303
Enteral nutrition 43*fc*, 301, 303, 304
    calculation 302
    contraindications to 39
Enteric encephalopathy 181, 182
Enterovirus 180
Enzyme-linked immunosorbent assay 105, 214
Epidemic typhus 213
Epigastrium 140
Epileptiform discharges 185
Epinephrine 114, 329
Erasmus Guillain-Barré syndrome respiratory insufficiency score 177
Erythroblastopenic crisis 104
Erythrocyte sedimentation rate 184, 185, 339
Escherichia coli 130
Esmolol 86
Esophageal dysmotility 338
Estimated blood volume 313
Estimated glomerular filtration rate 125
Estrogen replacement 205

Ethosuximide 323
Ethylenediaminetetraacetic acid 271
Etomidate 37, 257, 298
External ophthalmoplegia, acute 175
Extracellular fluid, base excess of 33
Extracorporeal membrane oxygenation 12, 54, 83
Exudate 316
Eye 228
    examination 154
    injuries 36
    movement, transient abnormalities of 212
    opening 173

F

Face, Legs, Activity, Cry, Consolability scale 308
Facial dysmorphism 254
Factor replacement therapy, dose of 100*t*
Fallot tetralogy 77
Fat 41, 301
    intralipids 301
Fatty acid oxidation defects 200
Fava beans 321
Febrile encephalopathy 180, 180*t*
    management of child with acute 182*b*
Febrile infection-related epilepsy syndrome 165
Febrile neutropenia 93
    management of 94*fc*
Febrile nonhemolytic transfusion reactions 101
Femoral artery 260
Femoral vein 131, 259
    catheterization 261*f*
Fenoldopam 87
Fentanyl 37, 254, 296, 298, 329
Ferritin 339
Fever 212
    causes of 209
    group, spotted 213
    induced refractory epileptic encephalopathy syndrome 184
Fibrin clots leading, formation of 91
Fibrinogen equivalent unit 13
Fibroelastosis, endocardial 80
Flaccid paralysis
    acute 175, 176*fc*, 178
    surveillance program, acute 177
Flecainide 323
Flucytosine 323
Fluid and metabolic
    complications 155*t*
    management 155*t*
Fluid
    and electrolyte loss 9
    attenuated inversion recovery 184
    bolus 182

fecal contents in 279
requirements 39
restoration 238
resuscitation 242
Flumazenil 37
Fluoroscopy 58
Folate 340
Follicle-stimulating hormone 203
Food
    caloric content of 301
    intake, improvement with 140
    type 301
Foreign body aspiration 58, 59fc
Fresh frozen plasma 92, 155, 157
Friedreich's ataxia 80
Fructose intolerance 153
Fungus 180
Furazolidone 321
Furosemide 81, 330

G

Galactosemia 153, 156
Gamma-aminobutyric acid 186
    A receptor 184
    B receptor 184
Gamma-glutamyl transferase 340
Gastric
    emptying 43
    lavage 219, 231
Gastroesophageal reflux 43
    disease 43, 150
Gastrointestinal
    bleed 143
    decontamination 219
        procedures 222
    obstruction, management of 150fc
    perforation 151
    tract 93, 100, 140
        disorders 137, 143
        pain 141t
Gastroschisis 271
Genital examination 204
Gentamicin 323
Gitelman syndrome 24
Glasgow coma scale 5, 145, 163, 173, 173t, 174, 179, 307, 308, 352
Glomerular filtration rate 133
Glomerulonephritis, acute 126
Glucagon 114
Glucocorticoid activity 317
Glucose 290, 340
    infusion rate 154, 155, 198
Glucose-6-phosphate dehydrogenase 97, 321
    deficiency 321

Glutamate decarboxylase 184, 186
Glycine receptor 184
Goal-directed therapy 14
Graft rejection 91
Gravity, specify 315
Great arteries, transposition of 73, 79
Gross motor function classification system 353
Growth hormone 114
Guillain-Barré syndrome 84, 177, 179fc

H

Hand-foot syndrome 104
Haptoglobin 340
Hashimoto encephalitis 184
Head
    injury 47, 172
    injury, protocol for management of 174, 174fc
Heart
    failure 79
        causes of 79t
        medical therapy in 83f
        congestive 18, 20, 23
    rate 8, 10, 85, 284, 285, 298, 326
        abnormalities 11
    sounds 74
Heated humidified high flow nasal cannula 51
Heavy metal toxicity 151
Hemarthrosis, acute 99
Hematemesis 143
Hematochezia 143
Hematological disorder 89
Hemochromatosis 28, 153, 156
Hemodialysis, intermittent 128, 135
Hemodynamic monitoring 290
Hemoglobin 105, 212, 320, 340
    abnormal 75
    amount of 344
    concentration 5, 6
Hemoglobinuria 211
Hemolytic uremic syndrome 91, 126, 130, 132fc
    atypical 130
    typical 130
Hemoperfusion 220
Hemophilia 100, 314
    emergencies 99
        management of 99, 100fc
Hemopneumothorax 274
Hemorrhage
    intracranial 197, 347
    pulmonary 190
    site of 100
Hemothorax 275
Heparin 330
    unfractionated 92

Hepatic based coagulopathy 153
Hepatic encephalopathy 153
　management of 155, 156*t*
　stages of 154*t*
Hepatic failure, causes of acute 153*t*, 153
Hepatic toxicity 231
Hepatitis
　A immunoglobulin M 154
　autoimmune 156
　B surface antigen 154
　C virus 154
Hepatorenal syndrome 156, 157
Hepatotoxic drugs 143
Hernia, incarcerated 149
Herpes simplex virus 156, 181
Human immunodeficiency virus 132
Humeral head 262
Hydralazine 87
Hydrocarbon 223*fc*
　poisoning 222
Hydromorphone 296
Hyperaldosteronism 24
Hyperammonemia, transient 200
Hyperchloremic metabolic acidosis 32*t*
Hyperglycemia 219, 315
Hyperglycinemia, nonketotic 200
Hyperhemolytic crisis 104
Hyperkalemia 26, 219
　causes of 26
　management of 27*fc*
　specific treatment of 118
Hyperlactatemia 211
Hyperlipidemia 315
Hypermagnesemia, maternal 28
Hypermetabolic response, management of 242
Hypernatremia 22
　causes of 22
　management of 23*fc*
Hyperoxia test 75
Hyperphosphatemia 28
Hyperproteinemia 315
Hypertension 128, 129, 132, 217, 306
　acute severe 84
　intracranial 157
　persistent pulmonary 76, 190
　pulmonary arterial 74
Hypertensive crisis, management of 86, 87*fc*
Hyperthermia 217
　malignant 26
Hyperventilate 170
Hypervolemia, features of 306
Hypnotics 37, 217
Hypocalcemia 28, 219
　management of 29*fc*
Hypogastrium 140

Hypoglycemia 114, 115*fc*, 155, 164, 211, 219
　correction of 204
　management of 114
Hypokalemia 24, 155, 219
　causes of 24
　management of 25*fc*
Hypomagnesemia 28
Hyponatremia 20, 155
　acute cases of 116
　causes of 20
　factitious 315
　treatment of 21*fc*
Hypoplastic left heart syndrome 79
Hypotension 19, 28, 155, 217
Hypotensive shock, management of 10*fc*, 210*fc*
Hypothalamic-pituitary-adrenal axis 118
Hypothermia 217
Hypovolemia 77
Hypoxic ischemic insult, acute 164
Hypoxic spells, circle of 77

I

Iliopsoas bleed 99
Illness, course of treatment of acute 105*fc*
Imipramine 323
Immunocompromised states 211
Immunofluorescence assay 214
Immunoglobulin
　A secretion 39
　G 185
　intravenous 167, 186
　M enzyme-linked immunosorbent assay 213
Infections 104, 197, 207, 263, 271, 347
Infiltrative disorders 120
Inflammatory bowel disease 140, 142
Inflammatory demyelinating polyradiculoneuropathy, acute 175
Ingestion, acute 224
Inhaled nitric oxide 53
Injury, mechanisms of 151
Inspired oxygen, fraction of 13, 30, 287
Insulin
　regular 332
　therapy 111
Intensive care unit 287
Intercostal drainage tube 275*f*
　insertion 274
Internal jugular vein 131
International League Against Epilepsy 164, 197
International System of Units 337
Intestinal obstruction 9, 141, 148, 257, 305
　causes of 149*t*
Intestinal signs 218
Intra-abdominal fluid paracentesis 253

Intra-abdominal masses 141
Intracardiac shunt, absence of 49
Intracranial bleed 99
Intracranial hypertension 157
    management of 155
Intracranial pressure 8, 92, 100, 157, 163, 170, 171, 174, 182, 241, 298
    causes of 169b
    clinical features of 170b
    increased 162, 169
    management of raised 171fc
Intracranial space occupying lesions 169
Intracranial vascular malformation 169
Intramuscular bleed 99
Intraosseous cannulation 262
    complications, prevention, and management of 263t
    contraindications of 262t
    site 263f
Intrapulmonary shunts 75
Intrathoracic airway obstruction 65
Intravascular volume depletion 305
Intravenous compatibility charts 328
Intravenous fluids, maintenance 300
Intubation 299
Intussusception 141, 149
Iron 230, 341
    level 231
    poisoning 230, 232fc
    serum 231
Isoniazid 31, 219
Isradipine 87

J

Japanese encephalitis virus 180
Jaundice 217
Jejunostomy 39
Jejunum 149
Joint bleed 107
Jugular vein, external 265

K

Kasabach-Merritt syndrome 91
Kawasaki disease 80, 214
Ketamine 37, 63, 254, 332, 257, 298
Ketones 301
Kidney
    biopsy 127
    disease 125, 132
    insensitivity of 120
    replacement therapy 126, 128
Kidney injury
    acute 125, 129
    classification of 125t
    evaluation of 127t
    management of 129fc
    severity 125
    causes of acute 126t
Kidney Disease: Improving Global Outcomes classification 125t
Krait 234

L

Labetalol 86
Lacrimation 228
Lactate 302, 341
    dehydrogenase 96, 132, 316, 341
Lactulose 156
Lamotrigine 323
Landry ascending paralysis 175
Large bowel obstruction 148
Laryngeal mask airway 8, 288, 311
Laryngeal nerve injury, recurrent 151
Laryngoscope blade 254
    sizes 311
    types 311
Laryngoscopy 255
Laryngotracheobronchitis 56
Lead 341
Lethargy 161
Leukemia
    acute lymphoblastic 96
    chronic lymphocytic 96
Leukomalacia, periventricular 347
Leukotriene inhibitor 64
Levocarnitine 81
Lidocaine 257, 268, 323
Lightening injuries 246
Lignocaine 268
Limb
    movements 196
    positioning of 269
    vascular compromise of 259
Lipase 341
Lipids 40
Lipogenesis 301
Lithium 323
Liver
    disease 143
    disorders 137
    failure 28
        acute management of 154t, 156t, 157fc
    function test 91, 141, 154, 199, 227, 230
    kidney microsome 154
    transplantation, King's college criteria for 157t
Lobectomy 274
Lorazepam 243, 297

Losartan 81
Lower airway respiratory obstruction 6, 47
Lower gastrointestinal bleed, approach to evaluation of 147*fc*
Lumbar puncture 36, 163, 184, 185, 353
 indications of 168
Lung
 carcinoma 116
 disease, chronic 52
 malformations 190
 sounds 4
 tissue 47
  disease 6
 ultrasound 252*f*
Luteinizing hormone 203

M

Magnesium 41
 sulphate 63
Magnetic resonance
 angiography 105
 imaging 100, 163, 181, 184, 185, 186, 247, 349
  interpretation 349*t*
Malaria 180, 214
 complicated 211
 diagnosis of 211
 parasite 168
 treatment of severe 212*fc*
Malignancy 84, 91
 chemosensitivity of 96
Mean airway pressure 15, 66, 67, 69, 157, 169, 171, 319
Mean cerebrospinal fluid production rate 353
Mean corpuscular volume 320
Measles 180
Mechanical ventilation 52, 65, 69*fc*
 noninvasive 52
Meckel's diverticulum 149
Meconium aspiration syndrome 67, 190
Melena 143
Menarche 203
Meningeal
 irritation 180
 irritation 180*t*
 signs 180
Meningitis 116, 194, 169
 bacterial 197
Meningoencephalitis, viral 181
Menstruation 140
Mental status, altered 14
Mesobuthus tamulus 237
Metabolic acidosis 30, 31, 31*t*, 155, 211, 219, 319
 management for 231
 severe 199
 treatment of 32

Metabolic alkalosis 30, 32, 155
Metabolic disease 164
Metabolic disorder, suspected 200*fc*
Metabolism, inborn error of 47, 164, 199
Metabotropic glutamate receptor 5 184
Methemoglobinemia 75
Methylene blue 321
Metoprolol 81
Microangiopathic disorders 91
Micropenis 202
Microscopic examination 96
Midazolam 254, 37, 243, 257, 259, 297, 298, 332
Miller Fisher syndrome 175
Milrinone infusion 239
Mineralocorticoid activity 317
Minimal map target 353
Minoxidil 87
Minute volume 66, 67
Miosis 228
Mixed venous oxygen
 content 319, 320
 tension 320
Monoclonal antibodies 61
Monroe-Kellie hypothesis 169
Morphine 37, 296, 333
Motion, equation of 65
Motor
 abnormalities 212
 axonal neuropathy, acute 175
 response 173
Mucosal damage 151
Murine typhus 213
Murmurs 74
Mycobacteria 180
Mycophenolate mofetil 132
Mycoplasma pneumoniae 175
Myelitis, transverse 183
Myeloid leukemia, acute 96
Myocarditis, viral 80
Myoclonic seizures 197

N

N-acetylcysteine 226
N-acetylglutamate synthetase 200
Naloxone 37
Naphthalene 321
Nares dilatation 190
Nasal
 blockade 56
 cannula, high-flow 48, 54, 223
 flaring 189
Nasogastric 43, 149, 150, 154
Nasopharyngeal airway 288
Necrotizing enterocolitis 139, 140, 150, 271

Neonatal intensive care unit 189
Nephritic syndrome 9, 305
Nephrotic syndrome 305
    management of edema in 306
Nerve conduction velocity 179
Neurological disorders 47, 73, 159
Neuromuscular disease 47, 74
Neuromuscular disorders 11
Neuromyelitis optica spectrum disorder 183
Neutropenia 93
Nicardipine 86
Nifedipine 87
Nitrates 217
Nitrofurantoin 321
Nitrogen ratio 41
Nitroglycerine 238
Nitrous oxide 37
N-methyl-D-aspartate receptor 184, 186
Nonimmunological reactions 101*b*
Noninvasive ventilation 223, 238, 295
Nonpoisonous snake 233*f*, 233*f*
Nonprotein calorie 41
Non-rebreather mask 51
Nonsteroidal anti-inflammatory
    drugs 26, 126, 143
Norepinephrine 333
Nortriptyline 324

O

Obstruction, radiological features of 148, 149*t*
Obstructive shock 6, 18
    investigations 19*fc*
    management of 19*fc*
Obtundation 161
Octreotide 145
Ocular decontamination 219
Ocular examination 85
Ocular signs 218
Oculocephalic responses 162
Oliguria 9
Omphalitis 271
Omphalocele 271
Oncological disorder 89
Opioid 296
    analgesic 257
    reversal 37
Optic
    nerve sheath diameter, measurement of 253
    neuritis 183
Optical coherence tomography 185
Oral hypoglycemic agent 219
Organ dysfunction syndrome, multiple 217
Organophosphate 217, 227, 228
    management of 229*fc*

Organophosphorus
    compounds 227
    poisoning 227
Ornithine transcarbamoylase 200
Orofacial dyskinesias 183
Orofacial-lingual movements 196
Orogastric 43, 150, 191
Oropharyngeal airway 288
Orthopedic manipulation 36
Oscillatory ventilation, high frequency 53, 54
Osmolar gap 319
Osteomyelitis 263
Oxidizing agents 321
Oxycodone 296
Oxygen
    arterial partial pressure of 73
    diffusion, impaired 74
    exposure, controlled 53
    partial pressure of 30, 77
    therapy 239
Oxygenation 52, 290
    index 34, 50
Oxyhemoglobin relation 34*t*

P

Packed cell volume 105, 198, 212
Packed red blood cell 10, 78, 83, 92, 101, 105, 128, 129, 136, 313
Pain
    location of 140
    sudden onset 139
    timing of 139
Painful episode, acute 104
Palivizumab 61
Palpate calves 264
Pancreatitis 91, 141
Pantoprazole 145
Papilledema 162
Para-aminosalicylic acid 321
Paracentesis
    abdominal 278
    needle 278
Paracetamol 226
Paralysis 258
Parapneumonic effusion 274
Parasitemia 211
Parathion 227
Parathyroid gland destruction 28
Parenchymal lung disease 68
Parenteral nutrition 301, 303
    maintenance of 41
Partial thromboplastin time 146
Patent ductus arteriosus 78, 79, 83
Peak expiratory flow rate 5, 64

Peak inspiratory pressure 53, 66, 67, 69
Pediatric acute respiratory distress syndrome 52
Pediatric advanced life support 15, 83, 240, 241, 247, 283
   evaluate, identify, and intervene cycle 7t
   systematic approach 7fc
Pediatric early warning score 291
Pediatric intensive care unit 15, 64, 84, 87, 125, 129, 154, 174, 240
   nutrition guidelines 302
Pediatric
   neurology charts 352
   stylet 254
Pediatric surgery 59
Pelvic inflammatory disease 140, 141
Percutaneous endoscopic gastrostomy 39
Pericardial effusion 273
Peripheral blood smear 85, 91, 132, 227
Peripheral cyanosis 75
Peripheral oxygen saturation 8, 10, 13, 34, 73, 105, 223, 229, 236, 291
Peripherally inserted central catheter 265
   care and maintenance 266
Peritoneal adhesions 149
Peritoneal dialysis 128, 134
   acute 133
   catheters 133
   low efficiency of 133
   prescription 134
Peritoneal fluid 141, 316
Peritonitis 139, 271
Petechiae 107
Petroleum distillate hydrocarbons 222
pH 31, 338
Phenobarbital 28, 324
Phentolamine 86, 341
Phenylketonuria 200
Phenytoin 28, 324
Phoenix sepsis
   criteria 13
   score 13t
Phosphorus 342
Pierre Robin sequence 190
Plasma
   ammonia 199
   loss 9, 305
   osmolality 319
Plasmodium falciparum 182, 211
Plateau pressure 53
Platelets 313
   and blood vessels, disorders of 107, 107t
Pneumonia 217
Pneumothorax 274
   needle aspiration of 277f
Poison 220
   antidotes 220t

Poisoning 217t, 219
   causes of 230
   suspected case of 217
Polymerase chain reaction 163, 181, 186, 213, 214
Polytrauma 91
Portex 311
Positive airway pressure
   bilevel 54, 223
   biphasic 48, 51
Positive end expiratory pressure 8, 48, 53, 66, 66, 67, 67, 69, 83, 157
Positive pressure ventilation, primary methods for 66
Positron emission tomography 184, 186
Potassium 41, 342
   levels and changes 27t
   oxalate 336
   serum 27
   sparing diuretics 26
   therapy 112
Povidone-iodine 265
Prazosin 239
Pressure
   necrosis 151
   ventilation 66
Primaquine 321
Primidone 324
Probenecid 321
Procainamide 324
Procedural sedation 36, 259, 296
Propofol 37, 257
Propranolol 145
Prostaglandin E1 76, 83
Protein 41
   cerebrospinal fluid 343
   intake 41
   losing syndromes 9, 305
   requirements 302
Prothrombin time 91, 102, 107, 108, 146, 155, 234
Protozoa 180
Protozoal diseases 214
Protriptyline 324
Proximal tibia 262, 263
Pruritus around mouth 16
Pseudohyponatremia 20
Pseudomonas 192
Pulmonary arterial pressure 320
Pulmonary arteriovenous fistula 75
Pulmonary capillary wedge pressure 320
Pulmonary embolism 19
   massive 18
Pulmonary end-capillary oxygen 320
Pulmonary hypertension, moderate-to-severe 61
Pulmonary index score for asthma, modified 62

Pulse 326
   oximetry 4, 5
   pressure 210
      narrowed 18
   rate 105
Pulseless
   electrical activity 283
   ventricular tachycardia 283
Pulsus paradoxus 18
Pupillary response 5, 355f
Pyomeningitis 181

Q

Quinidine 324
Quinine 182
Quinolones 126

R

Radial artery 268, 269
   cannulation 268
   puncture and cannulation, technique of 270f
Radiation 28
Radio-opaque central venous catheter 265
Random blood sugar 210, 212
Ranitidine 145
Rapid-sequence intubation 50, 63, 171, 257, 298
   drugs 298
   protocol for 258fc
   steps of 257
Rasmussen encephalitis 184
Raynaud phenomenon 338
Rectal bleed 140
Red blood cell 144, 234, 316, 320
Red flag signs 140
Refractory anasarca 306
Refractory status epilepticus, new-onset 165
Regurgitation 251
   pulmonary 79
Renal angina index 126
Renal disease, end-stage 130, 132
Renal disorders 123
Renal failure 236
   index 319
Renal function test 85, 91, 154, 224
Renal losses 24
Renal parenchymal disease 84
Renal replacement therapy 133, 135, 136fc, 259
   type of 136
Renal tubular acidosis 32
Renal vein thrombosis 126
Respiration 105
Respiratory
   abnormalities, assessment of 5

   compensation, determining adequacy of 319
   disorders 45
   distress 47, 48fc, 189, 190b, 191fc
      syndrome 67, 190
   failure 49
      acute 49, 51fc
   management 53
   muscle failure, primary 68
   pump failure 49, 68
   quotient 301
   rate 4, 66, 67, 191, 285, 291, 308
   tests 184
Retinol 343
Retraction 191
Rhabdomyolysis 245
Rheumatic carditis, acute 80
Rhinorrhea 228
Ribavirin 61
Rickettsia 180
Rickettsial disease 213
   approach to 214fc
Rifampicin 28
Ringer's lactate 150, 155
Road traffic accident 174
Rocuronium 254, 298
Rule of nine 242
Rumack-Matthew nomogram 225f
Russell's viper 234

S

Salbutamol 63
Salicylates 217, 324
Saline nebulization 60
Salt wasting features 203
Saphenous vein 265
Saw scaled viper 234
Scalp veins 265
Schofield-HW equation 302
Sclerodactyly 338
Sclerosis, multiple 183
Scorpion
   bite 217
      approach to 237
   sting
      envenomation, clinical grade of 238b
      treatment of 238fc
Scrub typhus 180, 181, 213
Sedation 36, 37t, 64, 290, 299
   levels of 36
   minimum 36
   protocol 38fc
   withdrawal 296
Sedatives 217, 296
   hypnotics 218

Seizures 47, 131, 153, 166, 183, 196, 198, 198*fc*
   electroclinical 196
   electrographic 196
   febrile 164, 168
   subtle 196
Sensation, loss of 36
Sensorium 210
Sensory axonal neuropathy, acute 175
Sepsis 9, 14, 28, 192
   culture negative 194
   early onset 194 fc
   late onset 195*fc*
Septic shock 13, 14
   early recognition of 14
   management of 15*fc*
Serum autoimmune studies 185
Serum cortisol level 118
Serum creatine phosphokinase 176
Serum electrolytes, pediatric early warning score 118
Sex determination 203*fc*
Sexual development 203
   disorder of 202, 203, 205
Shock
   distributive 6
   hypovolemic 6, 9
   management of 209, 231
   meningococcemia 182
   obstructive 6, 18
   septic 13, 14
Sickle cell
   crisis 104
      analgesics for 106*t*
   disease 104, 105*fc*, 140
Silverman-Andersen score 190*t*, 191
Sirolimus 324
Skin
   decontamination 219
   perfusion, changes in 14
   prep solution 276
Sleep disorder 183
Small bowel 149
Snake
   bite 217
      suspected 236*fc*
      treatment protocol 233
   envenomation 91
   nonvenomous 234*t*
   poisonous 233*f*
   venomous 233, 234*t*
Sodium 41
   abnormal 315
   bicarbonate 27
   deficit 20, 22
   fluoride 336
   fractional excretion of 315
   glucose cotransporter 2 83
   maintenance 20
   nitroglycerine 86
   nitroprusside 86, 239
Soft-tissue bleed 107
Solid tumors 91
Somatosensory evoked potentials 185
Somatostatin 145
Spironolactone 81
Splenic sequestration crisis 104
Splenorenal view 253*f*
Spondylodiscitis 151
Spontaneous circulation, return of 289
Staphylococcus aureus 192
   infection, methicillin-resistant 93
Status epilepticus 164
   management of 164, 166*t*
   type of 164
Stenosis, pulmonary 74, 79
Sterile
   blade 271
   draping 274, 276
Steroid 317
   synthesis 204
Stiff peritoneal dialysis catheter insertion 135
Stool specimen collection 177
Stupor 161
Stylet 257
Succinylcholine 298
Sucralfate 145
Suction apparatus 254
Sulfacetamide 321
Sulfamethoxazole prophylaxis 94
Sulfanilamide 321
Sulfasalazine 321
Sulfhemoglobinemia 75
Sulfisoxazole 321
Sulfonamides 126
Sulfoxone 321
Supportive care 166, 167
Sweating 217
Syndrome of inappropriate antidiuretic hormone 117*fc*, 247, 315
   secretion 116, 170
Systemic lupus erythematosus 338
Systemic steroids, recurrent 317
Systemic vascular resistance 77, 319

T

Tachycardia 9, 19, 77, 217
Tachypnea 9, 189, 217
   transient 190
Tacrolimus 325
Targeted temperature management 290

Telangiectasia 338
Tension pneumothorax 18, 276
Terbutaline 334
Terlipressin 145
Testosterone 205
Tet spells 77
Tetanus prophylaxis 236
Tetanus toxoid 236
Tetany 28
Tetraethyl pyrophosphates 227
Thalassemia 28
Theophylline 63, 325
Therapeutic drug monitoring 325
Thiopentone 50
Thoracentesis 253
Thoracic cavity 252
Thoracocentesis 276
Thoracotomy 274
Thrombin time 91
Thrombocytopenia 274, 278
Thrombocytosis 26
Thrombosed artery 268
Thrombotic microangiopathy 131
Thrombotic thrombocytopenic purpura 130
Thyroid stimulating hormone 184, 185
Tissue ischemia 26
Tobramycin 325
Tongue thrusting 196
Tonic seizures 196
Total anomalous pulmonary venous return 79
Total body sodium
   decreased 20
   increased 20
   normal 20
Total iron binding capacity 342
Total parenteral nutrition 42, 157, 265, 301
Toxidromes 218t, 227
Toxin 218t
Tracheoesophageal fistula 150, 190
Tracheostomy sizes tube 311
Transcranial magnetic stimulation 163
Transferrin 342
Transfusion reaction
   acute 101
   management of 102, 103fc
Transjugular intrahepatic portosystemic shunt
     procedure 146, 156
Transtubular potassium concentration gradient 25
Trauma
   abdominal 259
   score, revised 308
Traumatic brain injury 5, 169
Tricuspid regurgitation 79
Trigger 62, 66

Trimethoprim 94
Troponin 342
Trousseau sign 29
Tuberculosis 163
Tuberculous meningitis 180, 181
Tubular necrosis, acute 126, 128, 315
Tubulointerstitial nephritis 126
Tumor
   high-risk group 95, 96
   intermediate-risk group 95, 96
   low-risk group 95, 96
   lysis syndrome 95, 96
     management of 97fc
   risk groups, classification of 95t
Typhus group 213
Tyrosinemia 153, 156

U

Ultrasonography 10, 105, 149, 185, 251
   guidance for 268
   use of 251
Ultrasound, abdominal 148
Umbilical arterial catheter 309
Umbilical vein catheterization 271, 273f, 309
Universal precautions 268, 271, 278
   materials 276
Upper airway respiratory obstruction 6, 47, 257
Upper gastrointestinal bleed, evaluation of 146fc
Urea cycle defects 153
Urea nitrogen 342
Uremic encephalopathy 169
Ureteroenterostomy 31
Uric acid 343
   serum 199
Urinalysis 85, 224
Urinary electrolytes 32t
Urinary incontinence 228
Urinary tract infection 141, 142
Urine 141, 315
   electrolyte 32
   output criteria 125
   urea nitrogen 315
   volume 315
Urolithiasis 141
Urticarial reaction, moderate-to-severe 101

V

Vaginal culture 141
Valproic acid 325
Valvular stenosis 251
Vancomycin 182, 325
Vascular access 253, 271
Vascular malformations 169

Vaso-occlusive crisis 104
Vasopressin 145, 334
    anti-diuretic action of 120
    deficiency 120
Vasopressors 140
Vecuronium 254, 298, 334
Vena cava, inferior 10, 305
Venous blood gas 5, 6, 15, 34t, 210
Ventilation 290
    perfusion 105
Ventilator
    illustration 294
    modes of 66
    parameters 66
Ventricular apex
    left 74
    right 74
Ventricular dysfunction 52
Ventricular fibrillation 283
Ventricular hypertrophy
    criteria 327
    left 327
    right 327
Ventricular outflow tract, right 78
Ventricular septal defect 74, 79
Ventricular tachycardia 283
Ventriculomegaly 347
Video-electroencephalography recordings 196
Viper bites 234
Virologic Classification Scheme 178, 178fc
Virus 180

Visual evoked potentials 185
Vital signs, abnormal 14
Vitamin
    A 343
    B12 343
    D 343
    D3 343
    K 321
Voltage-gated potassium channel-complex 184, 186
Volvulus 149
Vomiting 140
    persistent 199
von Willebrand disease 107
Voriconazole 325

W

Water-soluble analog 321
Weaning 68
    conversion strategy for 296
Wheezing 217
White blood cell 96, 101, 176, 181, 316, 343
Whole bowel irrigation 220
Wilson disease 28
Winter formula 319
Wong-Baker Faces Pain Rating Scale 308f
Wound dressing 36

X

Xiphoid 190

EU GSPR Authorised Reprsentative
Logos Europe, 9 rue Nicolas Poussin
1700, La Rochelle, France
Phone: +33 (0) 6 67 93 73 78
E-mail: contact@logoseurope.eu

www.ingramcontent.com/pod-product-compliance
Ingram Content Group UK Ltd.
Pitfield, Milton Keynes, MK11 3LW, UK
UKHW060949220426
5322IPUK00033B/603